Clinical Handbook of Perinatal and Pediatric Respiratory Care

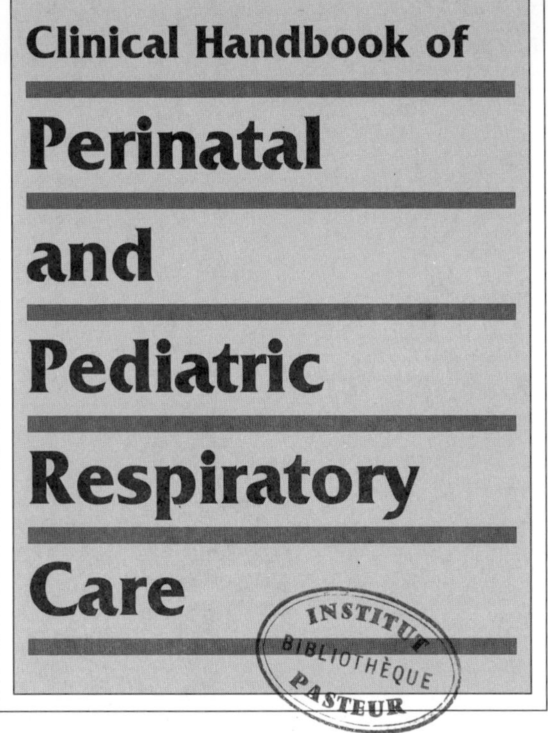

Sherry L. Barnhart, AS, RRT

Neonatal and Pediatric Respiratory Care Practitioner
Cardiopulmonary Services
Covenant Medical Center
Urbana, Illinois
Formerly, Education Coordinator and Assistant Director
Respiratory Care Services
Arkansas Children's Hospital
Little Rock, Arkansas

Michael P. Czervinske, BSRT, RRT

Manager, Cardiopulmonary Diagnostics
Departments of Respiratory Care and Cardiology
Tulane University Medical Center Hospitals and Clinics
New Orleans, Louisiana

W.B. SAUNDERS COMPANY

A Division of Harcourt Brace & Company

Philadelphia London Toronto Montreal Sydney Tokyo

W.B. SAUNDERS COMPANY
A Division of Harcourt Brace & Company

The Curtis Center
Independence Square West
Philadelphia, Pennsylvania 19106

Clinical Handbook of Perinatal and
Pediatric Respiratory Care ISBN 0–7216–6739–2

Printed in the United States of America

Last digit is the print number: 9 8 7 6 5 4 3 2 1

To those children who have taught us that courage comes in all sizes and that caring for others is one of life's greatest blessings.

Preface

This handbook was written to provide the health care professional and student with practical and current information concerning neonatal and pediatric respiratory care. It has been designed primarily for use in the clinical setting, and every attempt has been made to make it a working companion.

This handbook, which fits in the pocket of a lab coat, is within reach at all times—more convenient than bringing a textbook to the patient's bedside. Space has been provided for the clinician to insert institution-specific comments or updates, such as new policies and procedures concerning equipment or drugs. The handbook is spiral bound so that it is easier to fold and read when working at the bedside. For quick reference, each section begins with a list of the abbreviations that are found in that section, as well as an outline of the material.

The handbook contains 11 sections and an appendix. We believe that clinicians must develop skills for working with children and their families and become sensitive to their needs during hospitalization. Through an understanding of growth and development, the clinician can help children and their families cope during this stressful time; thus, we have addressed this aspect of care in Section 1. Section 2 provides information that assists the practitioner in obtaining an accurate medical history and performing physical assessment. Both conventional and high-frequency mechanical ventilation are covered in Section 3. The majority of clinicians that we questioned asked that the handbook include information on mechanical ventilation and stated that it is when working with mechanically ventilated patients that they most often find they need an at-the-bedside manual. It is for this reason that we placed this section early in the handbook. Sections 4 through 7 are devoted to neonatal and pediatric disease states and should be used as a quick reference or overview of disorders and how to treat them. Section 8 covers therapeutic procedures common to neonatal and pediatric respiratory care. Guidelines and explanations for diagnostic and monitoring techniques are provided in Section 9, and pharmacology is addressed in Section 10. Section 11 reviews the steps necessary in cardiopulmonary resuscitation and airway management of infants and children. Normal laboratory values for the neonatal and pediatric population are listed in the Appendix.

Portions of this handbook include both text and illustrations that also appear in the textbook, *Perinatal and Pediatric Respiratory Care.* This handbook is not intended to provide all concepts or theories related to the respiratory care of neonatal and pediatric patients. We refer the clinician and student to the textbook for a comprehensive discussion of perinatal and pediatric respiratory care.

Our sincere appreciation goes to some very special individuals at W.B. Saunders: Lisa Biello, Helaine Barron, and Amy Norwitz. We could not have completed this handbook without their guidance and remarkable patience.

Sherry L. Barnhart
Michael P. Czervinske

Contents

SECTION 1

Psychosocial Aspects of Neonatal and Pediatric Care

I. Psychosocial and Emotional Development

A. Newborn to 6 months of age
   1. Development
   2. Normal needs
   3. Response to hospitalization
   4. Needs during hospitalization

B. 6 months to 1 year of age
   1. Development
   2. Normal needs
   3. Response to hospitalization
   4. Needs during hospitalization

C. 1 year to 3 years of age (toddler)
   1. Development
   2. Normal needs
   3. Response to hospitalization
   4. Needs during hospitalization

D. 3 years to 6 years of age (preschool)
   1. Development
   2. Normal needs
   3. Response to hospitalization
   4. Needs during hospitalization

E. 6 years to 12 years of age (school age)
   1. Development
   2. Normal needs
   3. Response to hospitalization
   4. Needs during hospitalization

F. 12 years to 15 years of age (adolescence)
   1. Development
   2. Normal needs
   3. Response to hospitalization
   4. Needs during hospitalization

II. Parental Reactions to a Child's Hospitalization

A. Guilt and shame

B. Denial

C. Anger

D. Fear and panic

E. Anxiety and stress

F. Shock

When a child (neonatal or pediatric patient) is hospitalized, both the child and family encounter psychologic and emotional stress in addition to the physical stress the child is experiencing. It is imperative that health caregivers understand the need for a family-centered approach to caring for the child; the needs of not only the child should be addressed but also those of the parents and siblings. The purpose of this section is to outline the reactions of children and their families when a child is hospitalized and the specific needs each may have.

PSYCHOSOCIAL AND EMOTIONAL DEVELOPMENT

Newborn to 6 Months of Age

Development. Senses are fully developed at this age. The infant reacts to and initiates reactions from caregivers, gazes and smiles at faces, and startles at loud sounds. The baby is completely self-centered and believes an object-person exists only within the range of vision. The infant begins to become attached to the mother or primary caregiver.

Normal Needs. The infant acquires a sense of trust. Sucking is used for tension release and gratification. Touch is practiced through play, holding, and rocking (comforts and builds trust). Play is critical for development; the infant learns to imitate and derives pleasure from play. The hands and mouth are used to experience the environment.

Response to Hospitalization. The routines of the infant are disrupted, for example, the sleep-wake cycle and feeding schedule. Inappropriate stimulation is present (overstimulation from lights, sounds, procedures [many are painful rather than pleasant]) as is understimulation (lack of meaningful stimulation). The infant has a feeling of "not being in control," for example, he or she cannot hear himself or herself cry when intubated and is disturbed while sleeping.

Needs During Hospitalization. Parental participation (feeding, baths, play, changing diapers) is necessary during an infant's hospitalization, and minimal separation should be the rule. Stimulation (exercise, mobiles, family pictures, music) should be provided, with awareness of overstimulation (infants respond by averting gaze, yawning, turning away from stimulation source). Pain relief is necessary (infants *do* experience pain). Variable, nonpainful touch (stroking, hand placed on head, body massage with lotion) is helpful. Day and night cycles should be maintained. A variety of positions should be provided (foam, infant seats, blanket rolls may be used). Minimal auditory stimuli should be present and consistency in caregivers should be practiced.

6 Months to 1 Year of Age

Development. At this age, the baby is aware that his or her needs are met by others. There is a well-established attachment to the parents. There is resistance to doing what he or she does not want to do, and persistence is present. The baby communicates with sound and imitates others' actions. Intellectual reasoning begins at this age.

Normal Needs. Social interaction, a sense of security, and a security object (blanket, toy) are necessary for a child of this age. Play is also necessary for development. An emotional relationship (usually with the mother) is present; the absence of this relationship is damaging and may lead to lack of trust and withdrawal.

Response to Hospitalization. Separation is the strongest fear of a child this age. Reactions to separation can include crying, feeding disturbances, gastrointestinal upset, and withdrawal. He or she remembers pain from previous experiences and responds with anxiety. Stranger anxiety is also present.

Needs During Hospitalization. Parental participation (feeding, baths, changing diapers, play) is helpful. Separation should be kept to a minimum (separation is traumatic). Relief for pain should be provided. The child should be made familiar with equipment before procedures (stethoscope, manual percussor, aerosol mask). Play is used as a distraction from fear or pain.

1 Year to 3 Years of Age (Toddler)

Development. Negativism and resistive behavior are strong at this age. There is an increase in autonomy and self-control (walking, toilet training, feeding). There is an increase in language skills. The toddler is developing a sense of time.

Normal Needs. The toddler requires normal routines and consistency in the environment. Play is a form of communication and is used to develop motor skills. Limits must be set for the toddler to feel secure. The child of this age explores the environment. Simple explanations are required.

Response to Hospitalization. The toddler experiences separation anxiety (the child this age is at highest risk of emotional trauma from hospitalization) and believes any brief separation is permanent. Regressive behavior occurs because of separation anxiety (loss of bladder control, immature verbal communication). The performance of new skills becomes limited (feeding self, walking, toilet training). At this age, the child feels guilt and believes "bad" behavior caused the hospitalization and painful procedures. Toddlers wonder why their parents are not "rescuing" them; they believe their parents are angry with them. Physical restraints represent a loss of control; the child becomes frightened and resistant. The immature thought process of a child of this age magnifies the fear (equipment becomes monsters).

Needs During Hospitalization. Parental participation (feeding, baths, changing diapers) and minimal separation are necessary. Routines should be maintained and consistency in hospital caregivers should be provided. Familiar toys and activities should be available; play is needed to provide stimulation and prevent boredom. The child this age needs limits set. Self-expression and movement are necessary. Familiarity with equipment before procedures (stethoscope, aerosol mask, percussor) is helpful; dolls, toys, and puppets are used for simple explanations. Verbal and physical comfort (stroking, holding hand) helps during procedures. The child should be allowed to sit up or be held in the parent's lap. The ability to express fear, anger, and discomfort should be encouraged.

3 Years to 6 Years of Age (Preschool)

Development. The preschool child begins to test his or her independence. He or she is more trusting and less frightened of strangers. "Why" questions are asked and the child of this age wants to know cause and purpose; he or she believes there is a reason for everything. The 3- to 6-year-old child feels guilty if he or she has "bad" thoughts or wishes. Learning right from wrong begins now and these children are more aware of danger. The imagination develops and the preschool child has difficulty differentiating fantasy from reality. At this age, the child can wait for needs to be met.

Normal Needs. The child of this age requires expressive play with others and large-muscle movement. Simple explanations are best. The preschool child should be comforted when left alone or in the dark. Routines are necessary.

Response to Hospitalization. Separation from parents is painful at this age. Misconceptions about equipment and procedures are common; preschool children interpret procedures as hostile acts and view surgery as body mutilation. Hospitalization and pain are seen as punishment. Regressive behavior (soiling clothes, immature speech, thumb-sucking, strong parental attachment) may occur. An adhesive bandage (Band-Aid) is seen as a comfort.

Needs During Hospitalization. Parental participation (feeding, baths, therapy) is required at this age. Simple reassuring explanations concerning what will and will not happen and what will be felt prior to procedures should be provided, demonstrating with props, pictures, puppets, and dolls. Verbal comfort helps during procedures. Honesty from caregivers is important. Choices are given when possible (which adhesive bandage to use, which lobe of chest physical therapy to perform first). Expressions of anger, pain, or fear should be allowed (it is okay to cry during procedures or use dolls and toys for expression). Therapeutic play is beneficial (the child plays freely without being disturbed with medical procedures). Reexplanations should be provided and the child's understanding determined.

6 Years to 12 Years of Age (School Age)

Development. The school-aged child is proud of his or her accomplishments and follows set limits and rules. Independence and social skills increase, along with the ability to reason. These children have a tendency, however, to say they understand when they do not, and they are reluctant to ask questions.

Normal Needs. The school-aged child needs privacy. Acceptance by and relationships with peers are important, as is family contact. A balance between the need for independence and the desire for parental support must be achieved. The child this age feels in control of his or her body and activities. Rules and schedules are required.

Response to Hospitalization. The school-aged child fears losing control, feeling pain, body disfigurement, anesthesia (fear of not waking up), and death. Anxiety occurs because the child is separated from peer and school activities. Separation from parents is better tolerated at this age. Attention to his or her body causes self-consciousness, but the child of this age is more accepting of medical procedures. Sleep and eating disturbances may occur.

Needs During Hospitalization. Privacy is required; these children may not want parents present during procedures. They should be encouraged to express fears, anger, and anxiety (it is okay to cry). Coping techniques (relaxation, self-talk, imagery, breathing techniques) are helpful. Thorough explanations of procedures (using dolls, body outlines, and letting the child handle equipment) should be provided. Verbal comfort and explanations should be given during procedures. Contact with peers and siblings (visitation, telephone use, cards, letters) is useful. The school-aged child should continue homework. Parental support is important. A wide range of activities should be available and the child should maintain normal routines. Emphasis should be on normal aspects of activities, procedures, and body appearance. The child should be able to wear his or her own clothes, not hospital pajamas.

12 Years to 15 Years of Age (Adolescence)

Development. The adolescent is achieving independence from his or her parents. There is awareness of and planning for the future. There is also insecurity about body and self. Mood swings, unpredictable behavior, and depression can occur. Peers determine self-image. The adolescent is egocentric. He or she reacts to what is explained and how the explanations are given.

Normal Needs. Group interaction, a sense of self, peer acceptance, self-control, and honesty are required at this age.

Response to Hospitalization. Anxiety caused by separation from peers and lack of independence because of hospitalization can occur. An adolescent has fear of pain and body disfigurement and great concern as to how his or her appearance will be affected. There may be regressive behavior (withdrawal, demands, fear of being alone). Denial of illness and the need for medical care as well as irrational conclusions may be present. Sleep and gastrointestinal disturbances may occur.

Needs During Hospitalization. Contact with peers (liberal visitation, telephone use, cards, letters) is helpful. Privacy, an active role in his or her care, and a feeling of self-control are required at this age. Information on the illness, an explanation of procedures, and verbal comfort and explanation during procedures are helpful. Activities (television, music, books, puzzles, writing materials) should be provided and homework should continue. Emphasis should be on normal aspects of activities, procedures, and body appearance. The adolescent should be able to wear his or her own clothes and not hospital pajamas. There should be an awareness of the schedule for procedures (Tables 1–1 and 1–2).

PARENTAL REACTIONS TO A CHILD'S HOSPITALIZATION

Guilt and Shame

If the child's illness is due to a preventable accident, parents often feel they are responsible. Parents (especially

TABLE 1–1 Interventions to Minimize Auditory Stimuli in an Intensive Care Unit
Silence or reset alarms quickly
Maintain continuous "beeps" at minimal volume level (e.g., pulse oximetry)
Repair noisy equipment
Be aware of gas flow levels inside oxygen hoods
Minimize noise at bedside during medical rounds and shift report
Empty water in aerosol-ventilator tubing
Quietly close portholes on isolettes, drawers, cabinet doors
Quietly raise and lower bedrails
Prohibit placing equipment on top of isolettes
Prohibit tapping on isolettes
Provide low-volume music
Establish day and night cycles
Place signs to alert visitors and personnel to quiet times for patients ("Shh—I'm sleeping," "Quiet time is from 2 to 4").

mothers) of infants born prematurely or with congenital anomalies may wonder what they did that caused this to happen to their child (ate poorly, took medications, too much exercise). There may be a realistic reason for their guilt (drug abuse, neglect, inherited disorder).

Denial

Parents may be unable to accept a poor prognosis, the need for medical procedures, or the reality that an illness is chronic. Although they may understand the seriousness of the illness, they may not be able to deal with it at this time—denial helps them to function.

Anger

Anger is a common reaction and is often a manifestation of guilt. It may be directed at the spouse, staff members, God, or extended family. Parents may not want medical students or certain staff members caring for their child. They may question the competency of the staff and want extensive explanations to their questions. These parents often feel that

TABLE 1–2 Interventions to Assist in Providing a Child with a Healthy Medical Encounter

STRIVE FOR GOOD COMMUNICATION WITH THE CHILD AND PARENTS

Communicate at the child's eye level—sit, crouch, bend over to do this. Look directly at the child.

Listen to what the child says; look for meaning behind the words. Restate what you have heard.

Don't ignore the child when in a room with medical staff or adults. Make eye contact and talk with the child as well as with the parents.

Children often understand more than we think they do. Be careful what is said that they might overhear.

Use language that the child can understand. Don't talk "down" to the older child.

Minimize conflicting details.

Provide consistency in procedures.

FAMILIARIZE SELF WITH CHILD'S PERSONAL NEEDS

Call the child by the name he or she prefers, not necessarily the name on the chart.

Visit with the child when you do not have a procedure or treatment to do.

Respect the child's need for privacy. Close blinds, pull drapes, ask visitors to step out during procedures unless the child indicates otherwise.

Acknowledge the child's fears.

FAMILIARIZE AND PREPARE THE CHILD FOR PROCEDURES

Explain what will and will not occur and what may be felt.

Ask for questions.

FOSTER THE CHILD'S NEED FOR INDEPENDENCE, SELF-WORTH, AND SELF-SUFFICIENCY

Include the child in decision-making.

Allow the child choices only if they are available.

Reinforce appropriate feelings and behavior.

Be positive and use lots of praise.

Table continued on following page

TABLE 1–2 Interventions to Assist in Providing a Child with a Healthy Medical Encounter *Continued*

State suggestions or directions in a positive rather than a negative form. Refrain from using "don't."

TREAT EACH CHILD WITH RESPECT

Keep promises; this builds trust and security.
Do not subject the child to long delays.
Speak to the child during medical rounds-reports.

they have lost the ability to care for their child and are attempting to regain control.

Fear and Panic

Some parents may be overwhelmed with the fear that their child may die. Fear of the unknown (diagnosis, prognosis) may cause the parent to overreact to minor issues. Keeping the parent informed and providing supportive listeners (staff, support groups) are helpful.

Anxiety and Stress

Parents of ill children are often faced with multiple problems that cause stress. Lack of privacy, sleep deprivation, financial burden (medical care, need to be away from work, meals at hospital, lodging), travel to and from the hospital (often located far from home), hospital parking, other children to care for (who may also be hospitalized or may be at home), babysitters, the hospital–intensive care unit (ICU) environment, and the illness itself may cause anxiety and stress.

Shock

Premature birth, congenital anomalies, or critical illness in a newborn is hard for parents to accept when they have been eagerly anticipating the birth of a healthy child. Parents of children who are involved in trauma or a situation in which they suddenly become critically ill are often in a state of shock and may need assistance in coping with the situation (Table 1–3).

TABLE 1-3 Parental Needs During a Child's Hospitalization

Encouragement to maintain active role as parent; ability to help with tasks (baths, meals, applying adhesive bandages)
Reminder that they are still the parents; that their child is still theirs
Schedule of child's daily activities (physician rounds, therapy, naps, play, meals)
Frequent repetition of information with consistent explanations (allow parents to write down information so that they may refer to it later or relay it to other family members)
Time to ask questions and assimilate information
Assistance in forming realistic perceptions of the illness and hospitalization
Hospital guidelines concerning visitation, ICU policies, parking, cafeteria hours
Opportunities to meet and seek support from other parents (parents' lounge, parent support groups, diagnosis-related groups, parent coffee hour)
Care, concern, and respect from hospital staff (including waiting room hostesses, family advocates, and chaplains)
In-hospital facilities to eat, sleep, bathe, store belongings, wash clothing (ICU sleeping areas, in-room sleeping accommodations, cafeteria-snack bar open 24 hours, meal tickets)
Out-of-hospital accommodations for other family members (guest houses, Ronald McDonald house, special hotel rates, community resources)
Information on illness and medical procedures (videos, pamphlets, handbooks, resource center)
Preadmission orientation programs (handbook, hospital-ICU tours, videos)

ICU, intensive care unit.

Bibliography

Azarnoff P: Preparing children for the stress of hospitalization. Resident Staff Physician 1984; 30:56.

Betz CL, Hunsberger MM, Wright S: Family-Centered Nursing Care of Children, 3rd ed. Philadelphia, WB Saunders, 1994.

Ell KO, Reardon KK: Psychosocial care for the chronically ill adolescent: Challenges and opportunities. Health Soc Work 1990; 15:272.

Gorski PA: Developmental intervention during neonatal hospitalization—Critiquing the state of the science. Pediatr Clin North Am 1991; 38:1469.

Hazinski MF: Nursing Care of the Critically Ill Child, 2nd ed. St. Louis, Mosby-Year Book, 1992.

Hobbs N, Perrin JM: Issues in the Care of Children with Chronic Illness. San Francisco, Jossey-Bass, 1985.

Merenstein GB, Gardner SL: Handbook of Neonatal Intensive Care, 3rd ed. St. Louis, Mosby-Year Book, 1993.

Mott SR, James SR, Sperhac AM: Nursing Care of Children and Families, 2nd ed. Redwood City, CA, Addison-Wesley Nursing, 1990.

Revell GM, Liptak GS: Understanding the child with special health care needs: A developmental perspective. J Pediatr Nurs 1991; 6:258.

Stanford G, Thompson R: Child Life in Hospitals: Theory and Practice. Springfield, IL, Charles C Thomas, 1984.

Stein REK: Caring for Children with Chronic Illness. New York, Springer Publishing, 1989.

SECTION 2

History and Physical Assessment

I. History and Assessment of the Neonate

- A. Maternal history and risk factors
- B. Antepartum assessment
  1. Ultrasonography
  2. Amniocentesis
  3. Fetal heart rate monitoring
  4. Nonstress test
  5. Contraction stress test, oxytocin challenge test
  6. Fetal biophysical profile
- C. Newborn assessment
  1. Apgar score
  2. Gestational age
     - a. Ballard examination
     - b. Gestational age classification
     - c. Direct ophthalmoscopy
- D. Physical examination of the newborn
  1. Vital signs
     - a. Respiratory rate
     - b. Heart rate
     - c. Blood pressure
     - d. Temperature
  2. Color
  3. Head
  4. Chest
     - a. Retractions
     - b. Chest symmetry
     - c. Auscultation
  5. Abdomen
  6. Extremities
  7. Spine
  8. Neurologic assessment
     - a. Grasp reflex
     - b. Magnet reflex
     - c. Moro reflex
     - d. Normal muscle tone
     - e. Rooting reflex
     - f. Stepping reflex

II. History and Assessment of the Child

- A. Medical history
  1. Current illness
  2. Previous illnesses
  3. Birth history
  4. General health
  5. Nutritional status
  6. Activity level
  7. Family history
  8. Environment
- B. Physical examination of the child
  1. Respiratory rate and pattern

2. Skin
   a. Cyanosis
   b. Edema
   c. Subcutaneous emphysema
3. Head and neck
   a. Head bobbing
   b. Tracheal palpation
   c. Allergic facies
4. Nose and mouth
5. Chest
   a. Chest expansion and symmetry
   b. Retractions
6. Abdomen
7. Extremities
8. Respiratory sounds
   a. Snoring
   b. Stridor
   c. Wheezing
   d. Grunting
9. Auscultation
   a. Technique
   b. Crackles
   c. Wheezes
10. Cough
   a. Effective cough
   b. Cough characteristics
   c. Sputum production

Abbreviations

AF–amniotic fluid
AFV–amniotic fluid volume
AGA–appropriate for gestational age
BP–blood pressure
bpm–beats per minute
CDH–congenital diaphragmatic hernia
CF–cystic fibrosis
CST–contraction stress test
ET–endotracheal
FBM–fetal breathing movements
FHR–fetal heart rate
FTT–failure to thrive
IUGR–intrauterine growth retardation
LGA–large for gestational age
LTB–laryngotracheobronchitis
NST–nonstress test
PFT–pulmonary function test
PIE–pulmonary interstitial emphysema

RDS–respiratory distress syndrome
SGA–small for gestational age
TE–tracheoesophageal
UC–uterine contractions

HISTORY AND ASSESSMENT OF THE NEONATE

Maternal History and Risk Factors

Various factors place the mother at risk for the development of problems during labor and delivery. Infants of these high-risk mothers are often born with severe complications, including prematurity and respiratory distress. Table 2–1 lists common maternal risk factors and their effects on the neonate. Table 2–2 lists those risk factors that are often associated with the need for resuscitation at delivery.

Antepartum Assessment

Antepartum testing is beneficial in determining the status of the fetus and the ability of the fetoplacental unit to function during labor and delivery.

Ultrasonography

Ultrasound is used to (1) estimate gestational age and weight; (2) assess fetal development, anatomy, sex, movement, and position; (3) identify fetal abnormalities; (4) investigate obstetric complications; (5) assess the placenta; (6) assist in medical interventions (amniocentesis, fetal blood sampling, surgery); (7) detect fetal heart activity; and (8) determine the viability of a pregnancy (Fig. 2–1).

Amniocentesis

Using ultrasound as a guide, a needle is inserted intra-abdominally into the amniotic sac, and amniotic fluid (AF) is aspirated. Indications for amniocentesis include (1) advanced maternal age (>35 years), (2) suspicion of fetal malformations, (3) known familial hereditary diseases, (4) a previous child with a chromosomal defect, and (5) suspicion of inborn errors of metabolism. Information that may be obtained from amniocentesis includes fetal lung maturity (Table 2–3), chromosome analysis (Down's syndrome), DNA analysis (hemophilia), presence of meconium, and Rh isoimmunization.

Fetal Heart Rate Monitoring

The normal fetal heart rate (FHR) is 120 to 160 beats per minute. Common causes of bradycardia (<120 bpm) include

TABLE 2–1 Maternal Risk Factors

MATERNAL CONDITION	NEONATAL CONDITION	MATERNAL CONDITION	NEONATAL CONDITION
Diabetes mellitus	LGA infants	Rh incompatibility	Hydrops fetalis Neonatal anemia Kernicterus
Hypertension	Congenital anomalies		
Toxemia	Growth retardation	Fetal bradycardia	Fetal asphyxia
Preeclampsia	Premature delivery	Meconium staining	Fetal asphyxia
Maternal hypertension	SGA infants	Abruptio placentae	Fetal asphyxia
Maternal age <16 or >40 years	Spontaneous abortion Congenital anomalies Chromosomal defects	Placenta previa	Anemia Hypovolemia Fetal asphyxia
Previous fetal loss	Premature delivery Congenital anomalies	Syphilis Maternal sepsis (urinary tract infection, chorioamnionitis)	Congenital syphilis Premature delivery
Maternal smoking	SGA infants		

Table continued on following page

TABLE 2–1 Maternal Risk Factors *Continued*

MATERNAL CONDITION	NEONATAL CONDITION	MATERNAL CONDITION	NEONATAL CONDITION
Maternal drug or alcohol use	Cogenital anomalies Withdrawal syndromes SGA infants	In utero infections (toxoplasmosis, herpes simplex, cytomegalovirus, rubella)	Central nervous system and eye lesions Hepatosplenomegaly Microcephaly Cataracts Deafness Bone lesions Prolonged infection Encephalitis Petechiae Intracranial calcification
Breech presentation	Premature delivery Abnormal fetus (malformation)		
Oligohydramnios	Renal anomalies Pulmonary hypoplasia		
Polyhydramnios	Gastrointestinal obstruction Central nervous system abnormality Hydrops fetalis		

LGA, large for gestational age; SGA, small for gestational age.

TABLE 2–2 Risk Factors Associated with Resuscitation at Delivery

MATERNAL HISTORY
Previous premature births
Tobacco, alcohol, drug use
Hypertension
Diabetes mellitus
Epilepsy
Systemic lupus erythematosus
Renal disease
Age <16 years or >40 years
Underweight
Respiratory disease (asthma, CF)
Cardiovascular disease
Intrauterine abnormalities
OBSTETRIC COMPLICATIONS
Preeclampsia
Placenta previa
Abruptio placentae
Multiple gestation
Maternal sepsis
Oligohydramnios
Polyhydramnios
Dialysis
Abnormal fetal presentation
Malnutrition
Cord prolapse
Maternal hypotension
FETAL COMPLICATIONS
Prematurity
Postmaturity
Exposure to teratogenic agents
Intrauterine infections
Intrauterine growth retardation
Fetal distress
Macrosomia (>4500 g)

CF, cystic fibrosis

hypoxia, hypothermia, maternal drugs, and postmaturity. Common causes of tachycardia (>160 bpm) include hypoxia, maternal drug ingestion, sepsis (maternal and fetal), and prematurity.

Nonstress Test

The nonstress test (NST) is used to assess fetal well-being. With the mother positioned on her left side and monitoring

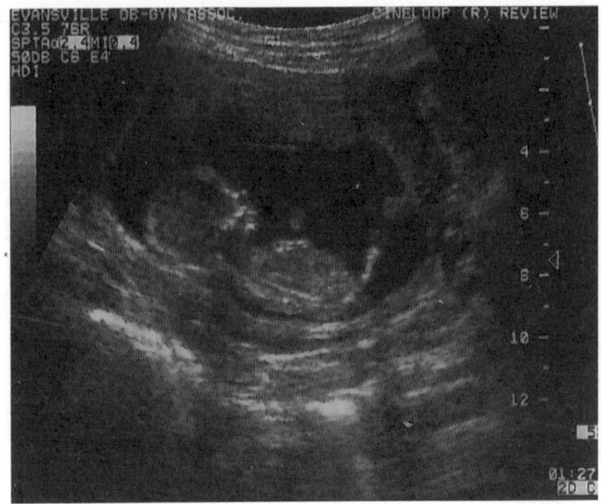

Figure 2–1 Ultrasound of a fetus at 14 weeks' gestational age.

devices attached to her abdomen, FHR and fetal movement are monitored for 20 to 60 minutes. FHR acceleration with fetal movement is considered a reactive test and is indicative of normal fetal status. If there is no FHR acceleration with fetal movement or if there is no fetal movement within a 20-minute period, the test is considered nonreactive, fetal

TABLE 2–3 Tests of Fetal Lung Maturity

TEST	PROCEDURE	INDICATES LUNG MATURITY
L:S ratio	Lecithin (component of surfactant) and sphingomyelin are compared	>2:1
Phosphatidylglycerol	A phospholipid in surfactant that is obtained from amniotic fluid	Present
"Shake test"	A 1:2 dilution of amniotic fluid to ethanol is shaken for 15 seconds	Ring of bubbles present

well-being is questioned, and a contraction stress test should be performed.

Contraction Stress Test, Oxytocin Challenge Test

The contraction stress test is used to assess the response of FHR to uterine contractions (UC). With the mother positioned on her left side and monitoring devices attached to her abdomen, FHR and UC are monitored. Nipple stimulation or oxytocin (intravenous pump) may be needed to induce contractions. The test is considered negative (the fetus normal) if there are no late decelerations in FHR during UC. If late decelerations occur during UC, the test is considered positive (abnormal) and may indicate poor fetal status and the need for delivery.

Fetal Biophysical Profile

An ultrasound is used to determine fetal well-being and is performed to assess fetal breathing movements (FBM), body movement, fetal tone, and amniotic fluid volume (AFV). The NST is used to measure reactive FHR. Each factor is scored as 2 or 0 (Table 2–4), with a total score derived. A total score of 0 or 2 indicates poor fetal well-being with asphyxia highly probable; immediate delivery or in-depth evaluation is recommended. A total score of 4 or 6 may indicate poor fetal well-being with asphyxia; repeat testing should be performed within 24 hours. A total score of 8 or 10 is considered normal, and the possibility of fetal asphyxia is minimal.

Newborn Assessment

Apgar Score

The Apgar score (Table 2–5) is determined at delivery and is used as an indicator of the degree of and response to resuscitation. The score is used at later dates to provide a clinical picture of the infant's condition at delivery. Each factor is scored as 0, 1, or 2, and the total score is derived. Scoring is usually performed at 1 minute and 5 minutes after delivery. If the score is less than 7, additional scores are taken at 5-minute intervals for 20 minutes or until the score is greater than 7. A score of 0 to 2 indicates the need for immediate resuscitation with endotracheal (ET) intubation, ventilation with 100% oxygen, and cardiac massage. A score of 3 to 4 indicates the need for ventilation with 100% oxygen; cardiac massage is needed if the heart rate is less than 60 beats per minute (bpm). A score of 5 to 7 indicates the need for oxygen via mask or mask-and-bag ventilation. A score of 8 to 10 is normal and does not require any special intervention.

TABLE 2–4 Biophysical Profile Scoring

BIOPHYSICAL VARIABLE	NORMAL (SCORE = 2)	ABNORMAL (SCORE = 0)
Fetal breathing movements	At least one episode of FBM of at least 30 seconds' duration in 30-minute observation	No FBM or no episode of >30 seconds in 30 minutes
Gross body movements	At least three discrete body-limb movements in 30 minutes (episodes of active continuous movement, considered as a single movement)	Two or fewer episodes of body-limb movements in 30 minutes
Fetal tone	At least one episode of active extension with return to flexion of fetal limb or trunk; opening and closing of hand considered normal tone	Either slow extension with return to partial flexion or movement of limb in full extension or absent fetal movement
Reactive FHR	At least two episodes of FHR acceleration of >15 bpm and of at least 15 seconds' duration associated with fetal movement in 20 minutes	Less than two episodes of acceleration of FHR or acceleration of <15 bpm in 40 minutes
Qualitative AFV	At least one pocket of AF that measures at least 1 cm in two perpendicular planes	Either no AF pockets or a pocket <1 cm in two perpendicular planes

Adapted from Manning FA, Lange IR, Morrison I, Harman CR: Fetal biophysical profile score and the nonstress test: A comparative trial. Obstet Gynecol 1984; 64:326.
FBM, fetal breathing movements; FHR, fetal heart rate; bpm, beats per mintue; AFV, amniotic fluid volume; AF, amniotic fluid.

TABLE 2–5 Apgar Scoring

	0	1	2
Heart rate	None	<100 bpm	>100 bpm
Respiratory rate	None	Weak, irregular	Strong cry
Color	Pale blue	Body pink, extremities blue	Completely pink
Reflex (irritability to suctioning)	No response	Grimace	Cry, cough, or sneeze
Muscle tone	Limp	Some flexion	Well flexed

bpm, beats per minute.

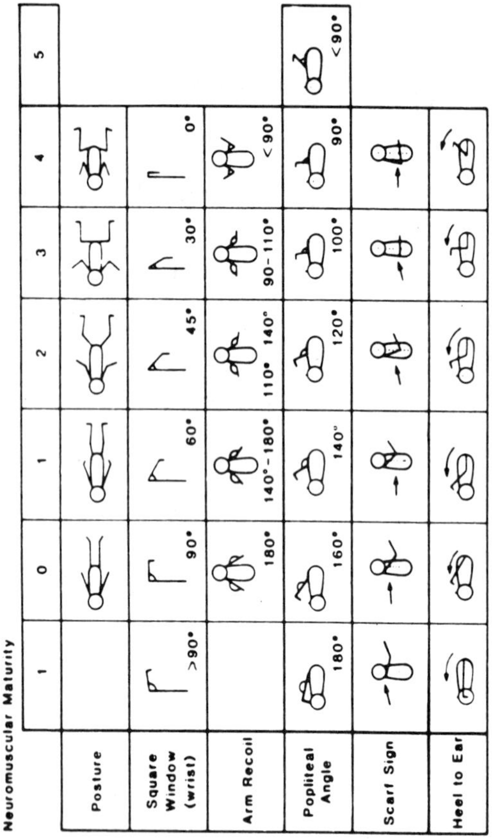

Neuromuscular Maturity

	1	0	1	2	3	4	5
Posture							
Square Window (wrist)	>90°	90°	60°	45°	30°	0°	
Arm Recoil		180°	140°-180°	110° 140°	90-110°	<90°	
Popliteal Angle	180°	160°	140°	120°	100°	90°	<90°
Scarf Sign							
Heel to Ear							

Figure 2–2 *See legend on opposite page*

Physical Maturity

Skin	sticky friable transparent	gelatinous red, translucent	smooth pink, visible veins	superficial peeling &/or rash. few veins	cracking pale areas rare veins	parchment deep cracking no vessels	leathery cracked wrinkled
Lanugo	none	sparse	abundant	thinning	bald areas	mostly bald	
Plantar Surface	heel-toe 40-50 mm: -1 < 40 mm: -2	> 50mm no crease	faint red marks	anterior transverse crease only	creases ant. 2/3	creases over entire sole	
Breast	imperceptible	barely perceptible	flat areola no bud	stippled areola 1-2mm bud	raised areola 3-4mm bud	full areola 5-10mm bud	
Eye/Ear	lids fused loosely: -1 tightly: -2	lids open pinna flat stays folded	sl. curved pinna; soft; slow recoil	well-curved pinna; soft but ready recoil	formed & firm instant recoil	thick cartilage ear stiff	
Genitals male	scrotum flat, smooth	scrotum empty faint rugae	testes in upper canal rare rugae	testes descending few rugae	testes down good rugae	testes pendulous deep rugae	
Genitals female	clitoris prominent labia flat	prominent clitoris small labia minora	prominent clitoris enlarging minora	majora & minora equally prominent	majora large minora small	majora cover clitoris & minora	

Maturity Rating

score	weeks
-10	20
-5	22
0	24
5	26
10	28
15	30
20	32
25	34
30	36
35	38
40	40
45	42
50	44

Figure 2–2 The Ballard score for estimating gestational age using scores derived from neurologic and physical signs. (From Ballard JL: New Ballard score, expanded to include extremely premature infants. J Pediatr 1991; 119:417–423.)

Gestational Age

Although a variety of conditions can hinder fetal growth and result in intrauterine growth retardation, gestational age is the principal determinant of newborn size. Assessment of gestational age should be performed on every newborn and may require consideration of several factors, including dating the last menstrual period, prenatal ultrasound findings, and postnatal physical and neurologic examinations.

Ballard Examination. This examination (Fig. 2–2) is commonly used and should be performed twice by two different examiners 30 to 42 hours after delivery (allows infant time to stabilize). The scores are totaled and gestational age is estimated using the maturity rating scale. Accuracy is plus or minus 2 weeks.

Gestational Age Classification. Once gestational age is determined, weight, length, and head circumference are plotted on a standard newborn grid and gestational age is classified as follows:

Small for gestational age (SGA): weight less than the 10th percentile for gestational age
Appropriate for gestational age (AGA): weight normal for gestational age
Large for gestational age (LGA): weight greater than the 90th percentile for gestational age

Direct Ophthalmoscopy. Examination of the lens with an ophthalmoscope is useful for determination of gestational age in infants between 27 and 34 weeks' gestation.

Physical Examination of the Newborn

Vital Signs

When monitoring vital signs, absolute numbers are not as important as the relative ranges and consideration of the clinical situation (Table 2–6).

Respiratory Rate. Irregular respirations should be noted. Periodic breathing is characterized by intermittent (groups of three or more) respiratory pauses for up to 10 seconds. Apnea is defined as cessation of breathing for longer than 15 seconds. A rate greater than 60 breaths per minute after the first hour of life indicates tachypnea and is an early sign of respiratory distress.

Heart Rate. Normal heart rates vary depending on gestational age. A rate less than 120 bpm indicates bradycardia, which is often associated with anoxia; however, the heart rate in term infants in deep sleep may decrease to 80 bpm.

TABLE 2-6 Normal Neonatal Vital Signs

RESPIRATORY RATE	HEART RATE	BIRTH WEIGHT	BLOOD PRESSURE	MEAN PRESSURE
30–60 breaths/min	120–170 beats/min	>600 g	45/20 mm Hg	25 mm Hg
		>1000 g	48/25 mm Hg	35 mm Hg
		>2000 g	50/30 mm Hg	40 mm Hg
		>3000 g	50/35 mm Hg	45 mm Hg
		>4000 g	65/40 mm Hg	50 mm Hg
		Newborn >12 hr	75/50 mm Hg	60 mm Hg

Blood pressure values from Versmold HT, Kitterman JA, Phibbs RH, et al: Aortic blood pressure during the first 12 hours of life in infants with birth weight 610 to 4220 grams. Pediatrics 1981; 67:607.

A rate greater than 170 bpm indicates tachycardia and is often the first sign of hypoxia; however, agitated infants may have rates greater than 200 bpm. Palpation of pulses may give valuable information: weak pulses suggest low cardiac output, bounding pulses are seen in left-to-right shunts, and delayed or weak pulses in lower extremities may indicate coarctation of the aorta.

Blood Pressure. Comparison of blood pressure in the upper and lower extremities is helpful in diagnosis; lower extremity pressures are usually slightly higher than those in the upper extremities. In the absence of data, an adequate mean blood pressure (BP) may be calculated:

$$\text{Adequate mean BP} = \text{gestational age} + 5$$

Temperature. Normal values are 97.6° F axillary and 99.6° F rectally.

Color

Skin color is an indicator of intravascular volume and perfusion status and is affected by both perfusion and natural complexion (Table 2–7).

Head

Bruising of the head and swollen eyes are common and result from pressures during birth. Fontanels and suture lines should be soft and not bulging. Unusual facies may suggest genetic abnormalities. Nasal patency is assessed by passing a catheter or alternately occluding each naris. Micrognathia (small lower jaw), microstomia (small mouth), and cleft palate are often associated with chromosomal defects. Excessive oral secretions may indicate tracheoesophageal (TE) fistula or esophageal atresia.

Chest

Retractions. Intercostal retractions are usually indicative of respiratory distress caused by reduced lung compliance. The seesaw effect of paradoxical respirations seen with subcostal retractions is indicative of airway obstruction.

Chest Symmetry. Bulging or asymmetry of the chest is found with congenital diaphragmatic hernia (CDH), diaphragm paralysis, phrenic nerve damage, ET tube malposition, enlarged heart, pulmonary hypoplasia, and pneumothorax.

Auscultation. Diminished breath sounds are often due to atelectasis, shallow respirations, respiratory distress syndrome (RDS), and pulmonary interstitial emphysema (PIE).

TABLE 2–7 Common Dermal Findings

FINDING	DESCRIPTION	CONDITION
Jaundice	Yellowish skin	Hyperbilirubinemia
True cyanosis	Centrally blue or dusky skin	Hypoxia
Acrocyanosis	Bluish hands and feet	Cold stress, ↓ circulation—normal for first few hours
Petechiae	Pinpoint hemorrhagic areas	Birth trauma, thrombocytopenia
Telangiectatic nevi	"Stork bites"—red flat areas	Capillary dilation, benign
Subcutaneous fat necrosis	Discrete firm masses in subcutaneous tissue	Trauma
Lanugo	Fine hair	More noticeable in preterm infants, benign
Sclerema	Hardening of the skin	Septicemia, shock, cold stress
Ruddy complexion	Deep reddish skin	Polycythemia or high hematocrit value
Ecchymoses	Bruising of various sizes	Birth trauma, disseminated intravascular coagulation

Table continued on following page

TABLE 2–7 Common Dermal Findings *Continued*

FINDING	DESCRIPTION	CONDITION
Mongolian spots	Irregular areas of pale blue over sacrum and buttocks	Benign, common in black and Asian infants
Strawberry hemangiomas	Bright red, flat spots 1–3 mm in diameter	Benign, usually resolve spontaneously
Milia	White papules <1 mm on forehead, chin, and nose	Distended sebaceous glands that disappear later
Erythema toxicum	Whitish pink papular rash	Cause unknown
Pallor	Pale or white skin	Blood loss or hypovolemia
Vernix caseosa	Whitish gray, cheese-like substance	More abundant on preterm infants
Mottled skin	Uneven color, blotchy	Decreased perfusion

Secretions or fluid in the airways often produces crackles. Stridor is often found with upper airway obstruction.

Abdomen

The normal shape of the abdomen at birth is slightly scaphoid, becoming more distended as the bowel fills with air. Distention is characterized by tightly drawn skin and suggests sepsis, obstruction, tumors, ascites, pneumoperitoneum, or necrotizing enterocolitis. A scaphoid, hollowed, or flat abdomen may indicate CDH. Omphalocele (opening in the abdominal wall into the umbilical cord with protrusion of the membranous sac that encloses the intestines) and gastroschisis (defect in the abdominal wall with protrusion of intestines that are not covered by peritoneum) are obvious defects that require immediate intervention.

Extremities

Extra digits (polydactyly) may be familial or associated with various syndromes and disorders (TE fistula). Syndactyly is abnormal fusion of the digits. Simian creases (a single transverse palmar crease) are found most often in Down's syndrome. Multiple fractures may indicate osteogenesis imperfecta.

Spine

Bony defects with tufts of hair or drainage of clear fluid near the base of the spine should alert one to underlying vertebral abnormalities (meningomyeloceles, encephaloceles).

Neurologic Assessment

The following are observed in normal term infants:

Grasp Reflex. A normal grasp reflex is seen when a finger placed in the palm of the infant's hand is grasped.

Magnet Reflex. A downcurving of the toes when a finger is pressed against the sole of the foot is normal.

Moro Reflex. When the head is allowed to fall back slightly, the infant will extend the extremities rapidly with open hands. This is followed by slow flexion back toward the body.

Normal Muscle Tone. The infant maintains extremities in a flexed position at rest. Poor tone is observed when the infant ''noodles through'' the examiner's hands.

Rooting Reflex. When the infant's lip and a corner of the cheek are stroked, the infant will turn with an open mouth toward that side.

Stepping Reflex. When the examiner suspends the infant and touches the top of the foot against a surface, the infant will lift the leg and then place it flat on the surface.

Table 2–8 lists physical and laboratory findings that may be considered "red flags" and should alert the examiner to further investigate the reason for the abnormality.

TABLE 2–8 "Red Flags" in Newborns

RESPIRATORY	RENAL
Respiratory rate >60 breaths/min	Edema
Grunting or retractions	No urine (anuria)
Cyanosis	↓ urine output (oliguria)
Apnea	No urine in first 24 hr
CARDIAC	**GASTROINTESTINAL**
Heart rate >170 or <90 beats/min	Abdominal distention
New murmur	Bile-stained vomitus
Cyanosis	Abdominal mass
Hypotension	Bloody stools
Decreased or no pulses	Failure to pass stool (48 hr)
GENERAL	**METABOLIC**
Lethargy	Vomiting
Poor feeding	Diarrhea
Infant "not acting right"	Jitteriness
Floppy	Seizures
Cord blood pH <7.2	Jaundice on first day
Low Apgar score	Hypoglycemia
SGA infants	
LGA infants	
Minor congenital anomalies	

Adapted from Ackerman NB, Curran JS: The newborn. *In* Kaye R, Oski FA, Bainars LA (eds): Textbook of Pediatrics. Philadelphia, JB Lippincott, 1988, p 414.
SGA, small for gestational age; LGA, large for gestational age.

HISTORY AND ASSESSMENT OF THE CHILD

Medical History

Information concerning the child's medical history and current illness is usually obtained from the parents, but questions may be directed to the child if his or her age is appropriate. Discussion should include the following areas.

Current Illness

Information should include symptoms, onset, duration, and treatment and response.

Previous Illnesses

Included in the history of previous illnesses should be those that did not require hospitalization as well as where, how, and when conditions were diagnosed; infections; contagious diseases and complications; surgeries; medication and therapy (past and current); rehabilitation; and pulmonary function tests (PFTs).

Birth History

This includes duration of labor, length of delivery, maternal complications (hypertension; sepsis; drug, alcohol, and tobacco use; bleeding), birth weight, length of gestation, Apgar scores, and neonatal history and complications (resuscitation, oxygen, mechanical ventilation, antibiotics required, excessive secretions).

General Health

Issues covered in a general health history should include status of immunizations, sleeping habits (need for frequent naps, insomnia), dental hygiene (tooth abscess), and general habits (tobacco, drugs, alcohol).

Nutritional Status

Appetite, recent weight gain or loss, food allergies, and the presence of respiratory distress or fatigue during feeding should be determined. Height and weight measurements should be compared with predicted values. Failure to thrive (FTT) should be considered in the child whose height or weight, or both, is less than the predicted range. Steroid use may result in a patient being normal in weight but much shorter than predicted for age.

Activity Level

Activities the child is involved in should be determined, including the type (competitive sports, travel). It should also be determined if the child is easily fatigued. School attendance (refusal to attend, poor scholastic performance, decreased class participation), exercise tolerance, and relationships with other children should be investigated.

Family History

The general health of the family should be determined, including the sex of the family members as well as their ages, health, recent illnesses, and previous sibling deaths. Medical information should include histories of asthma, CF, cancer, hypertension, $alpha_1$-antitrypsin deficiency, congenital heart disease, bronchitis, emphysema, and tuberculosis. Social and emotional characteristics should be investigated (happy, depressed, violent). Drug abuse by parents and general life style may cause certain situations or disorders to be suspected (AIDS, hepatitis, trauma, abuse, neglect).

Environment

Living conditions should be investigated, including pollution exposure (smokestacks, cigarette smoke, lawn-garden insecticides), home heating and airconditioning (wood-burning stoves, fireplaces), bedding (feathers, wool), plants, type of neighborhood, and crowded living conditions. The existence of animals (dogs, cats, birds, sheep, cattle) nearby and their health should be discussed, because some disorders (tularemia, psittacosis, histoplasmosis) are linked to contact with certain animals. The parent's work environment should be discussed if the child accompanies the parent to work.

Physical Examination of the Child

Respiratory Rate and Pattern

A child's respiratory rate and breathing pattern are often influenced by activities and sounds. Table 2–9 demonstrates the variability between the awake and sleep states at different ages. Abnormal breathing patterns include Kussmaul's respirations (diabetic ketoacidosis, salicylate overdose), Cheyne-Stokes respirations (congestive heart failure, intracranial hypertension), and Biot's breathing (brain damage).

Skin

Cyanosis. The skin color should be noted. Bluish skin and mucous membranes is referred to as cyanosis. Peripheral

TABLE 2-9 Respiratory Rates Per Minute in Normal Children (Both Sexes, Sleeping and Awake)

	SLEEPING			AWAKE		
Age	No.	Mean	Range	No.	Mean	Range
6–12 mo	6	27	22–31	3	64	58–75
1–2 yr	6	19	17–23	4	35	30–40
2–4 yr	16	19	16–25	15	31	23–42
4–6 yr	23	18	14–23	22	26	19–36
6–8 yr	27	17	13–23	28	23	15–30
8–10 yr	19	18	14–23	19	21	15–31
10–12 yr	11	16	13–19	17	21	15–28
12–14 yr	6	16	15–18	7	22	18–26

From Iliff A, Lee VA: Pulse rate, respiratory rate, and body temperature of children between two months and eighteen years of age. Child Dev 1952; 23:237.

cyanosis occurs in the extremities and central cyanosis involves the tongue and mucous membranes. Cyanosis will not be noticeable unless at least 5 g of reduced hemoglobin is present; thus, it may not be evident in the anemic child in spite of severe hypoxemia. Cyanosis may be located prominently in one area of the body; cyanosis of only the lower body is seen in coarctation of the aorta, whereas cyanosis of only the upper body is seen in transposition of the great arteries. When examining the child for cyanosis, there should be adequate lighting in the room.

Edema. Edematous skin may be categorized as pitting or nonpitting edema. If an impression remains when a finger is pressed firmly against the skin, the child has pitting edema, which is due to an increased amount of extracellular fluid. The child with a puffy appearance but in whom finger pressure does not leave indentations may have nonpitting edema.

Subcutaneous Emphysema. This is felt as a crackling sensation when the skin is pressed and is present most often around the neck, shoulders, and upper chest area. It is seen in cases of trauma and in barotrauma.

Head and Neck

Head Bobbing. When observed in infants, head bobbing results from contraction of the sternocleidomastoid muscle, which causes the head to bob forward in synchrony with each inspiration (Fig. 2–3). This is indicative of increased work of breathing.

Tracheal Palpation. This is performed to determine a normal midline trachea position (Fig. 2–4). During palpation, the patient must be positioned straight with the clinician directly in front of him or her so that vision is not directed more to one side than the other. Changes in volume or pressure on either side of the chest may cause the trachea to move. Lung collapse will pull the trachea toward the unaffected side. Pleural effusion or pneumothorax will exert pressure to push the trachea away from the affected side.

Allergic Facies. Atopic children or those with allergic rhinitis (often associated with asthma) have several characteristic facial features (Fig. 2–5). The dark bluish coloration under the eyes is called allergic shiners and is due to infraorbital venous congestion from edematous tissues. A bilateral fold of skin in the infraorbital region (just below the lower eyelid) is known as the Dennie's line. A transverse nasal crease runs at the junction of the cartilaginous and bony portions of the nose and is produced by the child's constant rubbing of the itchy, runny nose. The child's mouth is opened slightly, signifying some degree of nasal blockage and the need for mouth breathing.

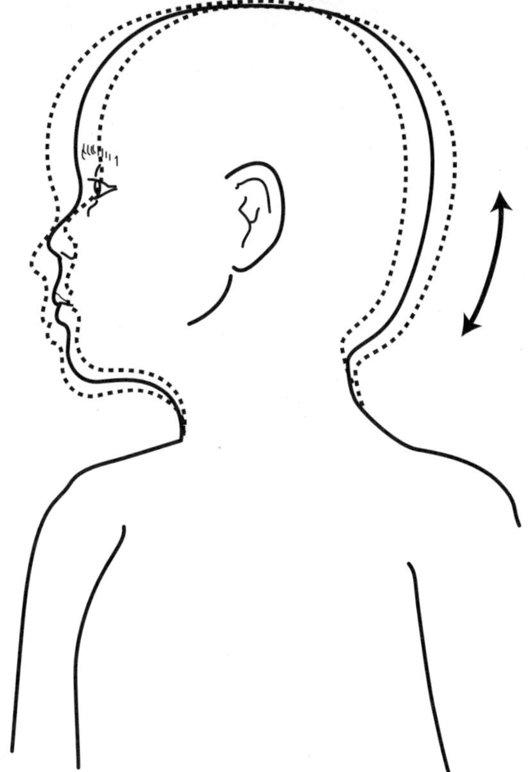

Figure 2–3 Head bobbing.

Nose and Mouth

Nasal patency and discharge (color and amount) should be noted. Patients with CF often have nasal polyps. Nasal flaring is a sign of respiratory distress and is an effort to reduce airway resistance. Fever may cause lips to be cracked or bleeding. Oral and dental hygiene should be noted. Children with a recent history of tooth abscess are susceptible to lung abscess. Foul-smelling breath may indicate a chronic infection such as foreign body obstruction in the nose, allergic rhinitis, bronchiectasis, lung abscess, sinusitis, and poor oral hygiene.

Chest

Chest Expansion and Symmetry. Several disorders may lead to decreased chest expansion or asymmetry, including scoliosis, kyphosis, kyphoscoliosis, atelectasis, pneumonia, hemidiaphragmatic paralysis, and rib cage trauma (flail chest). The shape of the chest and rib cage should be noted.

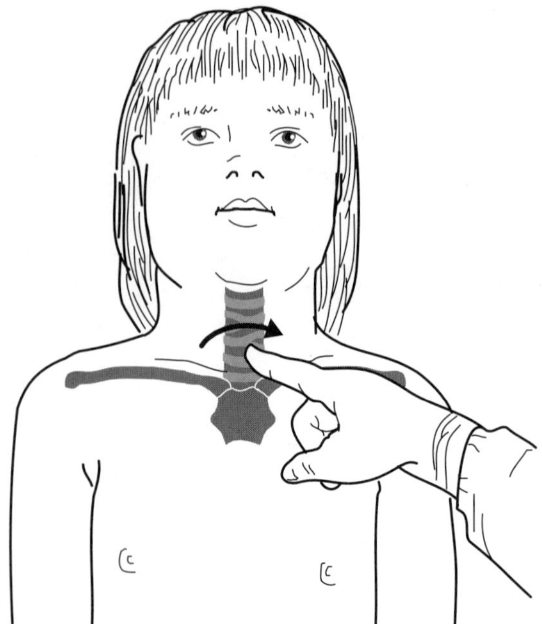

Figure 2–4 Technique for determining tracheal position in the older child.

An increase in the anteroposterior diameter may indicate chronic obstructive pulmonary disease (CF, asthma). A small rib cage may indicate thoracic dystrophy.

Retractions. Suprasternal retractions are observed in the space above the superior border of the sternum and are primarily related to upper airway obstruction disorders including laryngotracheobronchitis (LTB), epiglottitis, laryngomalacia, and postextubation laryngeal edema (Fig. 2–6). Intercostal retractions are observed between the ribs and are seen in obstructive or restrictive disorders, or both (Fig. 2–7). Subcostal (substernal, subdiaphragmatic) retractions are characterized by a drawing inward of the chest just below the lower border of the rib cage and sternum (Fig. 2–8). They usually indicate an upper airway obstruction. Retractions become more obvious as respiratory distress increases.

Abdomen

Several disorders may cause abdominal distention that results in restriction of diaphragm movement and respiratory distress; these disorders include ascites (fluid in the abdomen), hepatomegaly (enlarged liver), and abdominal masses.

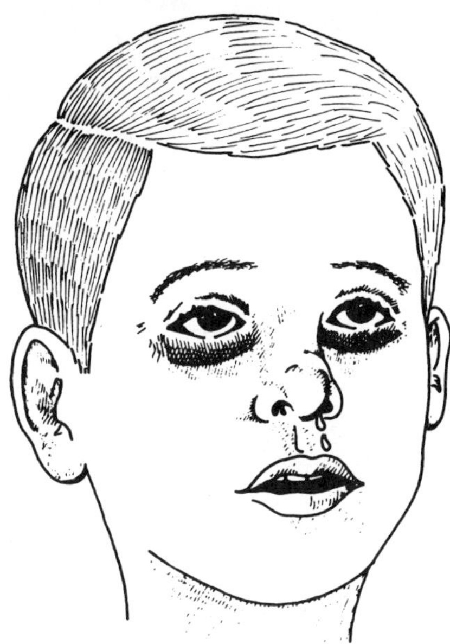

Figure 2–5 The allergic facies of an atopic child, usually with allergic rhinitis. Features include the dark areas under the eyes ("allergic shiners"), "Dennie's lines" below the lower eyelids, the transverse nasal crease, and the slightly opened mouth. (From Simons FEF: Chronic rhinitis. Pediatr Clin North Am 1984; 31:801–819.)

Extremities

The hands and feet should be observed for cyanosis, swelling or edema, and clubbing (Table 2–10). The nailbeds can be used to assess capillary refill. The palms and soles of the feet are often bluish and cold in infants.

Respiratory Sounds

Several respiratory sounds may be heard without using a stethoscope and may be due to mucosal edema or anatomic obstruction of the airway.

Snoring. Snoring sounds may indicate enlarged tonsils and adenoids and may be extremely loud during sleep (Table 2–11).

Stridor. Stridor is a sound produced from upper airway obstruction and is heard most often on inspiration, although it may be heard on expiration. It is commonly heard in epiglottitis, LTB, and postextubation laryngeal edema.

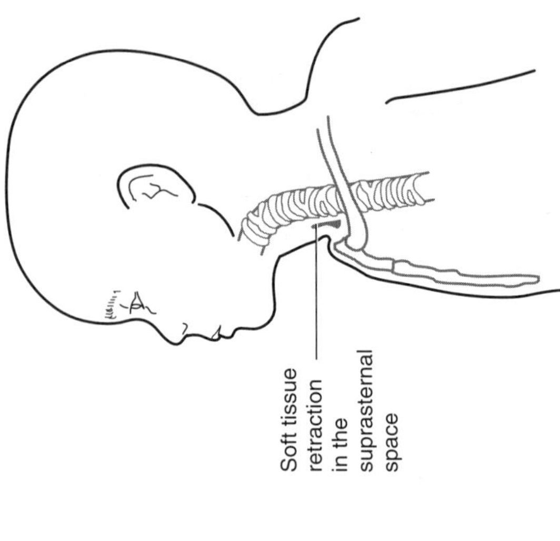

Figure 2–6 Suprasternal retractions. Soft tissue in the suprasternal space is retracted because of a high negative pressure, which is most often due to the patient's attempt to breathe against an airway obstruction.

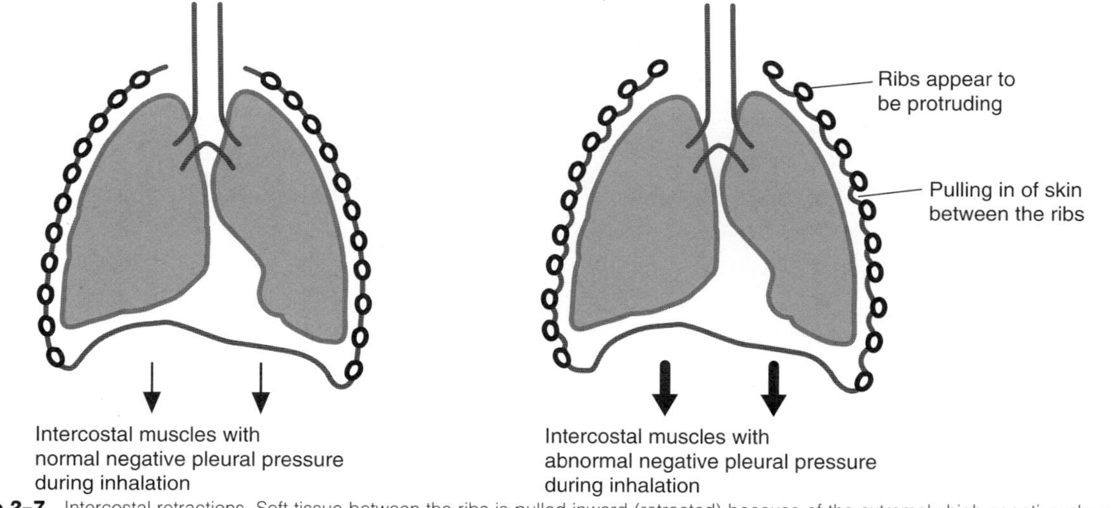

Figure 2–7 Intercostal retractions. Soft tissue between the ribs is pulled inward (retracted) because of the extremely high negative pleural pressure.

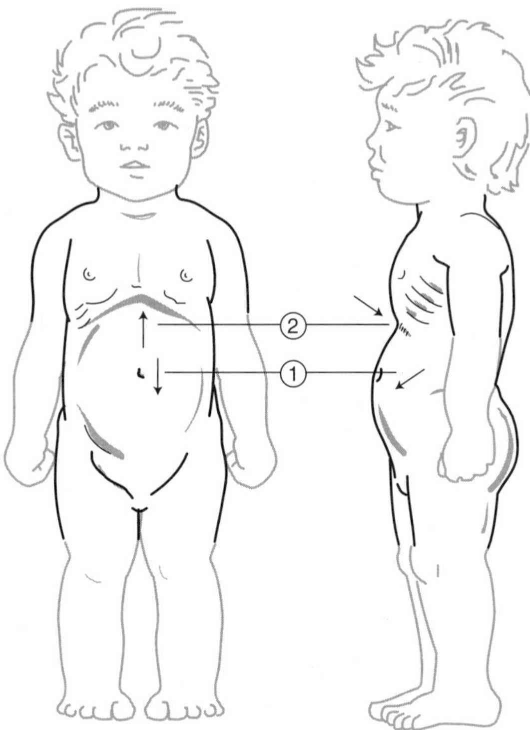

Figure 2–8 Subcostal/substernal retractions. Airway obstruction results in a pulling inward of the lower costal margins. The abdomen is protruding (1) and there is a sunken substernal notch (2). A seesaw movement of the chest and stomach is also present.

Wheezing. Wheezing may be heard on inspiration and expiration without a stethoscope and is typically due to hyperreactive airway disease (asthma). Table 2–12 lists other causes of wheezing.

Grunting. Grunting occurs with closure of the glottis during expiration and is an attempt to maintain lung volume. It is heard most often in pneumonia and atelectasis. The child who is no longer grunting or wheezing may not necessarily have improved lung volume and oxygenation but may instead be in respiratory failure. Further assessment should be performed to determine if there is truly an improvement.

Auscultation

Technique. Less anxiety may result if auscultation is begun on an infant's back when he or she is being held in the parent's arms. Techniques to obtain a deep breath in younger children include "blowing out birthday candles"

TABLE 2–10 Pulmonary and Nonpulmonary Diseases Associated with Clubbing

PULMONARY
Cystic fibrosis
Bronchiectasis
Empyema
Lung abscess
Extrinsic allergic vasculitis
Arteriovenous malformations
Bronchiolitis obliterans
Sarcoidosis
Chronic asthma
CARDIAC
Cyanotic congenital heart disease
Subacute bacterial endocarditis
Chronic congestive heart failure
GASTROINTESTINAL
Crohn's disease
Ulcerative colitis
Chronic dysentery
Small-bowel lymphoma
Cirrhosis
Polyposis coli

Adapted from Pasterkamp H: The history and physical examination. *In* Chernick V (ed): Kendig's Disorders of the Respiratory Tract in Children, 5th ed. Philadelphia, WB Saunders, 1990, p 74.

and a gentle "tickle" in the ribs or on the soles of the feet. Auscultation should be performed in an organized, routine fashion so that a segment is not "missed." It should be carried out over each lung segment for one to two complete breaths, with right and left lung segments compared together (rather than listening to the entire left lung before proceeding to the right lung).

Crackles. Crackles are noncontinuous sounds that may be described as coarse, fine, inspiratory, or expiratory. They may be produced by secretions in the airway or when alveoli are reinflated.

TABLE 2–11 Clinical Symptoms of Children with Heavy Nocturnal Snoring

NIGHTTIME MANIFESTATIONS
Enuresis
Restless sleep
Profuse nocturnal sweating
PROBLEMS WITH GROWTH AND NUTRITION
Anorexia
Poor weight gain
Nausea with and without vomiting
BEHAVIORAL AND LEARNING PROBLEMS
Aggression
Hyperactivity
Social withdrawal
MINOR MOTOR PROBLEMS
Clumsiness
Lack of coordination
OTHER
Frequent morning headaches
Excessive daytime somnolence

Adapted from Pasterkamp H: The history and physical examination. *In* Chernick V (ed): Kendig's Disorders of the Respiratory Tract in Children, 5th ed. Philadelphia, WB Saunders, 1990, p 71.

Wheezes. Wheezes are continuous sounds with a musical quality. They vary in pitch (high, low) and may be heard during inspiration and expiration. They are most often heard with spasm of bronchial smooth muscle, foreign body obstruction, or mucous plugging.

Cough

Effective Cough. Cough may be the most common respiratory complaint in children. It is unusual for infants and young children to expectorate mucus; most will not be able to until 6 years of age. When asked to cough, young children will either swallow the mucus or expectorate saliva only. However, the older toddler or preschooler with a chronic

TABLE 2–12 Causes of Wheezing and Stridor Other Than Asthma

MALFORMATIONS
Airway
Esophageal
Cardiovascular
INFLAMMATION
Tracheitis
Bronchiolitis
Bronchiectasis
Cystic fibrosis
COMPRESSION
Extrinsic
Intrinsic
EXTRATHORACIC DISEASE
Laryngitis
Epiglottitis
Laryngomalacia
Vocal cord paralysis
Peritonsillar abscess
Retropharyngeal abscess
OTHER
Psychogenic
Metabolic disturbances

From Pasterkamp H: The history and physical examination. *In* Chernick V (ed): Kendig's Disorders of the Respiratory Tract in Children, 5th ed. Philadelphia, WB Saunders, 1990, p 71.

lung disease such as CF may be able to effectively cough and expectorate mucus.

Cough Characteristics. A dry, nonproductive cough occurring mainly at night may indicate an allergic disorder. A consistent early morning cough that produces large amounts of sputum is characteristic of chronic lung disease (CF, bronchiectasis). Coughing during or after feeding or in association with swallowing may occur with aspiration due to a neuromuscular abnormality, congenital abnormalities of the upper airway, or gastroesophageal reflux. The barking seal cough is heard when there is obstruction or swelling in the glottic area (LTB, epiglottitis). Paroxysmal coughing may be heard in pertussis infections and foreign body aspiration.

Sputum Production. Volume, color, odor, and the presence or absence of blood in the sputum should be noted. Yellow-green sputum suggests retained secretions. A change in color may indicate that the child's normal flora is changing. Foul-smelling sputum may indicate a lung abscess or empyema. The presence of blood in the sputum (hemoptysis) is considered serious, depending on the frequency and volume of expectorated blood. Ingestion of red candy, cough syrup, and food containing red dye has resulted in mistaken diagnosis of hemoptysis in children. Reddish sputum may be seen in certain pneumonias and in pulmonary embolism.

Bibliography

Avery ME, First LR: Pediatric Medicine. Baltimore, Williams & Wilkins, 1989.

Battaglia FC, Lubchenco LU: A practical classification of newborn infants by weight and gestational age. J Pediatr 1967; 71:159.

Creasy RK, Resnik R: Maternal Fetal Medicine. Philadelphia, WB Saunders, 1994.

Cugell DW: Lung sound nomenclature. Am Rev Respir Dis 1987; 136:1016.

Druzin ML: Antepartum fetal heart rate monitoring—State of the art. Clin Perinatol 1989; 16:627.

Eigen H: The clinical evaluation of chronic cough. Pediatr Clin North Am 1982; 29:67.

Feingold M, Bossert WH: Normal values for selected physical parameters. Birth Defects 1974; 10:14.

Forgacs P: The functional basis of pulmonary sounds. Chest 1978; 73:399.

Garbaciak JA: Prematurity prevention: Who is at risk? Clin Perinatol 1992; 19:277.

Grundy H, Freeman RK, Lederman S, Dorchester W: Nonreactive contraction stress test: Clinical significance. Obstet Gynecol 1984; 64:337.

Hamilton PR, Hauschild D, Broekhuizen FF, Beck RM: Comparison of lecithin: sphingomyelin ratio, fluorescence polarization, and phosphatidylglycerol in the amniotic fluid in the prediction of respiratory distress syndrome. Obstet Gynecol 1984; 63:52.

Hansen-Flaschen J, Nordberg J: Clubbing and hypertrophic osteoarthropathy. Clin Chest Med 1987; 8:287.

Hittner HM, Hirsch NJ, Rudolph AF: Assessment of gestational age by examination of the anterior capsule of the lens. J Pediatr 1977; 94:455.

Iliff A, Lee VA: Pulse rate, respiratory rate and body temperature in children between two months and eighteen years of age. Child Dev 1952; 23:237.

Lepley CJ, Gardner SL, Lubchenco LU: Initial nursery care. *In* Merenstein GB, Gardner SL (eds): Handbook of Neonatal Intensive Care, 3rd ed. St. Louis, Mosby-Year Book, 1993, pp 76–99.

Manning FA, Lange IR, Morrison I, Harman CR: Fetal biophysical profile score and the nonstress test: A comparative trial. Obstet Gynecol 1984; 64:326.

Pasterkamp H: The history and physical examination. *In* Chernick V (ed): Kendig's Disorders of the Respiratory Tract in Children, 5th ed. Philadelphia, WB Saunders, 1990, pp 55–77.

Payne DK, George RB: Clubbing and hypertrophic osteoarthropathy: An overview. Respir Care 1985; 30:256.

Petres RE, Redwine FO: Ultrasound in the intrauterine diagnosis and treatment of fetal abnormalities. Clin Obstet Gynecol 1982; 25:753.

Sanders M, Allen M, Alexander GR, et al: Gestational age assessment in pre-term neonates weighing less than 1,500 grams. Pediatrics 1991; 88:542.

Tabsh K, Theroux N: A primer on biophysical evaluation of the fetus. *In* Pomerance JJ, Richardson CJ (eds): Neonatology for the Clinician. Norwalk, CT, Appleton & Lange, 1993, pp 13–22.

Vintzileos AM, Campbell WA, Nochimson DJ, Weinbaum PJ: Antenatal evaluation and management of ultrasonically detected fetal anomalies. Obstet Gynecol 1987; 69:640.

SECTION 3

Mechanical Ventilation

Abbreviations

A-C–assist-control
AMV–augmented minute ventilation
C–compliance
CMV–continuous mandatory ventilation
CPAP–continuous positive airway pressure
ECMO–extracorporeal membrane oxygenation
ETT–endotracheal tube

F–flow rate
f–respiratory frequency
F_{IO_2}–fraction of inspired oxygen
FRC–functional residual capacity
HFCV–high-frequency conventional ventilation
HFFI–high-frequency flow interruption
HFJV–high-frequency jet ventilation
HFOV–high-frequency oscillatory ventilation
HFPPV–high-frequency positive pressure ventilation
HFV–high-frequency ventilation
Hz–hertz
ICP–intracranial pressure
IMV–intermittent mandatory ventilation
IVH–intraventricular hemorrhage
MMV–minimum minute ventilation
P–pressure
$\bar{P}$aw–mean airway pressure
PCV–pressure-control ventilation
PEEP–positive end-expiratory pressure
PIP–peak inspiratory pressure
PSV–pressure-support ventilation
PVR–pulmonary vascular resistance
R–resistance
SIMV–synchronized intermittent mandatory ventilation
T–time
TCPV–time-cycled, pressure-limited ventilation
$\mathbf{T_e}$–expiratory time
$\mathbf{T_i}$–inspiratory time
$\mathbf{T_{total}}$–respiratory cycle time
VCV–volume-control ventilation
$\mathbf{V_D:V_T}$–dead space to tidal volume ratio
V/Q–ventilation to perfusion ratio
$\mathbf{V_T}$–tidal volume

CLASSIFICATION OF MECHANICAL VENTILATORS

Ventilator Classification Variables

Variables in classifying mechanical ventilators include

1. Portability—stationary, portable
2. Power source—electric, pneumatic, fluidic
3. Control circuit (power mechanism)—electric, pneumatic, fluidic, electronic
4. Circuit characteristics
   a. Single circuit in which the source gas is delivered to the patient—piston, direct gas source
   b. Double circuit in which the source gas is diverted to a delivery mechanism—bellows, inflation bags
5. Control variable used by ventilator to manipulate inspiration—pressure, volume, flow, time (Figs. 3–1 and 3–2)
6. Phase variable measured and used to initiate some phase of the ventilator cycle (Figs. 3–1 and 3–3)
   a. Trigger variable that causes inspiration to begin—pressure, volume, flow, time

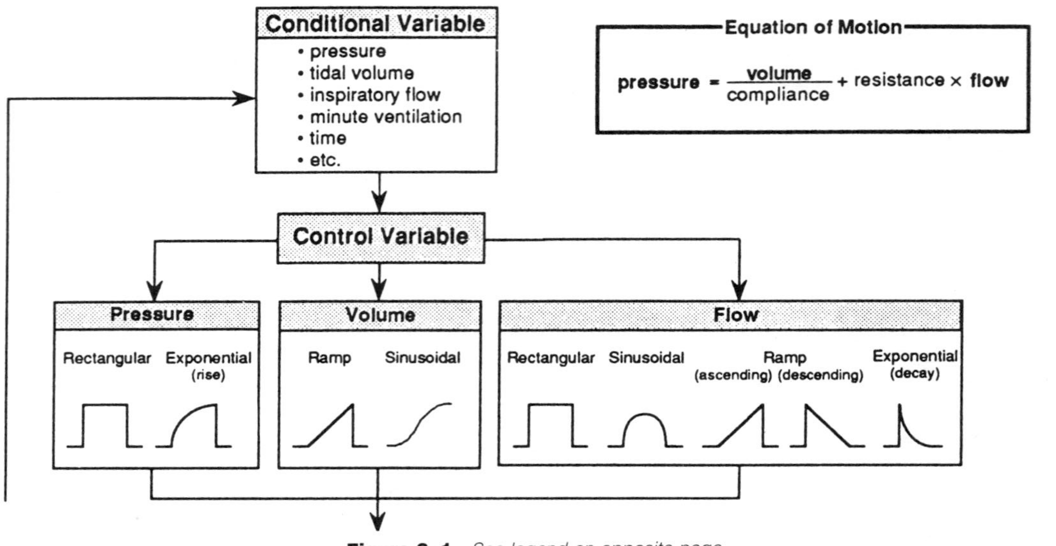

Figure 3–1 *See legend on opposite page*

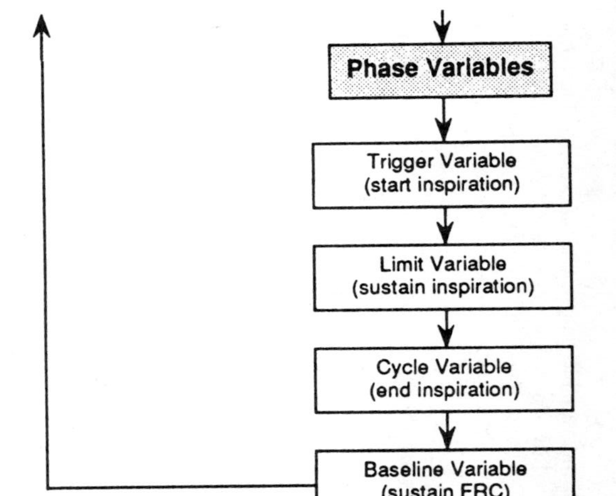

Figure 3–1 A new paradigm for understanding mechanical ventilators based on a mathematical model known as the equation of motion for the respiratory system. The model illustrates that during inspiration the ventilator can control only one variable at a time. The diagram shows common waveforms for each control variable. Pressure, volume, flow, and time are also used as phase variables that determine the characteristics of each ventilatory cycle. The diagram is drawn as a flow chart to emphasize that each breath may have a different set of control and phase variables, depending on the mode of ventilation used. (From Chatburn RL: Classification of mechanical ventilators. Respir Care 1992; 37:1009–1025.)

b. Limit variable that reaches a preset value before the end of inspiration—pressure, volume, flow, time
c. Cycle variable that when reached terminates inspiration—pressure, volume, flow, time

Modes of Ventilation

Ventilator modes used in the mechanical ventilation of neonatal or pediatric patients include

- Control mode: All breaths are delivered at a preset frequency, volume or pressure, and flow rate; the patient cannot trigger the ventilator into inspiration.
- Assist-control (A-C) mode: Ventilator delivers mandatory breaths at a set frequency, volume or pressure, and flow rate; the patient can trigger the ventilator and receive a mandatory breath.
- Intermittent mandatory ventilation (IMV) mode: Ventilator delivers mandatory breaths at a set frequency and volume or pressure; the patient is able to breathe spontaneously between mandatory breaths.
- Synchronized intermittent mandatory ventilation (SIMV) mode: Ventilator delivers breaths as in IMV but attempts to deliver the breaths in synchrony with the patient's inspiratory efforts.
- Pressure-control ventilation (PCV) mode: All breaths are delivered at a preset frequency and are pressure-limited and time-cycled.
- Pressure-support ventilation (PSV) mode: Spontaneous ventilation mode in which each breath must be patient-triggered; the patient's inspiratory effort is assisted up to a preset inspiratory pressure level.
- Continuous positive airway pressure (CPAP) mode: Spontaneous ventilation mode in which each breath must be patient-triggered; a constant level of positive airway pressure is maintained during the entire respiratory cycle.

Control and Phase Variables for Specific Ventilators

Table 3–1 lists the control and phase variables for ventilators commonly used with neonatal and pediatric patients.

CONTINUOUS POSITIVE AIRWAY PRESSURE (CPAP) AND POSITIVE END-EXPIRATORY PRESSURE (PEEP)

Terms used to describe the various applications of positive pressure on exhalation are listed in Table 3–2.

Text continued on page 57

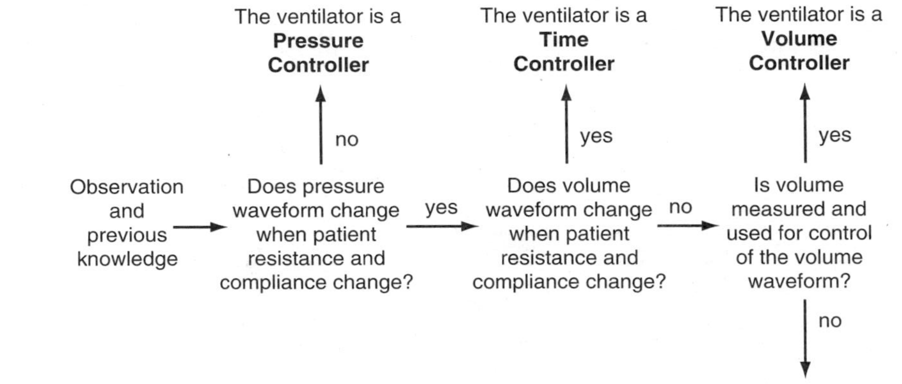

Figure 3–2 Criteria for determining the control variable during a ventilator-assisted inspiration. (From Chatburn RL: Classification of mechanical ventilators. Respir Care 1992; 37:1009–1025.)

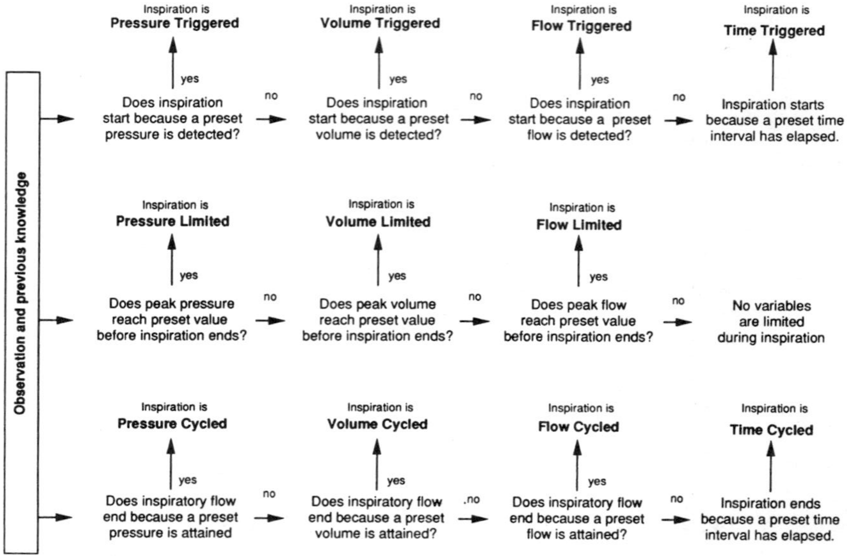

Observation and previous knowledge

Does inspiration start because a preset pressure is detected?
yes → Inspiration is **Pressure Triggered**
no → Does inspiration start because a preset volume is detected?
yes → Inspiration is **Volume Triggered**
no → Does inspiration start because a preset flow is detected?
yes → Inspiration is **Flow Triggered**
no → Inspiration starts because a preset time interval has elapsed. → Inspiration is **Time Triggered**

Does peak pressure reach preset value before inspiration ends?
yes → Inspiration is **Pressure Limited**
no → Does peak volume reach preset value before inspiration ends?
yes → Inspiration is **Volume Limited**
no → Does peak flow reach preset value before inspiration ends?
yes → Inspiration is **Flow Limited**
no → No variables are limited during inspiration

Does inspiratory flow end because a preset pressure is attained
yes → Inspiration is **Pressure Cycled**
no → Does inspiratory flow end because a preset volume is attained?
yes → Inspiration is **Volume Cycled**
.no → Does inspiratory flow end because a preset flow is attained?
yes → Inspiration is **Flow Cycled**
no → Inspiration ends because a preset time interval has elapsed. → Inspiration is **Time Cycled**

Figure 3–3 *See legend on opposite page*

Physiologic Effects

Pulmonary System. Chest wall compliance of the neonate is high, and the chest wall does not have sufficient elastic recoil to maintain an adequate functional residual capacity (FRC). Because of the resulting low-resting lung volumes, a neonate must begin each inspiration from a low-resting lung volume and generate high alveolar opening pressures with each breath. In the premature neonate, this, along with surfactant deficiency, results in an increase in the work of breathing, which may lead to respiratory distress, muscle fatigue, and apnea. Continuous positive airway pressure (CPAP) or positive end-expiratory pressure (PEEP) may stabilize the chest wall and reduce the work of breathing by

- Increasing mean airway pressure ($P\overline{aw}$)
- Preventing early terminal airway closure and atelectasis
- Improving ventilation to areas with a low V/Q ratio
- Potentially reducing airway resistance
- Improving ventilation and oxygenation
- Increasing FRC
- Increasing static lung compliance
- Providing collateral ventilation through the pores of Kohn
- Preventing alveolar collapse and reducing the consumption of surfactant (may enhance surfactant production via cholinergic mechanisms)
- Increasing alveolar pressure and pulmonary vascular pressure independent of interstitial pressure and forcing the movement of water into the interstitium of the lung (redistribution of lung fluid)

Figure 3–4 shows the effect CPAP has on a compliance curve.

Cardiovascular System. The lower the lung compliance, the lower the amount of positive pressure transmitted to the vascular system. CPAP or PEEP may increase intrathoracic pressure, which in turn may

- Reduce venous return and compromise cardiac output
- Decrease right ventricular preload and decrease cardiac output
- Decrease right ventricular end-diastolic volume and decrease stroke volume
- Reduce coronary perfusion and myocardial function

Text continued on page 62

Figure 3–3 Criteria for determining the phase variables during a ventilator-assisted breath. (From Chatburn RL: Classification of mechanical ventilators. Respir Care 1992; 37:1009–1025.)

TABLE 3–1 Control and Phase Variables for Specific Ventilators

Ventilator, Manufacturer	Mode	MANDATORY				SPONTANEOUS			
		Control	Trigger	Limit	Cycle	Control	Trigger	Limit	Cycle
Cub BP2001, Bear Medical Systems, Inc. Riverside, CA	CMV-IMV	P,F*	T†	P,F*	T	—	—	—	—
	CPAP	—	—	—	—	—	—	—	—
	SIMV‡	P,F*	T,F†	P,F*	T	—	—	—	—
	A-C	P,F*	T,F†	P,F*	T	n/a	n/a	n/a	n/a
Babylog 8000, Drager, Inc., Oaksdale, PA	CMV(IMV)	P,F*	T†	P,F*	T,P§	—	—	—	—
	A-C	P,F*	T,V†	P,F*	T,P§	n/a	n/a	n/a	n/a
	SIMV	P,F*	T,V†	P,F*	T,P§	—	—	—	—
	CPAP	—	—	—	—	—	—	—	—
Infant Star, Infrasonics, Inc., San Diego, CA	Continuous flow IMV	P,F*	T†	P,F*	T,P§	P¶	P¶	P¶	P¶
	Demand flow IMV	P,F*	T†	P,F*	T,P§	P¶	P¶	P¶	P¶
	Continuous flow CPAP	—	—	—	—	P¶	P¶	P¶	P¶

	Demand flow CPAP	—	—	—	—	P¶	P¶	P¶	P¶
	SIMV‡	P,F*	T,P†	P,F*	T,P§	P¶	P¶	P¶	P¶
	A-C	P,F*	T,P†	P,F*	T,P§	n/a	n/a	n/a	n/a
IV-100B, Sechrist Industries, Inc., Anaheim, CA	Vent	P,F*	T†	P,F*	T	—	—	—	—
	CPAP	—	—	—	—	—	—	—	—
V.I.P. Bird, Bird Products Corp., Palm Springs, CA	IMV	P,F*	T†	P,F*	T,P§	P¶	P¶	P¶	P¶
	A-C	F	T,P†	F	T,P§	n/a	n/a	n/a	n/a
	SIMV	F	T,P†	F	T,P§	P	P	P	P
	PSV**	—	—	—	—	P	P	P	F,T§
	Continous flow CPAP	—	—	—	—	P¶	P¶	P¶	P¶
	Demand flow CPAP	—	—	—	—	P	P	P	P
Bear 5, Bear Medical Systems, Inc., Riverside, CA	CMV	F	T†	F,V	T,P§	n/a	n/a	n/a	n/a
	Assist CMV	F	T,P†	F,V	T,P§	n/a	n/a	n/a	n/a
	SIMV-IMV	F	T,P†	F,V	T,P§	P¶	P¶	P¶	P¶
	AMV	F	T,P†	F,V	T,P§	P	P	P	P
	Time-cycled	F,P*	T†	F,P*	T,P§	—	—	—	—

Table continued on following page

TABLE 3–1 Control and Phase Variables for Specific Ventilators *Continued*

Ventilator, Manufacturer	Mode	MANDATORY				SPONTANEOUS			
		Control	Trigger	Limit	Cycle	Control	Trigger	Limit	Cycle
	CPAP	—	—	—	—	P¶	P¶	P¶	P§
	PSV**	—	—	—	—	P	P	P	F
Veolar, Hamilton Medical, Inc., Reno, NV	(S)CMV	F	T,P†	F,V	T,P§	n/a	n/a	n/a	n/a
	SIMV	F	T,P†,F‡	F,V	T,P§	P	P,F‡	P	F
	PCV-CMV	P	T,P†	P	T,P§	n/a	n/a	n/a	n/a
	PCV-SIMV	P	T,P†	P	T,P§	P	P,F‡	P	F
	Spontaneous	—	—	—	—	P	P,F‡	P	F
	MMV	—	—	—	—	P	P,F‡	P	F
	PSV**	—	—	—	—	P	P,F‡	P	F,T,P‡§
Wave Model, E200, Newport Medical Instruments, Inc.,	A-C (pressure)	P	T,P†	P	T,P§	n/a	n/a	n/a	n/a
	A-C (flow)	F	T,P†	F,V	T,P§	n/a	n/a	n/a	n/a
	SIMV (pressure)	P	T,P†	P	T,P§	P¶	P¶	P¶	P§

Newport Beach, CA	SIMV (flow)	F	T,P†	F,V	T,P§	P¶	P¶	P¶	P§
	Spontaneous	—	—	—	—	P¶	P¶	P¶	P§
	PSV**	—	—	—	—	P	P	P	F,P,T,V¶§
Servo 900C, Siemans Medical Systems, Inc., Piscataway, NJ	VCV	F	T,P	F,V	T,P§	n/a	n/a	n/a	n/a
	VCV + sigh	F	T,P	F,V	T,P§	n/a	n/a	n/a	n/a
	SIMV	F	T,P	F,V	T,P§	P	P	P	F,P
	SIMV + PSV	F	T,P	F,V	T,P§	P	P	P	F,T,P¶§
	PCV	P	T,P	P	T,P§	n/a	n/a	n/a	n/a
	PSV	—	—	—	—	P	P	P	F,T,P¶§
	CPAP	—	—	—	—	P	P	P	F,P

Adapted from Chatburn RL, Lough MD, Primiano FP Jr: Mechanical ventilation. *In* Chatburn RL, Lough MD (eds): Handbook of Respiratory Care, 2nd ed. St. Louis, Mosby-Year Book, 1990, pp 159–223.

* Applies if airway pressure does not reach set pressure limit.

† Breaths may be manually triggered.

‡ Available with upgraded system only.

§ Secondary or safety cycle variable.

¶ Applies if demand flow provided in addition to available continuous flow.

** May also be set in SIMV and CPAP modes.

P, pressure; F, flow; T, time; n/a, not applicable; —, ventilator does not respond; CMV, continuous mandatory ventilation; IMV, intermittent mandatory ventilation; CPAP, continuous positive airway pressure; SIMV, synchronized intermittent mandatory ventilation; A-C, assist-control; PSV, pressure-support ventilation; AMV, augmented minute ventilation; PCV, pressure-control ventilation; MMV, minimum minute ventilation; VCV, volume-control ventilation.

TABLE 3–2 Terms Used to Describe Positive Pressure

TERM	DEFINITION
CPAP	Application of positive airway pressure throughout the respiratory cycle to spontaneously breathing patients
EPAP	Application of positive airway pressure during exhalation to spontaneously breathing patients, with airway pressure becoming subatmospheric during inspiration
CDP	Application of either positive or negative pressure to maintain increased transpulmonary pressures throughout the respiratory cycle to spontaneously breathing patients
PEEP	Application of positive airway pressure during exhalation to a mechanically ventilated patient.

CPAP, continuous positive airway pressure; EPAP, expiratory positive airway pressure; CDP, continuous distending pressure; PEEP, positive end-expiratory pressure.

- Compress the pulmonary vasculature causing a rise in pulmonary vascular resistance (PVR)
- Shift the intraventricular septum to the left and inhibit left ventricular filling

CPAP may reduce PVR, resulting in less right-to-left shunting via a patent ductus arteriosus or foramen ovale, thus improving oxygenation.

Renal System. CPAP that reduces cardiac output may decrease renal perfusion and urine output. Changes in cardiac output may also stimulate the pituitary gland to secrete anti-diuretic hormone.

Intracranial Pressure. A reduced venous return can lead to an increase in intracranial pressure (ICP), which is a risk factor for intraventricular hemorrhage (IVH) in the preterm infant. However, an increased incidence of IVH has not been associated with nasal or endotracheal tube (ETT) CPAP. Caution should be used, and CPAP devices should *not* be secured around the circumference of the neck.

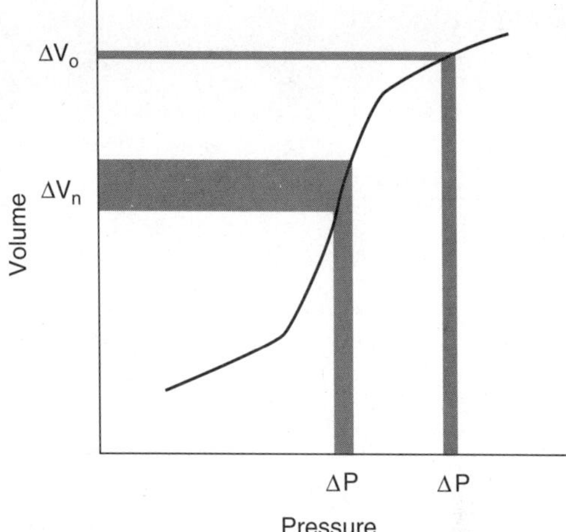

Figure 3–4 Compliance curve shows the effect of overdistention on tidal volume. ΔP is the same amount in each case. ΔV_n is normal compliance and tidal volume. Overdistention places the breath on the flat portion of the compliance curve, resulting in a smaller tidal volume, ΔV_o. The effect of the same level of CPAP-PEEP at various positions on the compliance curve can also be shown. Improved V_T occurs as CPAP-PEEP moves the change in pressure onto the steep portion of the curve. Overdistention occurs when CPAP-PEEP is applied at the top, flat portion of the curve. ΔP, oscillatory amplitude; CPAP, continuous positive airway pressure; PEEP, positive end-expiratory pressure; V_T, tidal volume.

Optimum Continuous Positive Airway Pressure and Positive End-Expiratory Pressure

The amount of pressure that produces maximum alveolar recruitment and FRC but produces the least amount of cardiac embarrassment, alveolar overdistention, and reduction in pulmonary capillary blood flow is considered the optimum level of CPAP or PEEP (best Pa_{O_2} and Pa_{CO_2} at the lowest F_{IO_2}, and possibly the best static lung compliance).

Indications for Continuous Positive Airway Pressure (Table 3–3)

Continuous Positive Airway Pressure Systems

Continuous Flow System. Figure 3–5 illustrates a continuous flow CPAP system using nasal prongs.

Carden Device. The Carden valve can be used to create resistance to expiratory flow and result in CPAP (Fig. 3–6). Gas flow enters the valve through one side port; the other

TABLE 3–3 Indications for Continuous Positive Airway Pressure

DECREASED FUNCTIONAL RESIDUAL CAPACITY
Pneumonia
Pneumonitis
Atelectasis
Pulmonary edema
Smoke inhalation
Meconium aspiration
Postoperative thoracotomy
Respiratory distress syndrome
Transient tachypnea of the newborn
Congenital heart defects with left-to-right shunting
HYPOTONIC AIRWAYS
Mixed apnea
Apnea of prematurity
Obstructive sleep apnea
Tracheobronchial malacia
OTHER
Physiologic CPAP
Weaning from mechanical ventilation

CPAP, continuous positive airway pressure.

port is attached to a proximal pressure manometer. The amount of flow through the valve is approximately equal to the amount of end-expiratory pressure (e.g., 5 L/min flow = 5 cm H_2O CPAP). Dead space volume is approximately 2 ml; adaptors may increase this. The Carden valve may be used continuously or during transport.

Nasal Mask Continuous Positive Airway Pressure. Nasal masks for CPAP delivery are commercially available. Masks should fit well, without leaks, covering the nose but not the mouth or eyes. They are held in place with a harness. Figure 3–7 is an example of a CPAP unit that uses a nasal mask; Figure 3–8 shows nasal masks with sizing gauges and spacers.

Continuous Positive Airway Pressure Failure

Clinical signs that indicate that CPAP therapy has failed are listed in Table 3–4. Mechanical ventilation is indicated if this occurs. If CPAP therapy has failed after being delivered with a mask, nasal prongs, or nasopharyngeal tube, the patient may be intubated and CPAP reinstituted.

MECHANICAL VENTILATION

Goals

The goals of mechanical ventilation (managing gas exchange) are

- To regulate the $Paco_2$—ventilation
- To regulate the Pao_2—oxygenation

Indications

Mechanical ventilation is indicated in an infant or child

- When respiratory failure has occurred secondary to a restrictive or obstructive process
- To reduce respiratory muscle fatigue
- To manage pulmonary or cerebrovascular function
- To normalize oxygen delivery to compensate for cardiac dysfunction
- To correct hypoventilation

Neonatal causes of respiratory failure and indications for mechanical ventilation are listed in Table 3–5. Pediatric situations in which mechanical ventilation is indicated are listed in Table 3–6.

Waveforms and Control Variables

Figures 3–9 through 3–14 illustrate the various waveforms and control variables used during the mechanical ventilation of neonatal and pediatric patients.

Formulas

Formulas that may be used during mechanical ventilation follow:

Effective V_T. Table 3–7 lists the steps needed to derive the effective V_T. Note: When correcting for circuit compliance, it is incorrect to refer to it as ''lost'' volume. The volume is

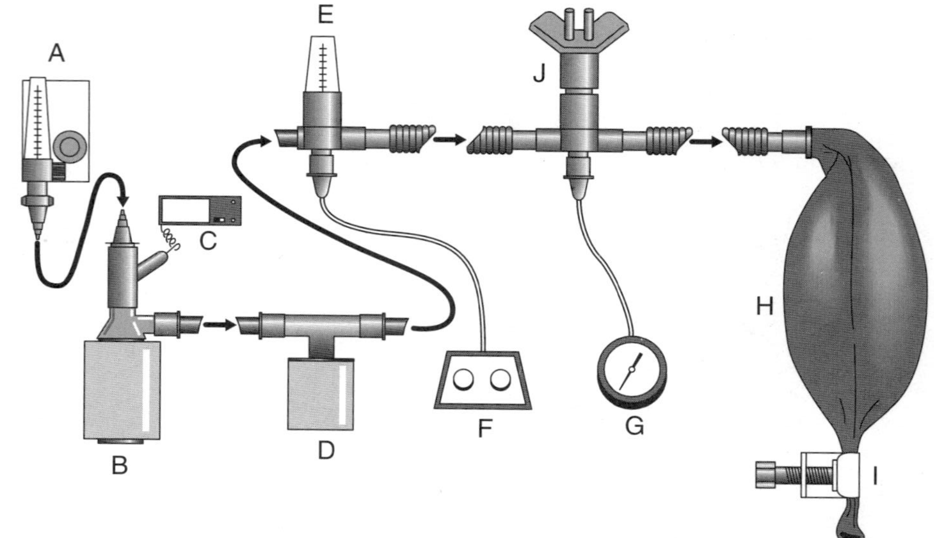

Figure 3–5 *See legend on opposite page*

compressed according to Boyle's law ($P_1V_1 = P_2V_2$). Monitoring exhaled volume does not correct for this phenomenon, since the volume going into the circuit is decompressed when it leaves the circuit. Monitoring volume at the airway with a pneumotachometer minimizes the error.

Desired FIO_2

desired FIO_2 = (desired PaO_2 × known FIO_2)/known PaO_2

Compliance (C)

C = change in volume/change in pressure (ml/cm H_2O)

Resistance (R)

R = change in pressure/change in flow (cm H_2O/ml/sec)

Note: Resistance increases inversely with the radius to the fourth power and proportionately with length.

During Constant Flow Ventilation

Tidal Volume (V_T)

$$V_T = V \times T_i$$

Mean Airway Pressure ($\overline{Paw}$)

$$\overline{Paw} = 1/2(PIP - PEEP) \times (T_i/T_{total}) + PEEP$$

During Time-Cycled, Pressure-Limited Ventilation

Tidal Volume (V_T)

$$V_T \; \alpha \; PIP \text{ and } T_i$$

Mean Airway Pressure ($\overline{Paw}$)

$$\overline{Paw} = [(PIP \times T_i)/T_{total}] + [(PEEP \times T_e)/T_{total}]$$

Time Constant (τ):

$$\tau = C \times R$$

Note: Set the minimum inspiratory or expiratory time 3 × τ

Setting Continuous Flow for a Time-Cycled, Pressure-Limited Ventilator or for Continuous Positive Airway Pressure

Flow = [(8 ml/kg × respiratory rate) × 3]/1000 = L/min

Monitoring During Mechanical Ventilation

Table 3–8 lists monitoring applications as they apply to pediatric mechanical ventilation.

Figure 3–5 Continuous flow CPAP system with nasal prongs; *A*, Blender or O_2-air gas flow. *B*, Heater-humidifier. *C*, O_2 analyzer. *D*, Water trap. *E*, Thermometer. *F*, High-low pressure alarm. *G*, Pressure manometer. *H*, Reservoir bag. *I*, Pigtail clamp. *J*, Nasal prongs.

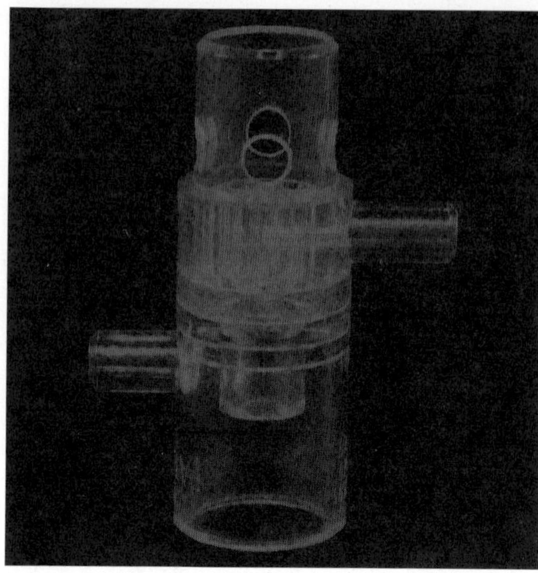

Figure 3–6 Dupaco Carden device (Carden valve). (Courtesy of MPI-Dupaco, Oceanside, CA.)

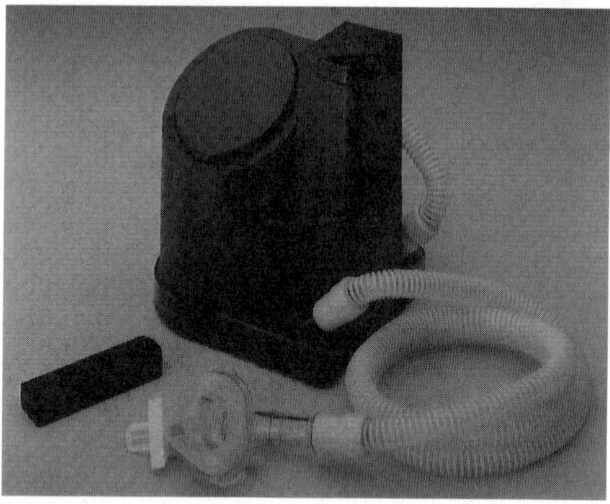

Figure 3–7 REMstar[R] Choice CPAP unit with nasal mask attached. (Courtesy of Respironics, Inc., Murrysville, PA. REMstar[R] is a registered trademark of Respironics, Inc.)

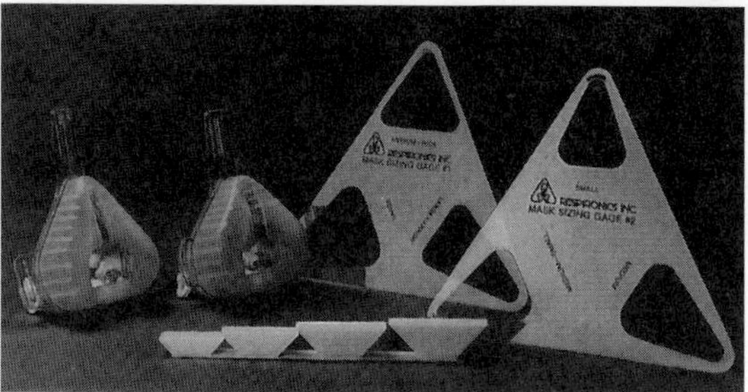

Figure 3–8 Nasal masks with sizing gauges and spacers. (Courtesy of Respironics, Inc., Murrysville, PA.)

Ventilator Settings and Adjustments

Table 3–9 suggests ventilator adjustments for ventilation of neonates. Tables 3–10 and 3–11 list ventilator strategies and adjustments that apply to pediatric patients. The advantages and disadvantages of volume and pressure control ventilation are compared in Table 3–12. Figure 3–15 demonstrates the effect of lung disease on the volume recruited by sustained inflation.

Air Leaks During Mechanical Ventilation

Uncuffed ETTs, tracheostomy tubes, and extrapulmonary air leaks are the most common causes of air leaks during mechanical ventilation. Accurate delivery and monitoring of the V_T are difficult. Air leaks may affect ventilator triggering mechanisms, especially pressure-triggered mechanisms. Reintubation is usually required if a patient is being volume-ventilated and the leak is greater than 15% to 20% of the tidal volumes or if the leak causes respiratory or hemodynamic instability. During pressure ventilation, leaks still occur, but

TABLE 3–4 Indicators of Continuous Positive Airway Pressure Failure

pH <7.25
Pa_{O_2} <50 mm Hg
Pa_{CO_2} >55 mm Hg
Fi_{O_2} >0.6
CPAP level >12 to 15 cm H_2O
Recurrent apnea and bradycardia

CPAP, continuous positive airway pressure.

TABLE 3–5 Causes of Respiratory Failure

PROBLEM AREA	POSSIBLE CAUSES	PROBLEM AREA	POSSIBLE CAUSES
Pulmonary	Respiratory distress syndrome (RDS)	Abnormalities of muscles of respiration	Phrenic nerve palsy
	Aspiration syndromes		Spinal cord injury
	Pneumonia		Myasthenia gravis
	Pulmonary hemorrhage		Werdnig-Hoffmann syndrome
	Pulmonary edema	Central problems	Apnea of prematurity
	Wilson-Mikity syndrome		Drugs; morphine, magnesium sulfate mepivacaine, meperidine
	Bronchopulmonary dysplasia		Seizures
	Pulmonary insufficiency of prematurity		Birth asphyxia
	Pneumothorax		Hypoxic encephalopathy
	Tumor		Intracranial hemorrhage
	Diaphragmatic hernia		Ondine's curse
	Chylothorax		Rapid eye movement sleep

	Congenital malformations (lobar emphysema, cystic adenomatoid malformation, lymphangiectasis)	Miscellaneous	Congestive heart failure
			Persistent fetal circulation
Airway	Laryngomalacia		Postoperative
	Choanal atresia		Tetanus neonatorum
	Pierre Robin syndrome		Extreme immaturity
	Micrognathia		Shock
	Nasopharyngeal tumor		Sepsis
	Subglottic stenosis		Hypoglycemia
			Electrolyte abnormalities
			Acid-base imbalance
			Infant botulism

From Goldsmith JP, Karotkin EH: Introduction to assisted ventilation. *In* Goldsmith JP, Karotkin EH (eds): Assisted Ventilation of the Neonate, 2nd ed. Philadelphia, WB Saunders, 1988.

TABLE 3–6 Clinical Indications for Mechanical Ventilation

RESTRICTIVE PROCESS
ARDS
Pneumonia
Flail chest
Bronchopleural fistula
Neuromuscular disorder
Myasthenia gravis
Muscular dystrophy
Guillain-Barré syndrome
OBSTRUCTIVE PROCESS
Asthma
Bronchiolitis
Cystic fibrosis
Bronchopulmonary dysplasia
HYPOVENTILATION
Sleep apnea
Overdose-poisoning
Postoperative recovery
INCREASED INTRACRANIAL PRESSURE
Infection
Head trauma
Near-drowning
Reye's syndrome
CARDIOVASCULAR DYSFUNCTION
Cardiac shunting
Circulatory collapse
Congestive heart failure
Postoperative cardiac surgery
Increased pulmonary vascular resistance

ARDS, adult respiratory distress syndrome.

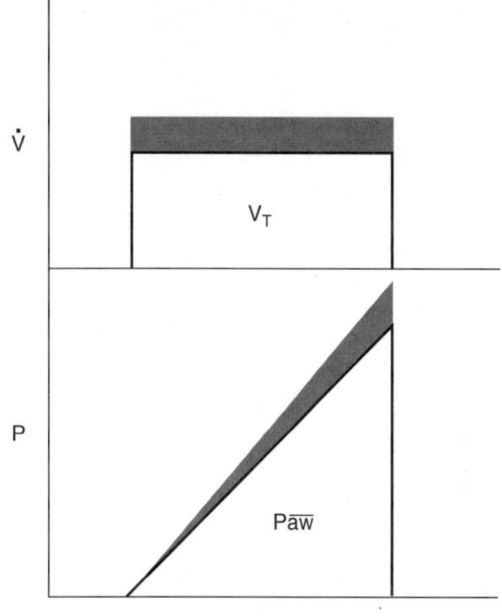

Figure 3–9 Flow ($\dot{V}$) and pressure (P) waveforms during constant flow-volume ventilation. The unshaded area below each waveform represents tidal volume (V_T) and mean airway pressure ($P\overline{aw}$). The shaded area represents the increase in V_T and $P\overline{aw}$ when flow is increased.

effective V_T may be improved by increasing flow and PIP. During volume ventilation, increasing V_T and monitoring the exhaled volumes may help improve the effective V_T. Effective V_T is not equal to the inflation volume or the exhaled volume.

Complications

Complications of mechanical ventilation are listed in Table 3–13.

HIGH-FREQUENCY VENTILATION

Types

High-Frequency Ventilation (HFV). HFV consists of mechanical ventilation using V_T less than or equal to dead space, delivered at supraphysiologic rates.

High-Frequency Conventional Ventilation (HFCV). HFCV consists of conventional pressure-limited infant venti-

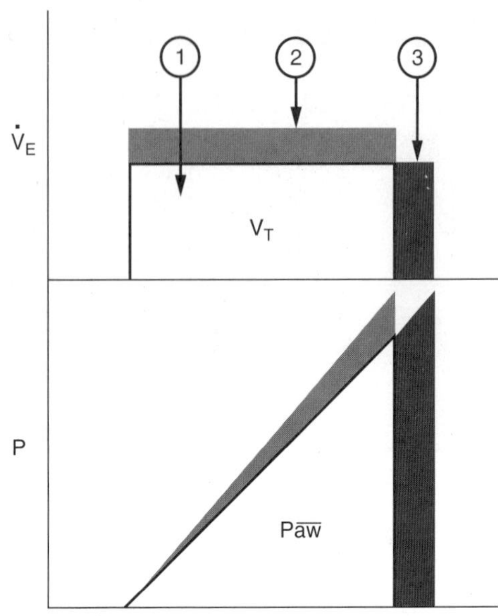

Figure 3–10 Control variables that affect minute ventilation ($\dot{V}_E$) by increasing the area under the flow waveform to increase V_T. Changes in ventilator settings affect the V_T and $P\overline{aw}$. *1,* Increase V_T or rate; PIP determines V_T but depends on pulmonary compliance and resistance. *2,* Increase VI; V_T increases with increases in flow. *3,* Increase T_i; V_T increases with increases in T_i. Also shown is the associated change in $P\overline{aw}$. V_T, tidal volume; $P\overline{aw}$, mean airway pressure; PIP, peak inspiratory pressure; VI, inspired volume per minute; T_i, inspiratory time.

lators using rates up to 150 breaths per minute (2.5 Hz). Exhalation is achieved by passive recoil.

High-Frequency Flow Interruption (HFFI). HFFI consists of the delivery of short, high-pressure, low V_T breaths administered proximal to the ETT. HFFI is frequently used in conjunction with conventional ventilation. Exhalation is achieved by passive recoil.

High-Frequency Jet Ventilation (HFJV). HFJV consists of the delivery of short jet bursts of gas distal to the proximal end of a triple-lumen ETT (using a modified triple-lumen tube or a jet catheter placed into the connector of a standard ETT) at rates of 4 to 11 Hz. Exhalation is achieved by passive recoil. HFJV is frequently used in conjunction with conventional ventilation.

High-Frequency Oscillatory Ventilation (HFOV). HFOV consists of the delivery of extremely small sine wave V_T at rates of 8 to 30 Hz, generated by a piston or speaker. Exhala-

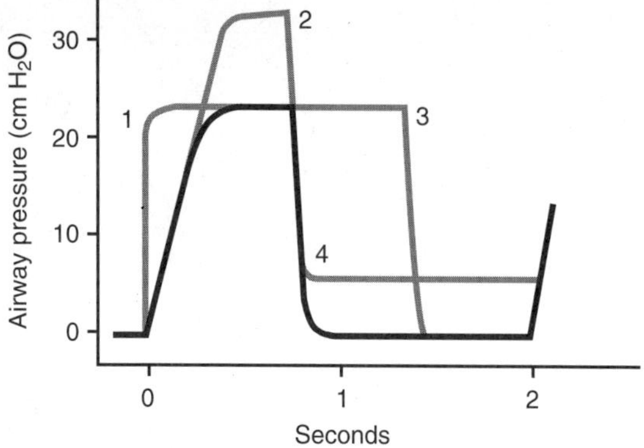

Figure 3–11 Four different ventilator setting increases that augment mean airway pressure: *1,* inspiratory flow; *2,* peak inspiratory pressure; *3,* I : E ratio; and *4,* positive end-expiratory pressure. (Redrawn from Harris TR: Physiological principles. *In* Goldsmith JP, Karotkin EH [eds]: Assisted Ventilation of the Neonate, 2nd ed. Philadelphia, WB Saunders, 1988, p 43; and Reynolds EOR: Pressure waveform and ventilator settings for mechanical ventilation in severe hyaline membrane disease. Int Anesthesiol Clin 1974; 12:259.)

tion is active. HFOV devices are generally not used in conjunction with conventional ventilation. A standard ETT is used with HFOV.

High-Frequency Devices Currently Available

Programmable Volumetric Diffusive Respirator (Bird Space Technologies, Sandpoint, ID). This device can provide conventional ventilation and HFV with passive exhalation. Adjustments can be made in the pressure amplitude, frequency, and inspiratory to expiratory ratio. It monitors airway pressure proximal to the ETT.

Infant Star HFV (Infrasonics, Inc., San Diego, CA). This device is a modification of the Infant Star neonatal ventilator. It can provide conventional ventilation or HFV with active exhalation, or both. Adjustments can be made in pressure amplitude and frequency when in the HFV mode. $\overline{Paw}$ is usually adjusted by altering the end-expiratory pressure on the conventional ventilator. This device monitors $\overline{Paw}$ proximal to the ETT.

Bunnell Life Pulse Ventilator (Bunnell, Inc., Salt Lake City, UT). This is an HFJV device. It requires a special ETT and pinch valve. Adjustments can be made in the peak airway pressure and rate and T_i. It monitors $\overline{Paw}$ in the trachea.

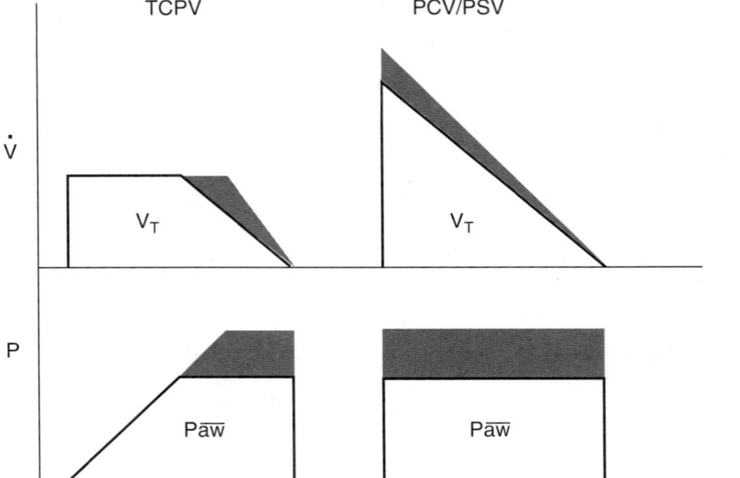

Figure 3–12 Waveforms comparing the mechanism of increasing tidal volume (V_T) by adjusting pressure limit during time-cycled pressure-limited ventilation (TCPV) to pressure-control or pressure-support ventilation (PCV/PSV). Flow changes during PCV/PSV, but only the length of time changes before flow decelerates during TCPV.

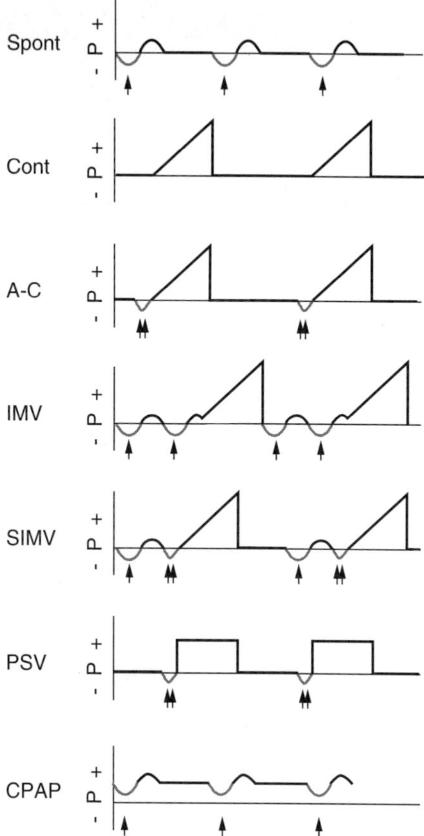

Figure 3–13 Pressure waveforms of seven modes of ventilation. *Single arrows* note spontaneous inspiratory efforts. *Double arrows* note ventilator breaths triggered by inspiratory efforts. Spont, spontaneous breathing; Cont, controlled ventilation; A-C, assist-control ventilation; IMV, intermittent mandatory ventilation; SIMV, synchronized intermittent mandatory ventilation; PSV, pressure-support ventilation; CPAP, continuous positive airway pressure.

SensorMedics Model 3100A (SensorMedics Corp., Yorba Linda, CA). This is an HFOV device. Adjustments can be made in the $\overline{Paw}$, pressure amplitude, ventilator frequency, and T_i percentage. It monitors $\overline{Paw}$ proximal to the ETT.

Humming II (Senko Medical Instruments, Tokyo, Japan). This is an HFOV device similar to SensorMedics Model 3100A. Adjustments can be made in the $\overline{Paw}$, ventilator frequency, and T_i percentage. It can produce sustained lung inflation. It monitors $\overline{Paw}$ proximal to the ETT.

Indications

HFV is used to achieve adequate gas exchange at the lowest peak and mean airway pressures in neonates in whom conventional ventilation has failed. Neonates with pulmonary interstitial emphysema may experience a more rapid resolution of emphysema with HFV than with conventional ventilation. It may reduce the occurrence of air leak syndromes, chronic lung disease, and the need for extracorporeal membrane oxygenation (ECMO).

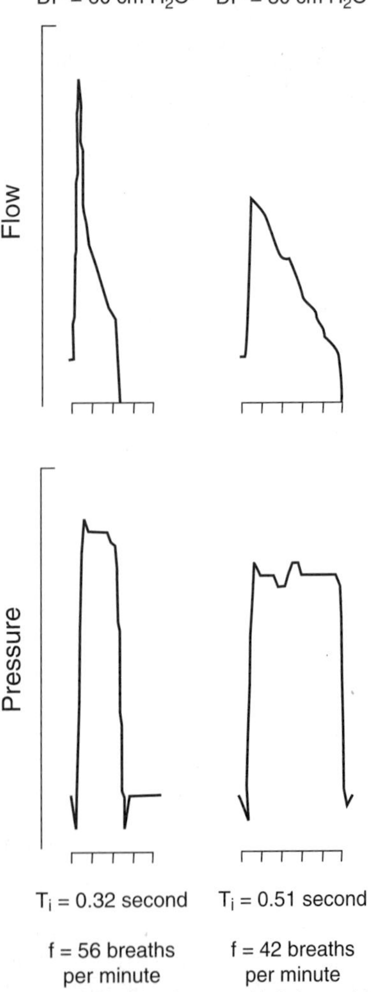

Figure 3–14 Waveforms and inflation variables comparing a high driving pressure (DP) (60 cm H_2O) and a low driving pressure (30 cm H_2O) to generate flow during pressure-support ventilation of an infant.

TABLE 3–7 Calculation of Effective Tidal Volume

$$V_{Teff} = V_{Tset} - [(P_{static}{}^{*} - PEEP) \times C_{circuit}]$$

DETERMINATION OF COMPLIANCE FACTOR OF CIRCUIT

(1) With the circuit assembled and connected to the ventilator, the patient connection to the circuit is occluded.

(2) A known volume of gas is delivered into the circuit via the ventilator and the resulting peak inspiratory pressure is noted.

(3) The resulting delivered volume is divided by the pressure to obtain the compliance factor of the circuit. This is generally 2 ml/cm H_2O for infant circuits and 3 to 4 ml/cm H_2O for larger circuits.

V_{Teff}, effective tidal volume; V_{Tset}, tidal volume set on ventilator; P_{static}, static (plateau) pressure measured during inflation; PEEP, positive end-expiratory pressure set on ventilator; $C_{circuit}$, compliance or compression factor of circuit.
* If static or plateau pressure measurement cannot be obtained because of airway leaks, the peak inspiratory pressure may be used as an approximation.

High-Frequency Ventilation Management

Table 3–14 is a generic list of oxygenation and ventilation strategies used during HFV ventilation. Sustained lung inflations are sometimes used to restore collapsed alveoli, whereas $\overline{Paw}$ is used to maintain lung recruitment (see Fig. 3–15). If poorly timed or controlled, sustained inflation may result in a decrease in cardiac output and blood flow to the brain, as well as in lung injury.

Adequate Inflation

Indicators used to determine adequate inflation during HFV include

- Chest x-ray findings
- Stomach wiggle
- Transcutaneous oxygen and carbon dioxide values
- Pulse oximetry saturation values
- Static compliance
- Indirect measures of cardiac output
- PaO_2:PAO_2 ratio

TABLE 3–8 Monitoring Applications in Pediatric Mechanical Ventilation

MEASURED VENTILATOR VARIABLES	SUPPLEMENTAL MONITORS
Effective tidal volume	Pulse oximetry
Minute ventilation	End-tidal carbon dioxide
Mean airway pressure ($\overline{Paw}$)	End-tidal carbon dioxide to $Paco_2$ gradient
Low-high PEEP	Pressure-volume loop
High peak pressure	Esophageal pressure
FIO_2	Transpulmonary pressure
Pause pressure	Dead space to tidal volume ratio
I:E ratio	Ineffective to effective tidal volume ratio
Pressure waveform	Work of breathing
Flow waveform	Pressure time product
Static compliance	Pressure time index
Respiratory time fraction	
Dynamic compliance	
Airway resistance	
Respiratory time constant	
Maximal inspiratory occlusion pressure	
Maximal expiratory occlusion pressure	
Maximal minute ventilation	
Vital capacity	

I:E, inspiratory to expiratory.

Complications

Complications that may be encountered during HFV include

- Air trapping
- Disconnection
- Tracheitis—may be the result of jet flow injury or reduced humidity
- Hypotension
- Intraventricular hemorrhage (IVH)

- Cardiac dysfunction:
  Reduced venous return
  Increased PVR
  Reduced cardiac output

TABLE 3-9 Suggested Neonatal Ventilator Adjustments

SETTING	ADJUSTMENT INCREMENT	ANTICIPATED RESULTS
FIO_2	2–5 (%)	Change in PaO_2
PIP	+1–2 (cm H_2O)	Increased PaO_2 Decreased $PaCO_2$
PEEP	+1–2 (cm H_2O)	Increased PaO_2 Decreased $PaCO_2$
T_i	+0.1–0.2 (sec) −0.1–0.2 (sec)	Increased PaO_2 Better synchronization
Rate	2–5 (breaths per minute)	Change in $PaCO_2$

PIP, peak inspiratory pressure; PEEP, positive end-expiratory pressure, T_i, inspiratory time.

TABLE 3–10 Pediatric Ventilator Strategies by Medical and Surgical Condition

CONDITION	VENTILATOR STRATEGY	RATIONALE
Apnea, hypoventilation	Intubation and PPV	Prevent respiratory acidosis
Neuromuscular disease	Pressure-support or negative-pressure ventilation	Decrease work of breathing
Restrictive lung disease (e.g., scoliosis, pulmonary hypoplasia)	Prolonged T_i or inspiratory plateau	Allow gas distribution
Upper airway obstruction	Artificial airway, usually with IMV	Maintain patent airway
Small airways disease (asthma, bronchiolitis, BPD)	Bronchodilation, prolonging T_e	Diminish air trapping
Alveolar disease; atelectasis; pulmonary edema	PEEP, inverse ratio ventilation	Improve lung volumes and hypoxemia

Flail chest	Moderate PEEP	Stabilize chest wall
Bronchopleural fistula	Minimum necessary PIP, PEEP, and T_i	Minimize air leak
Low-output state; cardiogenic shock	PPV with minimal PEEP necessary	Avert acidosis, decrease PVR
Pulmonary hypertension; elevated PVR	Elevated Po_2, hyperventilation	Pulmonary vasodilation
Left-to-right shunt—pulmonary hyperemia	Minimize Fio_2, moderately high PEEP; avoid hyperventilation	Increase PVR, reduce pulmonary blood flow
Fontan physiology (right atrium to pulmonary artery)	Low PIP and PEEP, early extubation	Minimize PVR
Pulmonary or pericardial hemorrhage	High PEEP	Tamponade bleeding

Adapted from Klem SA: Cardiovascular support—Mechanical. *In* Holbrook PR (ed): Textbook of Critical Care. Philadelphia, WB Saunders, 1993, pp 279–287.
PEEP, positive end-expiratory pressure; PPV, positive-pressure ventilation, T_i, inspiratory time; IMV, intermittent mandatory ventilation; BPD, bronchopulmonary dysplasia; T_e, expiratory time; PVR, pulmonary vascular resistance.

TABLE 3–11 Pediatric Ventilator Adjustments Related to Goals of Ventilation

Goal	Adjustment
Increase ventilation (decrease Pa_{CO_2})	Increase f Increase V_T (or PIP) Increase $\dot{V}$ Increase T_i
Increase oxygenation (increase $\overline{Paw}$)	Increase F_{IO_2} Increase PEEP Increase V_T (or PIP) Increase f Increase $\dot{V}$ Increase T_i

f, frequency; V_T, tidal volume; $\dot{V}$, minute volume; T_i, inspiratory time; F_{IO_2}, fraction of inspired oxygen; PEEP, positive end-expiratory pressure; PIP, peak inspiratory pressure; $\overline{Paw}$, mean airway pressure.

TABLE 3–12 Volume-Versus Pressure-Control Ventilation

PRESSURE		VOLUME	
Advantages	**Disadvantages**	**Advantages**	**Disadvantages**
Decelerating flow waveform allows for diffusion of gas during low-flow period of inflation	Higher initial flow and airway resistance, V_T changes with compliance changes	Constant flow during inflation cycle	V_T delivery equal throughout inflation cycle, less time for gas diffusion at end of inflation
Constant PIP during inflation, sustained alveolar opening pressure, lower PIP, improved $V_D : V_T$, improved distribution of gas exchange, improved ventilation and oxygenation	Higher $P\overline{aw}$, potential increase in pulmonary vascular resistance	Gas diffusion augmented with end-inspiratory pause (system with no leak)	Variable PIP during inflation

PIP, peak inspiratory pressure; V_D: V_T, dead space to tidal volume ratio; V_T, tidal volume; $P\overline{aw}$, mean airway pressure.

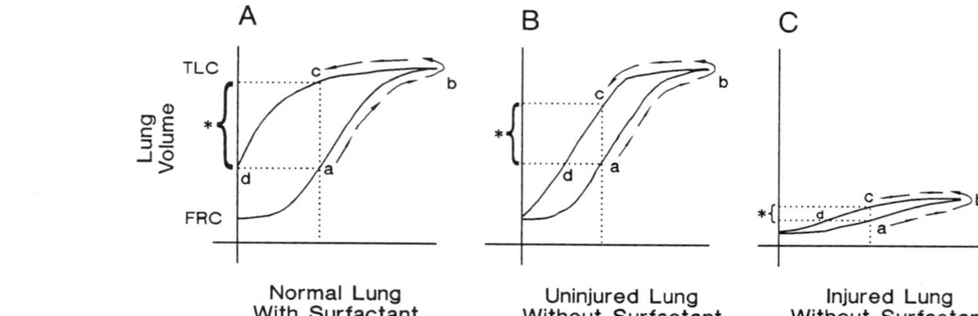

Figure 3–15 Effect of lung disease on the volume recruited by sustained inflation (SI). *A*, Pressure-volume (P-V) curve characteristic of a normal lung with surfactant. Total lung capacity (TLC) is normal, and good stability is demonstrated during deflation. *B*, P-V curve of a surfactant-deficient lung without pulmonary injury. It demonstrates a TLC similar to that in *A*, but deflation stability is poor. *C*, P-V curve of a surfactant-deficient lung with pulmonary injury. It demonstrates reduced TLC and poor deflation stability. On each P-V curve, point *a* is the position prior to an SI; point *b* is peak inflation; point *c* is the position at the end of inflation if the preinflation airway pressure (Paw) is equal to the postinflation Paw; and point *d* occurs if preinflation Paw is greater than postinflation Paw. (From Gerstmann DR, deLemos RA: High-frequency ventilation: Issues of strategy. Clin Perinatol 1991; 18:563.)

TABLE 3–13 Complications of Mechanical Ventilation

OVERDISTENTION

Air leaks
- Pneumothorax
- Pneumomediastinum
- Pneumopericardium
- Pneumoperitoneum
- Subcutaneous emphysema

Excessive $\overline{Paw}$

Reduced ventilation

Increased work of breathing

Increased anatomic dead space

Decreased static compliance

Increased leak around ETT

Difficulty in weaning

CARDIOVASCULAR COMPROMISE

Reduced cardiac function
- Decreased cardiac output
- Decreased venous return
- Ventricular septal distention
- Increased PVR
- Reduced pulmonary and cardiac blood flow
- Vascular shunting changes (may be used therapeutically)

ALTERATIONS IN CEREBRAL BLOOD FLOW

Increased ICP and IVH

Reduced cerebral blood flow (may be used therapeutically)

OXYGEN TOXICITY

Retinopathy of prematurity

Bronchopulmonary dysplasia

UNDERVENTILATION

Inadvertent disconnection

Inadvertent extubation

Mainstem bronchus intubation

Kinking of ETT

Plugging of endotracheal-tracheostomy tube

Respiratory muscle fatigue

Mechanical, electrical, or source gas failure

Operator error

Table continued on following page

TABLE 3–13 Complications of Mechanical Ventilation *Continued*

RENAL DYSFUNCTION
Alterations in renal blood flow rate
Inappropriate antidiuretic hormone secretion
Fluid retention
INFECTION
Pneumonia
Sepsis
Aspiration
Tracheitis

$P\overline{aw}$, mean airway pressure; ETT, endotracheal tube; PVR, pulmonary vascular resistance; ICP, intracranial pressure; IVH, intraventricular hemorrhage.

TABLE 3–14 Generic Oxygenation and Ventilation Strategies for Use During High-Frequency Ventilation in Patients With Diffuse Lung Disease

OXYGENATION STRATEGIES			
Pa_{O_2}	Increased	Normal	Decreased
Lung inflation	Normal	Normal	Normal
Primary response	Decrease F_{IO_2}	None	Increase F_{IO_2}
Secondary response	None	None	None
Pa_{O_2}	Increased	Normal	Decreased
Lung inflation	Decreased	Decreased	Decreased
Primary response	Increase $P\overline{aw}$	Increase $P\overline{aw}$	Increase $P\overline{aw}$
Secondary response	Decrease F_{IO_2}	None	Increase F_{IO_2}

Table continued on following page

TABLE 3–14 Generic Oxygenation and Ventilation Strategies for Use During High-Frequency Ventilation in Patients With Diffuse Lung Disease *Continued*

OXYGENATION STRATEGIES			
Pa_{O_2}	Increased	Normal	Decreased
Lung inflation	Increased	Increased	Increased
Primary response	Decrease $P\overline{aw}$	Decrease $P\overline{aw}$	Decrease $P\overline{aw}$
Secondary response	Decrease F_{IO_2}	None	Increase F_{IO_2}
VENTILATION STRATEGIES			
Pa_{CO_2}	Increased	Normal	Decreased
Primary response	Increase OA	None	Decrease OA
Secondary response	Decrease frequency	None	Increase frequency

OA, oscillator amplitude

Bibliography

AARC Clinical Practice Guideline: Application of continuous positive airway pressure to neonates via nasal prongs or nasopharyngeal tube. Respir Care 1994; 39:817–823.

Abraham E, Yoshihara G: Cardiorespiratory effects of pressure control ventilation in severe respiratory failure. Chest 1990; 98:1445–1449.

American College of Chest Physicians: Consensus Conference on Mechanical Ventilation. Chest 1993; 104:1835–1859.

Boros SJ, Mammel MC, Coleman JM, et al: Neonatal high-frequency jet ventilation: Four years experience. Pediatrics 1985; 75:657.

Boros S, Matalon S, Ewald R, et al: The effect of independent variations in inspiratory-expiratory ratio and end expiratory pressure during mechanical ventilation in hyaline membrane disease: The significance of mean airway pressure. J Pediatr 1977; 91:794.

Carlo WA, Martin RJ: Principles of assisted ventilation. Pediatr Clin North Am 1986; 33:221.

Cavanaugh K, Bloom BT: Combined HFV and CMV for neonatal air leak. Respir Management 1990; 20:43.

Chatburn R: Principles and practice of neonatal and pediatric mechanical ventilation. Respir Care 1991; 36:569–593.

Chatburn R: A new system for understanding mechanical ventilators. Respir Care 1991; 36:1123–1155.

Chatburn RL, Lough MD, Primiano FP Jr: Mechanical ventilation. *In* Chatburn RL, Lough MD (eds): Handbook of Respiratory Care, 2nd ed. St. Louis, Mosby-Year Book, 1990, pp 159–223.

Clark RH: High frequency ventilation. J Pediatr 1994; 124:661–670.

Cleary JP, Bernstein G, Heldt GP, et al: Improved oxygenation during synchronized vs. intermittent mandatory ventilation in VLBW infants with respiratory distress: A randomized crossover design. Pediatr Res 1993; 33:1226A.

Czervinske MP: Continuous positive airway pressure. *In* Koff PB, Eitzman D, Neu J (eds): Neonatal and Pediatric Respiratory Care. St. Louis, CV Mosby, 1988, pp 225–245.

Gerstmann DR, deLemos RA: High-frequency ventilation: Issues of strategy. Clin Perinatol 1991; 18:563.

Goldsmith JP, Karotkin EH: Introduction to assisted ventilation. *In* Goldsmith JP, Karotkin EH (eds): Assisted Ventilation of the Neonate, 2nd ed. Philadelphia, WB Saunders, 1988.

Goldsmith LS, Greenspan JS, Rubenstein D, et al: Immediate improvement in lung volume after exogenous surfactant: Alveolar recruitment versus increased distention. J Pediatr 1991; 119:424–428.

Guilleminault C, Mino-Murcia G, Heldt G: Alternative treatment to tracheostomy in obstructive sleep apnea syndrome: Nasal continuous positive airway pressure in young children. Pediatrics 1986; 78:797–802.

Hall SV, Johnson E, Hedley-Whyte J, et al: Renal hemodynamics and function with continuous positive-pressure ventilation in dogs. Anesthesiology 1974; 41:452–461.

Hess D: Pediatric and neonatal respiratory care: Some implications for adult respiratory care. Respir Care 1991; 36:489–511.

Jonson B, Ahlström H, Lindroth M, et al: CPAP: Modes of action in relation to clinical application. Pediatr Clin North Am 1980; 27:687–697.

Keszler M, Davis J, Spitzer A, et al: "High-volume" strategy of high-frequency ventilation in the treatment of newborns with uncomplicated RDS. Presented at the Tenth Conference on High-Frequency Ventilation of Infants, Snowbird, Utah, April, 1993.

Lain DC, DiBenedetto R, Morris SL, et al: Pressure control inverse ratio ventilation as a method to reduce peak airway pressure and provide adequate ventilation and oxygenation. Chest 1989; 95:1081.

Miller MJ, Difiore J, Strohl K, et al: Effects of Nasal CPAP on supraglottic and total pulmonary resistance in preterm infants. J Appl Physiol 1990; 68:141–146.

Rennie JM, South M, Morley CJ: Cerebral blood flow velocity variability in infants receiving assisted ventilation. Arch Dis Child 1987; 62: 1247–1251.

Reynolds EOR: Pressure waveform and ventilator settings for mechanical ventilation in severe hyaline membrane disease. Int Anesthesiol Clin 1974; 12:259.

Saunders RA, Milner AD, Hopkins IE, et al: The effects of continuous positive airway pressure on lung mechanics and lung volumes in the neonate. Biol Neonate 1976; 29:178–186.

Shapiro B: Clinical Application of Respiratory Care. St. Louis, CV Mosby, 1991, pp 335–364.

Smith RA, Rasanen JO, Downs JB: Flow, pressure, and time modifications. Contemp Management Crit Care 1990; 1:15–28.

Spearman C: Egan's Fundamentals of Respiratory Care. Chicago, Year Book Medical, 1982.

Suter PM, Fauley HB, Isenberg MD: Optimum end-expiratory airway pressure in patients with acute pulmonary failure. N Engl J Med 1975; 292:284–289.

Vender J: Complications and physiologic alterations of positive airway pressure therapy. Anesth Clin North Am 1987; 5:807–817.

Walker AM, Brodecky VA, dePreu ND, et al: High-frequency oscillatory ventilation compared with conventional mechanical ventilation in newborn lambs: Effects of increasing airway pressure on intracranial pressures. Pediatr Pulmonol 1992; 12:11.

SECTION 4

Pediatric Pulmonary Disorders

I. **Laryngotracheobronchitis**
II. **Epiglottitis**
III. **Bronchiolitis**
IV. **Bronchiectasis**
V. **Cystic Fibrosis**
VI. **Alpha$_1$-Antitrypsin Deficiency**
VII. **Asthma**
VIII. **Pneumonia**
IX. **Pleural Effusion**
X. **Lung Abscess**
XI. **Atelectasis**
XII. **Sarcoidosis**
XIII. **Pulmonary Alveolar Proteinosis**
XIV. **Pulmonary Hemosiderosis**
XV. **Pulmonary Hemorrhage**
XVI. **Pulmonary Embolism**
XVII. **Immotile Cilia Syndrome**
XVIII. **Tuberculosis**
XIX. **Fungal Disorders**
  A. Aspergillosis
  B. Blastomycosis
  C. Coccidioidomycosis
  D. Cryptococcosis
  E. Histoplasmosis
XX. **Sudden Infant Death Syndrome**
XXI. **Adult Respiratory Distress Syndrome**
XXII. **Near-Drowning**
XXIII. **Foreign Body Aspiration**

Abbreviations

ABG–arterial blood gas
AD–autogenic drainage
AP–anteroposterior
ARDS–adult respiratory distress syndrome
BPD–bronchopulmonary dysplasia
CF–cystic fibrosis
CHD–congenital heart disease
CNS–central nervous system
CPAP–continuous positive airway pressure
CPT–chest physical therapy
CVA–cerebrovascular accident
DFA–direct fluorescent antibody
D_{LCO}–diffusing capacity of carbon monoxide
ECMO–extracorporeal membrane oxygenation

ED–emergency department
ELISA–enzyme-linked immunosorbent assay
ET–endotracheal
FET–forced expiratory technique
FEV–forced expiratory volume
FTT–failure to thrive
HFCC–high-frequency chest compression
Hib–*Haemophilus influenzae* Type B
ICP–intracranial pressure
ICU–intensive care unit
IV–intravenous
LTB–laryngotracheobronchitis
MDI–metered dose inhaler
OR–operating room
PE–pulmonary embolism
PEEP–positive end-expiratory pressure
PEFR–peak expiratory flow rate
PEP–positive expiratory pressure
PFT–pulmonary function test
PVR–pulmonary vascular resistance
RSV–respiratory syncytial virus
RV–residual volume
SIDS–sudden infant death syndrome
SPAG–small-particle aerosol generator
SVN–small-volume nebulizer
TB–tuberculosis
TLC–total lung capacity
V/Q–ventilation to perfusion

LARYNGOTRACHEOBRONCHITIS

Laryngotracheobronchitis consists of inflammation of tissue in the larynx, trachea, bronchi, and bronchioles, resulting in edema, increased secretions, and airway narrowing.

Etiology

Parainfluenza Types I and II, influenza Types A and B, and respiratory syncytial virus (RSV) are the most common causes. Bacterial infection is rare. Transmission is by direct contact.

Incidence

It occurs most often in children 3 months to 3 years of age and is more common in boys. Late fall to early winter is the seasonal peak.

Diagnosis

The diagnosis is suggested by the history and physical examination and is confirmed by a lateral neck x-ray film.

Clinical Presentation

History. A coryzal prodrome is present for 1 to 3 days, along with rhinitis, malaise, and poor appetite. Symptoms are worse at night.

Physical Examination. The examination reveals stridor, a barking cough, hoarseness, low-grade fever (or the patient is afebrile), tachypnea, nasal flaring, supraglottic and substernal retractions, and decreased breath sounds. Agitation and crying worsen stridor; stridor may decrease with fatigue or severe obstruction. Cyanosis, tachycardia, and restlessness occur with hypoxia.

Neck X-ray Findings. Variable subglottic narrowing is present, with a wider air column on expiration than on inspiration. Thickened vocal cords, a normal epiglottis, a classic ''pencil tip'' or ''steeple sign'' (tapering of upper airway) in the subglottic region, and distention of the hypopharynx are also seen.

Arterial Blood Gas Analysis. Oxygenation should be assessed noninvasively with pulse oximetry to reduce anxiety. Arterial blood gas (ABG) analysis is usually not warranted unless respiratory failure and hypercapnia are suspected.

Management

The major goal of management is to stabilize the airway and reduce respiratory distress. The child is kept calm and quiet, and anxiety is minimized. Hospitalization is recommended if there are severe airway obstruction symptoms, symptoms present in the morning, or underlying upper airway lesions. Chest physical therapy (CPT) is usually avoided during the acute phase, as anxiety during therapy may increase respiratory distress.

Home Care. A cool-mist vaporizer is used. Alternatively, all hot water taps can be turned on in a closed bathroom. Mist tent or ''croup'' tent therapy is administered in the hospital.

Humidification. The goal is to provide moisture to inflamed mucosae.

Oxygen Therapy. Humidified oxygen via hood or tent is indicated if hypoxemia is present. Helium-oxygen therapy has been used successfully to improve airflow in some patients.

Aerosol Therapy. Racemic epinephrine is given via small-volume nebulizer (SVN) to reduce airway edema. It may be administered every 30 minutes. The clinician monitors for tachycardia. Rebound worsening may occur.

Monitoring. The clinician observes oxygen saturation with pulse oximetry (continuous if hypoxemia present), respiratory rate and pattern, degree of retractions, breath sounds, pitch of stridor, and color.

Airway Management. Endotracheal intubation (ET) is indicated with severe obstruction and impending respiratory failure (hypercapnia, respiratory fatigue). The ET tube should be one-half to one size smaller than that indicated by patient age. Intubation should be performed in a controlled setting (i.e., operating room [OR] or intensive care unit [ICU]). A mist-oxygen tent or hood is used while the patient is intubated. A T-tube set-up is not used because it may cause undue pull on the ET tube. Mechanical ventilation is rarely indicated except in cases of oversedation during intubation. The patient should be restrained to prevent self-extubation. Extubation usually takes place 48 to 72 hours later when the child is afebrile, minimal secretions are present, and an air leak develops around the ET tube. Bronchoscopy may be used to evaluate the airway. Preparations to reintubate the patient should be made prior to extubation; obstruction may recur 12 to 48 hours following extubation. Tracheostomy is needed in rare cases in which extubation fails.

Steroids. Although controversial, the antiinflammatory effects of dexamethasone may decrease mucosal edema and the need for racemic epinephrine treatments.

Complications

Atelectasis, pneumonitis, and pulmonary edema may occur.

Spasmodic Laryngotracheobronchitis

This form of LTB presents at night with symptoms similar to those of viral LTB, but the patient is afebrile and has no history of a viral prodrome. The cause may be allergic in nature. Recovery is usually within 6 hours; treatment is rarely needed.

Membranous Laryngotracheobronchitis–Bacterial Tracheitis

This condition is potentially life-threatening; it is usually due to *Staphylococcus aureus, Streptococcus pneumoniae,* or *Haemophilus influenzae*. Acute airway obstruction results from necrosis and sloughing of airway mucosa, with a pseudomembrane forming along the trachea. Membranous laryngotracheobronchitis-bacterial tracheitis appears clinically similar to viral LTB. Although the condition progresses rapidly, the child appears more toxic and fails to respond to racemic epinephrine. Bronchoscopy may confirm the diagnosis.

Treatment consists of tracheal suctioning, airway management (usually intubation), antibiotic therapy, and ICU monitoring. Extubation usually takes place 1 week following intubation.

EPIGLOTTITIS

Epiglottitis is a medical emergency that is characterized by acute upper airway obstruction caused by bacterial inflammation of the epiglottis. Complete airway obstruction may occur within minutes or 2 to 5 hours.

Etiology

H. influenzae Type B (Hib) is the most common cause.

Incidence

Epiglottitis occurs most often in children 2 to 6 years of age. There is a decreased incidence since the introduction of an Hib vaccine. This condition is seen in any season, and rarely recurs.

Diagnosis

The diagnosis is suggested by the history and physical examination. It is confirmed by a lateral neck x-ray film (taken with child sitting upright). Since complete airway obstruction may occur suddenly and without warning, the diagnosis must be made quickly and assumed in patients with the classic presentation.

Clinical Presentation

History. There is an acute onset of respiratory distress progressing rapidly over a few hours. No history of upper respiratory tract infection is present. The patient may complain of a sore throat.

Physical Examination. The examination may show stridor, a barking cough, a muffled voice, high fever, bradypnea, supraglottic and substernal retractions, decreased breath sounds, drooling, and dysphagia. The child is irritable or lethargic and sits upright in a tripod position with the jaw protruding and the neck hyperextended in an attempt to keep the airway open. Cyanosis, listlessness, and bradycardia are signs of hypoxia.

Lateral Neck X-ray Findings. A thickened epiglottis (thumb sign) and aryepiglottic folds and a normal subglottic area are seen.

Airway Visualization. A cherry-red, swollen epiglottis and edema of the arytenoids and aryepiglottic folds are seen. Visualization should be performed quickly prior to intubation. *Direct visualization is performed only by personnel skilled in emergency airway management (including tracheostomy) in a controlled setting with equipment readily available* (i.e., emergency department [ED], OR, ICU).

Management

The first priority of management is to establish a stable artificial airway. Racemic epinephrine is not indicated. Examinations and diagnostic tests that may upset the child are postponed until an airway is in place. The child is kept calm and quiet and is allowed to sit in the most comfortable position with a parent. He or she is not forced to lie supine, as complete obstruction may result.

Airway Management. The child and parents are transported to the OR or ICU accompanied by a physician skilled in airway management. Emergency airway equipment is available during transport. If time permits, intubation is performed after general anesthesia. The ET tube is one size smaller than that indicated by the patient's age. Gagging may cause laryngospasm and complete obstruction, requiring a tracheostomy. Light sedation and restraints reduce the risk of self-extubation. Extubation is performed when an air leak develops around the ET tube—usually within 48 to 72 hours. Reintubation equipment should be readily available during extubation.

Oxygen and Humidity. Humidification of the airway in epiglottitis is similar to that in LTB. Oxygen is rarely needed. CPT is not indicated. Oxygenation is monitored with pulse oximetry.

Mechanical Ventilation. Mechanical ventilation is used only until the patient regains consciousness following anesthesia.

Antibiotic Therapy. A combination of ampicillin and chloramphenicol, cefotaxime, or ceftriaxone is given. Rifampin is given prophylactically for the family and other exposed individuals.

Complications

Complications include atelectasis, pneumonitis, pulmonary edema, subglottic stenosis and webs following extubation, hypoxic ischemic encephalopathy due to severe airway obstruction, and meningitis associated with bacteremia (Table 4–1).

BRONCHIOLITIS

Viral inflammation of the bronchioles, producing airway edema and mucus plugging, constitutes bronchiolitis. Airway obstruction leads to atelectasis and hyperinflation (ball-valve effect); ventilation/perfusion (V/Q) mismatch results in hypoxemia. Increased work of breathing is due to decreased compliance and increased airway resistance. Pneumonia may develop, with formation of hyaline membranes, destruction of respiratory epithelium, and necrosis of lung parenchyma.

Etiology

Bronchiolitis is most often caused by RSV. Adenovirus, parainfluenza Types 1 and 3, influenza, and enterovirus causes are less common. Rarely the cause is *Mycoplasma.* Transmission is by direct contact with contaminated surfaces. Strict handwashing, gown and glove precautions, and having patients cared for by the same personnel during an epidemic reduce the infection rate.

Incidence

This condition occurs in children 1 month to 2 years of age, the highest incidence being in the 1- to 6-month-old infant. Epidemics occur between October and April. Cross-contamination is frequently seen in hospitals and daycare settings. Hospitalized infants and staff working with infants are at highest risk. Passive smoking (older siblings, parents) increases the risk.

Diagnosis

Diagnosis is by clinical presentation, patient age, and RSV identification via enzyme-linked immunosorbent assay (ELISA).

TABLE 4–1 Differential Diagnosis of Laryngotracheobronchitis and Epiglottitis

	LARYNGOTRACHEOBRONCHITIS	EPIGLOTTITIS
Age	3 months–3 years	2–6 years
Cause	Viral (parainfluenza, RSV)	Bacterial (*Haemophilus influenzae* Type B)
History	Gradual onset (2–3 days) Previous cold symptoms	Acute onset (few hours) Complaint of sore throat
Symptoms	Stridor Barking cough Fever variable Hoarse voice No position preferred Retractions Irritable Does not appear acutely ill	Stridor Minimal cough High fever Muffled voice Prefers sitting upright with chin forward Retractions Drooling Anxious Appears acutely ill
X-ray findings	Subglottic narrowing	Swollen epiglottis (thumb sign)

RSV, respiratory syncytial virus.

Clinical Presentation

History. The history includes otitis media, a cough, a viral prodrome, or a family member with an upper respiratory tract infection.

Physical Examination. Symptoms may include tachypnea (>60 breaths per minute), labored and shallow respirations, wheezing, a hacking cough, marked intercostal retractions, nasal flaring, prolonged expiration, restlessness, poor appetite, dehydration from poor fluid intake, a variable fever, cyanosis, and tachycardia with hypoxia.

Chest X-ray Findings. Diffuse hyperinflation, a flattened diaphragm, bulging intercostal spaces, and patchy infiltrates may be seen. Some infants have a normal radiograph.

Arterial Blood Gas Analysis. Hypoxemia is common; hypercarbia and acidosis are rare.

Management

Home Care. Home care consists of careful monitoring, increased fluid intake, acetaminophen for fever, upright positioning in an infant seat, and instructions to contact the physician if the child's clinical state deteriorates (e.g., increased work of breathing, apnea, cyanosis, decreased fluid intake).

Indications for Hospitalization. If moderate to severe respiratory distress, cyanosis, tachypnea greater than 60 beats per minute, a $Pa{O_2}$ determination of less than 60 mm Hg, hypercarbia, or fatigue is present, the infant should be hospitalized. In addition, an infant younger than 2 months of age or one with an underlying cardiac, pulmonary, or immunodeficiency disorder should be hospitalized.

Oxygen Therapy. Forty percent oxygen given by hood usually corrects hypoxemia. Oxygenation is monitored with pulse oximetry, transcutaneous monitors, or ABG determinations, or a combination of these methods.

Aerosol Therapy. A trial of beta-agonists is given, although bronchodilator use is controversial and the response unpredictable. Ribavirin (antiviral agent) is aerosolized continuously via a small-particle aerosol generator (SPAG) for 18 to 20 hours per day; it is indicated for high-risk infants with underlying conditions such as cystic fibrosis (CF), bronchopulmonary dysplasia (BPD), and congenital heart disease (CHD) and for those with hypoxemia and hypercarbia.

Mechanical Ventilation. Mechanical ventilation is indicated in cases of clinical deterioration, apnea, or respiratory failure, or a combination of these conditions. Ribavirin may be given in-line with some ventilators.

Hydration. Fluid intake is increased with oral or intravenous (IV) fluids.

Complications

Sudden apnea is common in infants younger than 6 months of age. Dehydration is present from decreased fluid intake resulting from respiratory distress. Pneumonia, pneumothorax, persistent wheezing, hyperinflation, abnormal pulmonary function, and airway hyperreactivity may be seen. There is a strong association between bronchiolitis and the development of asthma. Death occurs secondary to respiratory failure.

BRONCHIECTASIS

Dilatation of the bronchi with associated inflammation and mucus accumulation is called bronchiectasis. Pooled secretions become infected, causing further airway scarring.

Etiology

Obstruction of the bronchioles with retained secretions and infection is believed to cause dilatation of the bronchi. Predisposing factors include infections (pertussis, measles, adenovirus, pneumonia), immotile cilia syndrome, CF, bronchial obstruction (foreign body, tuberculosis [TB], tumors), right middle lobe syndrome, and asthma. A small percentage of patients have congenital bronchiectasis.

Incidence

The incidence is low, most likely because of improved treatment of airway obstruction and respiratory tract infections.

Diagnosis

Thoracic computed tomography is used most often for diagnosis, although the pattern of bronchiectasis is most strikingly seen with bronchography.

Clinical Presentation

The onset may be acute following an infection or may be progressive in patients with CF. Lower lobes are most frequently involved. A chronic, productive cough; wheezing and crackles; hemoptysis; dyspnea; and clubbing of the nails are common symptoms. The chest radiograph is unremarkable, or it may reveal cystic changes.

Management

Aggressive CPT is needed to facilitate clearance of secretions. Antibiotic therapy is directed at specific pathogens. Surgical excision of the abnormal pulmonary segment may be performed in patients who are unresponsive to aggressive therapy and who experience recurrent severe illness, failure to thrive (FTT), or significant hemoptysis.

Complications

Complications are rare and the prognosis is good.

CYSTIC FIBROSIS

CF is an inherited autosomal recessive disease of exocrine gland function, which is characterized by abnormal, thick, tenacious secretions that cause disturbances in multiple organ systems.

Pulmonary disturbances include excessive secretions that cover cilia. Mucus plugging of small airways occurs early in life. Airway obstruction and dilatation lead to V/Q mismatch, hypoxemia, chronic infection, hyperinflation, bronchiectasis, airway collapse, pulmonary hypertension, cor pulmonale, and respiratory failure. Chronic lung injury tends to accelerate in the second decade of life. Some patients may have airway hyperreactivity.

Gastrointestinal disturbances include pancreatic insufficiency in 85% of patients, which leads to maldigestion and small bowel obstruction. Focal biliary cirrhosis is present in 15% of patients. Portal hypertension is common.

Reproductive disturbances are present in 97% of males, who have abnormal development in the vas deferens, leading to obstructive azoospermia and sterility. Abnormal vaginal secretions may lead to infertility in females.

Etiology

The CF gene has been mapped to chromosome 7 and produces an abnormal protein, cystic fibrosis transmembrane conductance regulator (CFTR).

Incidence

CF is the most common lethal hereditary disease affecting whites; the incidence is approximately 1 in 2500 births. The incidence in blacks is 1 in 17,000 births, in Native Americans it is 1 in 80,000 births, and in Asians it is 1 in 90,000 births. It is estimated that 1 in 20 whites carries the gene for CF. The male to female ratio is 1.3 : 1. Couples with the CF gene have a 1 in 4 chance of having a child with CF. A mother with CF has a 1 in 40 chance of having a child with CF; the child will carry the CF gene.

Diagnosis

The pilocarpine iontophoresis method is used to collect sweat. A sweat chloride determination greater than 60 mEq/L is positive for CF. False negative results can occur in edema and hypoproteinemia. False positive results can occur in malnutrition, laboratory error, and various metabolic and endocrine conditions, including hypothyroidism. To confirm the diagnosis, two positive sweat test results and blood testing for mutational analysis of the CFTR gene are required (Table 4–2).

TABLE 4–2 When to Suspect Cystic Fibrosis in Infants and Children
Newborn with initial meconium passed >30 minutes after birth
Newborn with intestinal obstruction
Infant with tachypnea, retractions, chronic cough
Infant with hypoprothrombinemia
Infant with hypoproteinemia when on soybean formula
Infant with unexplained hyponatremia
Meconium ileus
Rectal prolapse
Steatorrhea
Failure to thrive
Chronic diarrhea; bulky, greasy, foul-smelling stool
Diagnosis of asthma and clubbing of digits
Chronic sinusitis and nasal polyposis
Cirrhosis of the liver, portal hypertension
Siblings of CF patient
Parent with CF
Celiac disease suspected or diagnosed

CF, cystic fibrosis.

Clinical Presentation

The majority of CF patients present with recurrent pneumonias, chronic cough, diarrhea with malodorous stools, and malnutrition.

Infancy. Symptoms in infancy include FTT, meconium ileus (small intestinal obstruction by thick meconium) in 10% of cases at birth, abdominal distention, diarrhea, bronchiolitis, pneumonia, and prolonged jaundice.

Physical Examination. The following symptoms may be seen on physical examination: productive cough (especially in the morning) with large amounts of mucopurulent secretions, clubbing of fingers and toes, decreased exercise tolerance, a nasal voice, increased anteroposterior (AP) chest diameter (barrel chest), tachypnea, dyspnea, decreased breath sounds with crackles, and bulky, greasy and foul-smelling stools.

Pulmonary Function Testing. Results of initial pulmonary function tests (PFTs) are characteristic of obstructive lung disease. There is a restrictive component in late stages. There is an increased residual volume (RV) and RV: total lung capacity (TLC) ratio. The following are reduced: FEV_1, FEV_1 : TLC ratio, forced expiratory flow between 25% and 75%, and reduced vital capacity, peak flow rate, and diffusing capacity of carbon monoxide (DL_{CO}).

Chest X-ray Findings. Progressive air trapping, bronchiectasis (upper lobes common), atelectasis, cyst and abscess formation, and cavitations may be seen on the radiograph.

Arterial Blood Gas Analysis. The ABG analysis shows progressive hypoxemia and normal $Paco_2$ levels until the advanced stages, when hypercarbia occurs as a result of chronic respiratory failure.

Sputum Culture. The clinical severity often correlates with the level of infection. *S. aureus* is usually colonized first. All patients eventually acquire *Pseudomonas aeruginosa. H. influenzae, Escherichia coli,* and *Klebsiella pneumoniae* are common. *P. cepacia* is resistant to multiple drugs and is usually associated with advanced disease.

Gastrointestinal Manifestations. Symptoms include a distended abdomen; bulky, greasy, and foul-smelling stools; rectal prolapse; gastroesophageal reflux; cholelithiasis, and a meconium ileus equivalent.

Indications of Pulmonary Exacerbation. Signs include increased cough and sputum production, low-grade fever, abnormal breath sounds, malaise, exercise intolerance, dyspnea, poor appetite, deterioration in PFT results, and abnormal changes in the chest radiograph.

Management

Because of the variability of the disease, treatment should be individualized.

Oxygen Therapy. Oxygen is given to improve Pa_{O_2}, reduce pulmonary hypertension, and prevent the development of cor pulmonale. It may be used at night and with exercise. It is often given continuously including at home, in the late stages of disease.

Aerosol Therapy. Aerosols are used to administer medications including bronchodilators, mucolytics, antibiotics, and rhDNase. Bronchodilator therapy is given prior to secretion clearance techniques to improve mucus clearance and prevent therapy-induced bronchospasm.

Secretion Clearance. The goal is to mobilize and remove tenacious secretions and thereby decrease the risk of infection. CPT, autogenic drainage (AD), forced expiratory technique (FET), positive expiratory pressure (PEP), high-frequency chest compression (HFCC), physical exercise, and vigorous coughing are included. These therapies are often performed on a daily basis at home. Older patients may exhibit poor compliance with daily therapy; these patients may be able to substitute or add an individually tailored aerobic exercise program.

Antibiotic Therapy. Chronic infection is controlled with antibiotics. Hospital or home therapy with 10 to 14 days of IV administration of antibiotics is given during acute exacerbations. Hospitalization is required when the patient fails the outpatient regimen. Daily prophylactic therapy is controversial.

Mechanical Ventilation. Ventilation is used postoperatively with surgical procedures; maximal preoperative assessment and pulmonary management should be available. Mechanical ventilation is usually avoided as treatment for respiratory failure in advanced disease because of the poor prognosis for weaning and extubation.

Lung Transplantation. Transplantation is used in patients with advanced disease and a poor life expectancy. Bilateral single lung transplants are used most often. There are a limited number of organs available.

Gastrointestinal Therapy. The goal of this therapy is to treat pancreatic insufficiency and improve nutrition. Patients with steatorrhea take variable doses of supplemental pancreatic enzymes (Pancrease) with meals and snacks. It is available in powder form (for infants) and capsules. Adverse effects include abdominal distention and cramping, bloating, and diarrhea. Fat-soluble vitamins and high-calorie diets are recommended (Table 4–3).

Complications

As the life span increases, complications of the disease are seen more frequently.

Bronchiectasis. This is found in the majority of CF patients. Surgical resection of the affected lobe may be indicated in severe cases.

Hemoptysis. This condition usually occurs during pulmonary exacerbations with coughing; it may occur during sleep. Mild hemoptysis is less than 30 ml/24 hr; massive hemoptysis consists of greater than 300 ml/24 hr. Massive hemoptysis may be fatal with the first episode and has a high incidence of recurrence. Treatment includes bed rest, antibiotic therapy,

TABLE 4–3 Drugs Commonly Used in Cystic Fibrosis

BRONCHODILATORS
Salbutamol
Albuterol
Terbutaline
Metaproterenol
Fenoterol
Ipratropium bromide
Theophylline
ANTIINFLAMMATORY AGENTS
Cromolyn sodium
Nedocromil
MUCOLYTICS
N-acetylcysteine
Recombinant human deoxyribonuclease

blood replacement, clotting defect correction, bronchoscopy or angiography to determine hemorrhage site, and bronchial artery embolization (Geofoam, Ivalon) if hemorrhage is massive. CPT is discontinued until the bleeding stops.

Atelectasis. The upper and middle lobes are affected most often. Treatment is with antibiotics and CPT. Lobar collapse is a poor prognostic sign.

Spontaneous Pneumothorax. Air trapping and bullae formation lead to rupture and release of air into the pleural space. Pneumothorax most often affects older patients with advanced disease; approximately 19% of patients are older than 13 years of age. Treatment may include chest tube placement, chemical pleurodesis with quinacrine via the chest tube, pleurectomy, pleural abrasion, or a combination of these treatments. Fifty percent of patients may have recurrence.

Cor Pulmonale. Right ventricular hypertrophy develops with progressive hypoxemia. Right ventricular failure may indicate the terminal stage of disease. Treatment includes oxygen therapy, fluid restriction, digoxin, and diuretic therapy.

Otolaryngologic Problems. Problems include nasal polyps, sinusitis, otitis media, and rhinitis.

Allergic Bronchopulmonary Aspergillosis. Acute deterioration in PFT results is seen with this condition. Treatment is with long-term steroids.

Gastrointestinal Problems. Problems include rectal prolapse, cholelithiasis, gastroesophageal reflux, and meconium ileus equivalent (intestinal obstruction in older child).

Diabetes Mellitus. This occurs in 15% of CF patients by 18 years of age.

Hypertrophic Pulmonary Osteoarthropathy. This is a syndrome consisting of arthritis, clubbing, and periosteitis (usually of long tubular bones). It is seen with advanced disease. Symptoms include joint pain and swelling, especially in hands, wrists, knees, and ankles. Treatment consists of antiinflammatory drugs for joint pain.

Salt Depletion. Depletion occurs during warmer seasons in infants; dehydration occurs in older patients during vigorous work or exercise.

Prognosis

The prognosis improves with early diagnosis and treatment. Disease progression is highly variable, even among siblings. Ninety-five percent of patients eventually die of cor pulmonale. The CF Patient Registry 1992 data list a median survival of 29.4 years. The major cause of morbidity and mortality is severe and recurrent respiratory infection.

ALPHA$_1$-ANTITRYPSIN DEFICIENCY

Alpha$_1$-antitrypsin deficiency is an inherited autosomal recessive disease characterized by emphysema and elastin destruction in the lungs.

Diagnosis

Gene analysis is used to detect the deficiency.

Clinical Presentation

Increasing dyspnea with exercise, clubbing of the digits, and minimal or no cough or sputum production are common symptoms. Chest x-ray findings reveal hyperaeration. PFT results indicate obstructive lung disease (increased residual volume) and reduced diffusing capacity of carbon dioxide (DL_{CO}). Hepatic disease with cirrhosis occurs in some patients.

Management

Bronchodilators are used only when benefit is apparent, and CPT is used if secretions are present. Patients should avoid exposure to forms of air pollution, including cigarette smoke (active or passive), as these toxins accelerate lung disease.

ASTHMA

Asthma is a reactive airway disease in which the small airways hyperreact to stimuli. Reaction is characterized by bronchospasm, mucosal edema, and excess mucus production, all of which produce varying degrees of airway obstruction, increased resistance to airflow, and hyperinflation. These result in V/Q mismatch, hypoxemia, and increased work of breathing.

Etiology

Asthma is believed to be genetically transmitted, IgE antibody-mediated, or induced by chemical mediators, or a combination of these factors.

Incidence

The estimated incidence of asthma is 5% to 10%. An increased prevalence, hospitalization rate, and death rate have been seen in recent years. The majority of children have an onset between 4 and 5 years of age. Asthma ranks first in causes for school days missed. The risk of the development of asthma increases if there is a family history of asthma or allergies, the parents smoke, or the child has had episodes of bronchiolitis.

Diagnosis

The diagnosis is based on history, physical examination, and laboratory findings. Table 4–4 lists laboratory findings useful in the diagnosis.

Clinical Presentation

The hyperreactivity response varies among patients, and exacerbations are classified as mild, moderate, or severe, based on clinical features (Table 4–5).

Physical Examination. Examination reveals respiratory distress; accessory muscle used; suprasternal, intercostal, and subcostal retractions; head bobbing; an increased AP diameter of the chest; crackles (secretions); wheezes (bronchospasm); chest pain; cough that may induce gagging and vomiting; poor exercise tolerance; prolongation of expiration; and "allergic shiners." Patients with severe asthma may not wheeze if airflow is too diminished to generate a wheeze.

Chest X-ray Findings. X-rays show markedly hyperinflated lungs with a flattened diaphragm, atelectasis, infiltrates, and an increase in perihilar markings.

Arterial Blood Gas Analysis. Hypoxemia is universal. Hypocarbia is seen in early stages. A normal $PaCO_2$ determination indicates impending respiratory failure, and hypercarbia indicates respiratory failure.

Indications of Impending Respiratory Failure. Symptoms include obvious exhaustion, rising $Paco_2$ levels (normal or hypercarbia), a "silent chest," and a decreased level of consciousness.

Management

Oxygen Therapy. All patients are presumed to be hypoxemic and should receive oxygen via cannula or mask.

Text continued on page 117

TABLE 4–4 Laboratory Findings in Asthma

TEST	POSSIBLE FINDINGS IN ASTHMA	COMMENTS
Complete blood count	Leukocytosis (occasional)	Induced by infection, epinephrine administration, "stress" (?)
	Eosinophilia (frequent)	Varies with medication, time of day, adrenal function; not necessarily related to "allergy"; often higher in "intrinsic" than "extrinsic" asthma
Sputum examination	White or clear with small yellow plugs	—
	Eosinophils	Present in both "intrinsic" and "extrinsic" asthma
	Charcot-Leyden crystals	Derived from eosinophils
	Creola bodies	Clusters of epithelial cells
	Curschmann's spirals	Threads of glycoprotein
Nasal smear	Eosinophils	Predominance suggests concomitant nasal allergy in children
	Lymphocytes, PMNs, macrophages	Predominant cells in upper respiratory infections
	PMNs with ingested bacteria	Suggests rhinitis or sinusitis

Quantitative serum immunoglobulin levels IgG, IgA, IgM, IgE	Often normal; may be abnormal	Various patterns seen
	Sometimes elevated in "allergic" asthma; often normal	
	Presence of *Aspergillus* precipitin	Suggestive but not diagnostic of bronchopulmonary aspergillosis
Sweat test	Normal in asthma	Performed to rule out cystic fibrosis (CF), especially in infants with growth retardation, recurrent pneumonia, or both; positive result does not rule out asthma, which can coexist with CF
Chest x-ray film	Hyperinflation, atelectasis, infiltrates, pneumomediastinum, pneumothorax	Should be done once in every asthmatic child; should always be considered on hospitalization for asthma
Lung function tests	Decreases in FEV_1, FVC, $FEF_{50-75\%}$, PEFR, and FEV_1/FVC	Useful for following course of disease and response to treatment
Response to β_2 bronchodilators	15% improvement in FEV_1 or PEFR, or both	Safest diagnostic test for asthma
Exercise tolerance tests	Decrease in lung function after 6 minutes of exercise	Useful to diagnose asthma in children; results often abnormal when resting lung function is normal

Table continued on following page

TABLE 4–4 Laboratory Findings in Asthma *Continued*

TEST	POSSIBLE FINDINGS IN ASTHMA	COMMENTS
Bronchial challenge tests		
Methacholine inhalation (Mecholyl) test, histamine inhalation test	20% fall in FEV_1 in asthmatic	Should be performed only by specialist, occasionally used to diagnose asthma
Antigen inhalation test	20% fall in FEV_1 immediately after challenge; possible delayed response 6–8 hours later	Potentially dangerous—can induce anaphylaxis; should be performed only by specialist; rarely necessary
Allergy skin tests	Positive reactions if patient is allergic to factors tested	Performed to identify potential allergic factors in asthma; only the likely factors (indicated by history) should be tested for
RAST	Same significance as allergy skin tests	More expensive than allergy skin tests

From Bierman CW, Pearlman DS (eds): Allergic Diseases from Infancy to Adulthood, 2nd ed. Philadelphia, WB Saunders, 1988.
PMN, polymorphonuclear neutrophils; RAST, radioallergosorbent test.

TABLE 4–5 Estimation of Severity of Acute Exacerbation in Children With Asthma

SIGN, SYMPTOM	MILD	MODERATE	SEVERE
Peak expiratory flow rate	70%–90% predicted or baseline	50%–70% predicted or baseline	<50% predicted or baseline
Respiratory rate	Normal to 30% above mean	30%–50% increase above mean	>50% increase above mean
Alertness	Normal	Normal	May be decreased
Dyspnea	Absent or mild, speaks in complete sentences	Moderate, speaks in phrases or partial sentences	Severe, speaks only in single words or short phrases
Accessory muscle use	No intercostal to mild retractions	Moderate intercostal retractions with tracheosternal retractions, use of sternocleidomastoid muscles, chest hyperinflation	Moderate intercostal retractions, tracheosternal retractions with nasal flaring during inspiration, chest hyperinflation
Color	Good	Pale	Possibly cyanotic

Table continued on following page

TABLE 4–5 Estimation of Severity of Acute Exacerbation in Children With Asthma *Continued*

SIGN, SYMPTOM	MILD	MODERATE	SEVERE
Auscultation	End-expiratory wheeze only	Inspiratory and expiratory wheezing	Breath sounds inaudible
Oxygen saturation (opt)*	>95%	90%–95%	<90%
$P_{CO_{2(opt)}}$	<35 mm Hg	<40 mm Hg	>40 mm Hg

From Provisional Committee on Quality Improvement: Practice Parameter: The office management of acute exacerbations of asthma in children. Pediatrics 1994; 93:119–126.

* Oxygen saturation values will have to be adjusted for altitude. These values assume that the patient is at sea level.

Aerosol Therapy. Aerosols are used to administer bronchodilating agents, antiinflammatory agents, and cromolyn sodium.

CPT. Therapy is not indicated during severe attacks. It is given only if secretions are excessive and the patient is well hydrated.

Endotracheal Intubation. Mask-bag ventilation may be nearly impossible. Intubation is necessary for the child in respiratory failure; it carries a high risk for the asthmatic patient, as vagal stimulation may worsen bronchospasm.

Mechanical Ventilation. Ventilation is indicated if respiratory failure develops. A volume-cycled ventilator with a long time constant for exhalation is required (high flow, short inspiratory time, low rates to maximize expiratory time). Sedation and paralysis are often necessary to decrease the risk of barotrauma.

Hydration. IV fluids are critical, but overhydration should be avoided because pulmonary edema may develop.

Management for Mild Exacerbation. Treatment consists of albuterol by SVN (use oxygen flow) at 0.1 mg/kg/dose (minimum of 1.25 mg) or two to four puffs by metered dose inhaler (MDI) repeated every 20 minutes for 1 hour as needed. The patient with a peak expiratory flow rate (PEFR) greater than 80% of predicted normal may be discharged home where albuterol treatments should be given every 4 hours while the child is awake.

Management for Moderate Exacerbation. Oxygen is given by Venturi mask or cannula to keep $Sa{O_2}$ at greater than 92%. Albuterol is given by SVN (use oxygen flow) at 0.15 mg/kg/dose or 0.03 ml/kg/dose (maximum of 5 mg or 1 ml) repeated every 20 minutes for 1 hour. If PEFR is less than 80% of predicted normal, the child should be hospitalized, systemic steroids instituted, albuterol administration repeated, and oxygen therapy maintained. IV fluid should be given for hydration. An aminophylline infusion is started.

Management for Severe Exacerbation. The patient is admitted to the ICU if the $F{IO_2}$ is greater than 0.6, the $Pa{CO_2}$ level is greater than 40 mm Hg, and the patient needs aerosolized bronchodilators more often than every 2 hours. Continuous aerosol nebulization may be indicated if the patient is not responsive to every-1-hour therapy. Continuous monitoring should be performed with pulse oximetry and a cardiac monitor. Intubation with mechanical ventilation is instituted if the child's condition deteriorates. IV isoproterenol may be instituted.

Complications

Respiratory failure, atelectasis, pneumothorax, pneumomediastinum, and death can ensue.

PNEUMONIA

Pneumonia is an infection of the lung parenchyma caused by bacteria, viruses, parasites, fungi, or rickettsiae.

Etiology

Approximately 80% of pneumonias in children are viral in nature, with RSV most frequent. Parainfluenza virus (Types 1, 2, and 3) is also seen in children. Pneumonia from influenza virus is common in children younger than 2 years of age. Adenovirus is common in the late summer and early fall and occurs most often in children less than 2 years of age. *Streptococcus pneumoniae* is the most common cause of bacterial pneumonia in children. *H. influenzae* infection is rarely seen in children younger than 5 years of age. This infection has rapidly declined since the institution of the Hib vaccination. *Staphylococcus aureus* is an aggressive pneumonia that may be rapidly fatal. *Chlamydia pneumoniae* and *Mycoplasma pneumoniae* infections occur most often in school-aged children and young adults. Fungi are an uncommon cause of pneumonia in immunocompetent patients.

Incidence

The incidence of the pathogens associated with pneumonia varies, with some seen year-round, whereas others have seasonal peaks.

Diagnosis

Viral pneumonia is diagnosed based on epidemiology as well as laboratory testing, including ELISA and direct fluorescent antibody testing (DFA). A definitive diagnosis is more difficult in bacterial pneumonia. Tests used for diagnosis include sputum cultures, blood cultures, and the detection of bacterial antigens in urine. Chlamydial penumonia is diagnosed by culture of the organism from the nasopharynx or by serologic testing. The diagnosis of *Mycoplasma* pneumonia is confirmed by culturing the organism in the nasopharynx via direct culture or DNA probe.

Clinical Presentation

Symptoms vary and often depend on the pathogen involved.

Physical Examination. Wheezes, crackles, and decreased breath sounds may be auscultated. Respiratory distress with nasal flaring, grunting, and retractions is common. Fever, shaking chills, dry or productive cough, tachypnea, malaise, and upper respiratory symptoms may also be seen.

Chest X-ray Findings. X-rays may reveal patchy or interstitial infiltrates or lobar or segmental consolidation.

Management

Antiviral therapy with ribavirin may be indicated in pneumonia caused by RSV. Antibiotic therapy is indicated in bacterial infections.

Oxygen Therapy. Oxygen is given to treat hypoxemia.

Aerosol Therapy. Bronchodilating agents and some antibiotics may be delivered.

CPT. Patients with retained secretions may benefit from CPT.

Complications

Empyema, pneumothorax, lung abscess, respiratory failure, shock, and death may ensue.

PLEURAL EFFUSION

Pleural effusion consists of an abnormal amount of fluid retained in the pleural space. The underlying disorder and degree of effusion determine the respiratory dysfunction. Large effusions will decrease lung volumes and impair gas exchange, resulting in hypoxemia and increased respiratory distress.

Etiology

Various infections may cause pleural effusions (Table 4–6).

Diagnosis

Pleural effusions may be suspected clinically when there is an area of decreased-intensity breath sounds on chest auscultation with dullness to percussion over the area. When an effusion is found on chest film, a thoracentesis is per-

TABLE 4–6 Infecting Organisms That May Cause Pleural Effusions

AEROBIC BACTERIA
Staphylococcus aureus
Haemophilus influenzae
Streptococcus pneumoniae
Streptococcus pyogenes
Group A, beta-hemolytic streptococci
ANAEROBIC BACTERIA
Bacteroides species
Peptostreptococcus species
Peptococcus species
Fusobacterium species
TUBERCULOSIS
Mycobacterium tuberculosis
VIRUSES-MYCOPLASMA
Adenovirus
Parainfluenza
Mycoplasma pneumoniae
FUNGI—FUNGUS-LIKE
Coccidioides immitis
Actinomyces species
Nocardia species
PARASITES
Paragonimus species
Cysticercus species
Amebiasis (hepatic)
Echinococcosis

formed to obtain pleural fluid for laboratory analysis (Tables 4–7 through 4–9).

Clinical Presentation

Physical Examination. Symptoms usually correlate with the size of the effusion; small effusions present with fewer symptoms. Chest pain, chest wall tenderness, dyspnea, pain with coughing or deep breathing, crackles and decreased breath sounds on auscultation, and dullness to percussion may also be seen.

TABLE 4–7 Potential Causes of a Transudative Pleural Effusion

Congestive heart failure
Nephrotic syndrome
Cirrhosis or liver failure
Acute glomerulonephritis
Hypoproteinemia
Myxedema
Sarcoidosis
Peritoneal dialysis

Chest X-ray Findings. Pleural effusion is present. The lateral decubitus position often allows smaller effusions to be detected. The chest film may not return to normal for months.

Management

Antibiotic therapy is given. Drainage of fluid may be indicated and is accomplished by chest tube placement or repeated thoracentesis.

Complications

Complications are rare; most are related to thoracentesis or chest tube placement and include pneumothorax, hemorrhage, and infection.

TABLE 4–8 Potential Causes of an Exudative Pleural Effusion

Parapneumonic effusion or empyema
Pulmonary embolism
Neoplasm
Collagen vascular disease
Trauma
Drug hypersensitivity
Lung transplant rejection
Chylothorax
Gastrointestinal disease
Lymphatic disease
Postcardiac injury syndrome

TABLE 4–9 Analyses Commonly Performed on Pleural Fluid

Total protein
Lactate dehydrogenase
Cell counts and differential cell count
pH
Cytology
Studies for infection
- Gram stain, bacterial culture
- Acid-fast stain and culture
- Fungal stains and culture

Glucose
Amylase

LUNG ABSCESS

A circumscribed, thick-walled cavity within the lung that contains purulent material is called a lung abscess. Compression by the abscess leads to V/Q mismatch, hypoxemia, and respiratory distress.

Etiology

Pathogens that cause lung abscess include viruses, bacteria, fungi, and protozoa. A primary abscess is one that develops in a healthy child. A secondary abscess is one that develops in a child who has an underlying disorder (Table 4–10).

Incidence

Lung abscess is uncommon except in immunocompromised patients.

Diagnosis

Chest radiography or computed tomography is used to obtain a diagnosis.

Clinical Presentation

The patient presents with fever, malaise, cough, chest pain, dyspnea, hemoptysis, foul-smelling breath, tachypnea,

TABLE 4–10 Conditions Predisposing to the Development of Secondary Lung Abscess in Children

CONDITION	EXAMPLES
Serious infection	Bronchopneumonia Meningitis Osteomyelitis Septicemia Infected eczema Septic arthritis Abdominal wall abscess Peritonsillar abscess Endocarditis
Immunodeficiency or immunosuppression disorder	Measles Burns Prematurity Blood dyscrasias Leukemia Hepatitis Dysgammaglobulinemia Nephrotic syndrome Chronic granulomatous disease Steroid therapy Malnutrition
Condition leading to repeated aspiration	Seizure disorders Mental deficiency Altered consciousness Dysphagia Periodontitis Riley-Day syndrome
Other (miscellaneous or rare)	Cystic fibrosis Misplaced central nervous catheter $Alpha_1$-antitrypsin deficiency Foreign body in respiratory tract Eroded foreign body in the esophagus

From Asher MI, Beaudry PH: Lung abscess. *In* Chernick V (ed): Kendig's Disorders of the Respiratory Tract in Children, 5th ed. Philadelphia, WB Saunders, 1990, p 430.

retractions, crackles, and decreased breath sounds on auscultation.

Management

Antibiotic therapy is usually sufficient. Drainage of the abscess is rarely needed.

Complications

Complications are uncommon.

ATELECTASIS

Atelectasis is closure or collapse of a segment, lobe, or lobes of the lung. Collapse causes V/Q mismatch, resulting in hypoxemia, decreased lung compliance, and hypoventilation. Secretions accumulate and increase the risk of infection.

Etiology

Table 4–11 lists causes of atelectasis.

Diagnosis

Chest x-ray films obtained with both lateral and posteroanterior views are needed; evidence of volume loss confirms the diagnosis.

Clinical Presentation

Symptoms vary with the severity of collapse and may include tachypnea, nasal flaring, grunting, retractions, low-grade fever, dyspnea, and cough. Breath sounds may be decreased with occasional wheezing. Lower lobes are more often involved in children; right upper lobe involvement is seen in intubated infants. The right middle lobe is affected most often in asthmatic patients and may be recurrent (right middle lobe syndrome).

Management

Therapy depends on the cause and severity. Bronchodilators and CPT may aid in preventing or removing mucus. Mobility, incentive spirometry, and coughing are used to prevent and treat atelectasis. Nasal or mask continuous positive airway pressure (CPAP) is used in some patients. Mechanical ventilation is indicated in patients who experience respiratory failure.

Complications

Complications are rare, and most patients respond to therapy. If the underlying cause of the atelectasis is severe

TABLE 4–11 Causes of Atelectasis in Infants and Children

INTRABRONCHIAL OBSTRUCTION
Foreign body
Mucus plugs
Cystic fibrosis
Asthma
BRONCHIAL WALL DAMAGE OR DISEASE
Airway stenosis
Airway inflammation and edema due to aspiration or inhalation injury
Airway edema
Bronchial tumors
Granuloma
Papillomas
EXTRINSIC BRONCHIAL COMPRESSION
Tumors
Lymph nodes
Cardiomegaly
Vascular rings
Lobar emphysema
SURFACTANT DEFICIENCY OR DYSFUNCTION
Hyaline membrane disease
ARDS
Pneumonia
Pulmonary edema
Near-drowning
COMPRESSION OF NORMAL LUNG TISSUE
Chylothorax
Hemothorax
Pneumothorax
Tumors

From Hazinski TA: Atelectasis. *In* Chernick V (ed): Kendig's Disorders of the Respiratory Tract in Children, 5th ed. Philadelphia, WB Saunders, 1990, p 510.

(e.g., foreign body aspiration, trauma), complications may increase.

SARCOIDOSIS

Sarcoidosis is a chronic granulomatous disorder that affects the lungs, skin, liver, lymph nodes, and eyes. Respiratory involvement includes an intense alveolitis.

Etiology

The cause of sarcoidosis is unknown.

Incidence

It is rare in children and is most common in adults 20 to 40 years of age.

Diagnosis

The diagnosis is established when clinical and radiographic findings are associated with granuloma formation in more than one organ or when a positive Kveim-Siltzback skin test result is obtained.

Clinical Presentation

Physical Examination. Findings reveal a dry, hacking cough; fatigue; fever; bone, joint, chest, and abdominal pain; dyspnea; and crackles, wheezing, and decreased breath sounds on auscultation.

Chest X-ray Findings. Bilateral hilar lymph node enlargement is the most common finding; fibrosis with bullae formation and pulmonary infiltrates may be seen in advanced disease.

Management

No specific treatment exists. Corticosteroids may relieve symptoms and suppress inflammation.

Complications

Most children improve, although some deaths have been reported.

PULMONARY ALVEOLAR PROTEINOSIS

Pulmonary alveolar proteinosis is a syndrome characterized by progressive dyspnea and cough; proteinaceous material is found within the alveoli.

Etiology

The cause of this condition is unknown. Overproduction of surfactant-like material by the Type II cell, dysfunction of the alveolar macrophages, and response to injury to the macrophage may be factors.

Incidence

This condition is rare in children.

Diagnosis

Changes on chest x-ray film may be diagnostic.

Clinical Presentation

Dyspnea, cough (may be productive), cyanosis, fatigue, weight loss or FTT, and crackles may be present. Chest x-ray film reveals a feathery perihilar increase similar to that in pulmonary edema.

Management

Aerosol therapy with proteolytic enzymes is given. Bronchopulmonary lavage is indicated if symptoms progress.

Complications

Progressive filling of the alveoli and infection increase the mortality rate in children.

PULMONARY HEMOSIDEROSIS

Pulmonary hemosiderosis is an accumulation of iron (in the form of hemosiderin) in the lungs that leads to impaired diffusion, airway obstruction, and decreased compliance.

Etiology

The cause is usually unknown, or pulmonary hemosiderosis may result from pulmonary hemorrhage and sensitivity to cow's milk, and it may occur in association with Goodpasture's syndrome (glomerulonephritis).

Incidence

Pulmonary hemosiderosis occurs most often in children and young adults.

Diagnosis

The presence of siderophages in sputum, bronchial washings, or gastric aspirate confirms the diagnosis. Biopsy is not without risks.

Clinical Presentation

The patient may have iron deficiency anemia, hemoptysis, respiratory distress with cyanosis and tachypnea, and fever. The chest x-ray film varies, revealing diffuse infiltrates, massive involvement with atelectasis and emphysema, pneumonia, and an appearance similar to that of pulmonary edema.

Management

Treatment may include oxygen therapy, CPAP or positive end-expiratory pressure (PEEP) via mechanical ventilation, blood transfusions, a hypoallergenic diet with milk restriction, and immunosuppressant drug therapy.

Complications

Massive hemoptysis, respiratory failure, shock associated with massive intrapulmonary hemorrhage, and death may occur.

PULMONARY HEMORRHAGE

Hemorrhage into the lungs may lead to airway obstruction, severe hypoxemia, and hypovolemia.

Etiology

Table 4–12 lists causes of pulmonary hemorrhage and hemoptysis in children.

Diagnosis

The diagnosis may be determined through bronchoscopy, angiograms, and computed tomography and magnetic resonance imaging scanning.

Clinical Presentation

Dyspnea, tachypnea, tachycardia, hypoxemia, hemoptysis, and chest pain may be seen.

Management

Treatment depends on the degree of bleeding and may include oxygen therapy; airway management, including intubation and suction; mechanical ventilation; blood replacement; bronchopulmonary lavage with iced saline; selective embolic occlusion of the vessels; and surgical resection.

Complications

Aspiration, asphyxia, shock, respiratory failure, and death may occur.

PULMONARY EMBOLISM

Pulmonary vascular obstruction by an embolus with alveoli ventilated despite decreased perfusion, resulting in increased alveolar dead space, is called a pulmonary embolism (PE). Wheezing occurs from bronchoconstriction of small airways that are no longer perfused. Pulmonary vascular obstruction causes increased pulmonary vascular resistance (PVR) and increased work for the right ventricle.

Etiology

Risk factors include bacterial endocarditis, the presence of a central venous catheter, sickle cell anemia, heart disease, trauma, and surgery. Neither age nor sex is a risk factor for children.

TABLE 4–12 Causes of Pulmonary Hemorrhage and Massive Hemoptysis in Pediatric Patients

CATEGORY	NEONATAL PERIOD	INFANCY	CHILDHOOD	ADOLESCENCE
Congenital or acquired cardiopulmonary abnormalities	Left ventricular failure with: Hyaline membrane disease Oxygen toxicity Bacterial pneumonia Aspiration Kernicterus Intracranial hemorrhage Prematurity Other problems, e.g., congenital cardiac lesions	Bronchogenic cysts Gastroenteric cysts	Pulmonary sequestration Bronchogenic cysts Congenital arteriovenous fistula (may be part of Osler-Weber-Rendu syndrome)	Congenital cardiac lesions: Tetralogy of Fallot Eisenmenger's complex Pulmonic valve stenosis Mitral valve stenosis Various shunting procedures for pulmonic stenosis Congenital pulmonary vein stenosis Pulmonary arterial stenosis Pulmonary embolism Pulmonary sequestration

Infections and their complications	Bacterial pneumonia Sepsis (?disseminated intravascular coagulation)	Pulmonary abscess (uncommon)	Pulmonary abscess—bacterial Mycoses: Mucormycosis—opportunistic organism Intracavitary aspergillosis (fungus ball) associated with preexisting pulmonary disease, e.g., cystic fibrosis Allergic bronchopulmonary aspergillosis (occasionally seen in asthmatics) Parasitic diseases, e.g., paragonimiasis	Cystic fibrosis Bronchiectasis
Immunologically mediated diseases	Not reported	Uncommon	Goodpasture's syndrome Immune complex–mediated glomerulonephritis Allergic bronchopulmonary aspergillosis Henoch-Schönlein purpura	Goodpasture's syndrome Systemic lupus erythematosus Periarteritis nodosa Wegener's granulomatosis Henoch-Schönlein purpura

Table continued on following page

TABLE 4–12 Causes of Pulmonary Hemorrhage and Massive Hemoptysis in Pediatric Patients *Continued*

CATEGORY	NEONATAL PERIOD	INFANCY	CHILDHOOD	ADOLESCENCE
Neoplasms				
Malignant	Not reported	(Uncommon) Primary Metastatic: Sarcoma Wilms' tumor Osteogenic sarcoma	Bronchial adenoma—carcinoid, cylindroma, mucoepidermoid	Bronchial adenoma Sarcoma
Benign	Not reported	Angiomas	Hemangioma	Hemangioma
Miscellaneous causes	Congenital hyperammonemia	Heiner's syndrome Pulmonary compression injury	Idiopathic pulmonary hemosiderosis Heiner's syndrome Retained foreign body Pulmonary compression injury	Pulmonary compression injury Pulmonary alveolar proteinosis Retained foreign body

From Firth JR, McGeady SJ, Smith DS: Pulmonary hemorrhage and massive hemoptysis. *In* Chernick V (ed): Kendig's Disorders of the Respiratory Tract in Children, 5th ed. Philadelphia, WB Saunders, 1990, p 967.

Incidence

PE is uncommon in children; there is a 3.7% total incidence in the pediatric population.

Diagnosis

Although the clinical presentation does not provide the diagnosis, PE should be considered in the child presenting with acute onset of respiratory distress and cardiogenic shock. A perfusion scan (technetium) is performed; if results are abnormal, a ventilation scan is performed. The differential diagnosis includes cardiac tamponade, cardiomyopathy, and pericarditis.

Clinical Presentation

Physical Examination. Tachypnea is the most common symptom. Other symptoms include pleuritic chest pain, dyspnea, cough, hemoptysis, sweats, diaphoresis, tachycardia, and cyanosis. Breath sounds may include wheezes and crackles.

Chest X-ray Findings. X-rays are usually abnormal, demonstrating infiltrates, atelectasis, and pleural effusion.

Arterial Blood Gas Analysis. ABG determinations are usually normal or are seen with respiratory alkalosis (due to hyperventilation) and hypoxemia (due to V/Q mismatch).

Management

Oxygen Therapy. Oxygen is given to treat the hypoxemia.

Mechanical Ventilation. Ventilation may be instituted to ensure adequate oxygenation and effective ventilation.

Pharmacologic Support. Anticoagulation therapy is begun immediately with IV heparin, followed by warfarin (Coumadin), which is continued for several months. Thrombolytic therapy (streptokinase, urokinase) may be used instead of heparin in patients with massive PE who are hemodynamically unstable. (Absolute contraindications to thrombolytic therapy are active internal bleeding, a cerebrovascular accident (CVA) within 2 months, and intracranial processes.) Dopamine or dobutamine is given to support the blood pressure and improve cardiac output.

IMMOTILE CILIA SYNDROME

Immotile cilia syndrome is a rare autosomal recessive disorder in which the cilia lining the respiratory tract do not function with the normal forward thrust, resulting in impaired mucociliary clearance. Secretions accumulate in dependent portions of the lungs and become infected. Kartagener's syndrome consists of immotile cilia, situs inversus (left-to-right reversal of the position of the heart and intestinal structures), chronic sinusitis, and bronchiectasis.

Diagnosis

Immotile cilia syndrome should be considered in patients with chronic rhinitis, sinusitis, otitis, and bronchitis, especially if other family members are affected also. The diagnosis is confirmed by electron microscopy of the cilia and of ciliated cells from nasal or bronchial biopsies.

Clinical Presentation

The common presentation is chronic or recurrent rhinitis, sinusitis, otitis, bronchitis, and a productive cough. Digital clubbing may be observed with bronchiectasis. The chest radiograph is typical for bronchial wall thickening and hyperinflation; situs inversus, bronchiectasis, atelectasis, and pneumonia occur in about 50% of patients. Males are often infertile because the sperm tails tend to have the same defect as the cilia, causing decreased sperm motility.

Management

There is no means to improve the defective cilia; therefore, treatment focuses on reducing the volume of pooled secretions. Postural drainage with or without percussion, along with an antihistamine decongestant and bronchodilator, is performed daily or during exacerbations. Antibiotic therapy is provided during exacerbations. Cigarette smoke (active or passive) is avoided. Surgical excision of an involved lung segment is considered if the disease is poorly controlled and localized to a single area.

TUBERCULOSIS

Pulmonary infections with *Mycobacterium tuberculosis* leads to pulmonary lesions that may progress into lymph nodes, bronchi, and the lung parenchyma. Pneumonia and airway obstruction with atelectasis or air trapping develop.

Children have a higher incidence of the extrapulmonary forms of TB, such as meningitis.

Etiology

Inhalation and deposition of *M. tuberculosis* into the lungs cause tuberculosis. An infected individual transmits it through aerosolized droplets by coughing, sneezing, laughing, or singing. Congenital TB is rare.

Incidence

There is a higher incidence in minority groups, those living in crowded conditions, and malnourished or immunocompromised patients.

Diagnosis

The tuberculin skin test is the principal diagnostic test. The diagnosis is confirmed by culture of sputum or gastric aspirates.

Clinical Presentation

TB is largely asymptomatic in children older than 1 year of age.

Physical Examination. Examination reveals low-grade fever, mild cough, weight loss, night sweats, FTT in infants, wheezing, decreased breath sounds, tachypnea, bone tenderness, and hepatosplenomegaly.

Chest X-ray Findings. All lobes are at equal risk of being involved. Lesions may be segmental. Cavitation is rare in children. Hilar adenopathy, hyperaeration, atelectasis, and localized pleural effusions may be present.

Management

Contagious individuals are isolated. Antimicrobial therapy and bronchoscopy may be performed to remove secretions and reexpand atelectatic areas.

Complications

Complications include pleural effusion, miliary TB (formation of multiple lesions), meningitis, and TB of the bones and joints, kidney, skin, and heart.

FUNGAL DISORDERS

Fungal respiratory infections resemble tuberculosis clinically. Most infections are treated with amphotericin B and resolve spontaneously.

Aspergillosis

Occurring most often in immunocompromised patients, infection with *Aspergillus fumigatis* (airborne spores) may lead to invasive disease that is often fatal. Nosocomial infection in hospitals has been reported, especially when construction is ongoing, because dust can carry the spores. Patients with leukemia, Hodgkin's disease, and heart, kidney, and bone marrow transplants are at higher risk of infection. Clinical features are fever, cough, dyspnea, chest pain, and round, patchy infiltrates on chest x-ray film that do not respond to antibacterial therapy. Attempts to identify the pathogen are often difficult. Bronchoscopy with bronchial washings and open lung biopsy are considered the best diagnostic tools. "Fungal balls" are sometimes resected.

Blastomycosis

Caused by the organism *Blastomyces dermatitidis,* blastomycosis occurs most often in the midwestern and central southern states of the United States, surrounding the Mississippi and Ohio rivers. The natural habitat of the organism is believed to be moist soil. Diagnosis is made by culturing sputum, skin, or lesions. The clinical presentation is one of pneumonia similar to that seen in TB; cavities may develop in the lungs.

Coccidioidomycosis

The fungus *Coccidioides immitis* is found most often in Central and South America and the western and southwestern United States. The spores are common in dust and are spread through digging and windstorms. The diagnosis is made through skin tests or antibody detection. Clinical features include fever, cough, chest pain, and skin rash. Chest radiography may reveal patchy infiltrates, hilar adenopathy, and large cavitary lesions.

Cryptococcosis

Cryptococcus neoformans is found in soil contaminated by bird feces (usually pigeons) and is inhaled and deposited in the lungs. Immunocompromised patients and those with chronic pulmonary disease are at higher risk of infection. Patients may be asymptomatic; clinical features are similar to those of TB and include fever, malaise, chest pain, dyspnea, weight loss, and night sweats. The appearance of the chest radiograph varies and may demonstrate infiltrates with nodular lesions, round opacities, or hilar lymph node enlargement. Diagnostic tools include sputum culture, bronchoscopy, and open lung biopsy.

Histoplasmosis

The fungus *Histoplasma capsulatum* is found in certain soils, and infection occurs by inhalation and deposition of the spores into the lungs. Soil in shady locations contaminated with bird and bat feces is often colonized with the fungus. Patients with AIDS are at high risk of infection. The diagnosis is made through sputum culture. Patients may be asymptomatic, present with flu-like symptoms, or demonstrate pulmonary infiltrates on chest radiography. Complications include dissemination to other organs, meningitis, pericarditis, and pleural effusion.

SUDDEN INFANT DEATH SYNDROME

Sudden infant death syndrome (SIDS) is the leading cause of death in infants between 1 week and 1 year of age. It is best defined as the sudden and unexpected death of an infant for which a death scene investigation, review of the history, and a postmortem examination fail to reveal a sufficient cause.

Incidence

Table 4–13 lists risk factors associated with SIDS.

Prevention Measures

Improving the general health of the mother and infant, improving compliance with home monitoring, breast feeding infants, positioning infants on their sides instead of prone, and decreasing maternal smoking may all help prevent SIDS.

ADULT RESPIRATORY DISTRESS SYNDROME

Adult respiratory distress syndrome (ARDS) is a syndrome of acute disruption of the pulmonary microvascular endothelium leading to respiratory failure as a result of

TABLE 4–13 Risk Factors Associated With Sudden Infant Death Syndrome

INFANT RISK FACTORS
Male sex
African-American race
Prematurity
Low birth weight
Bottle feeding
Prone position
Winter season
Small for gestational age
Exposure to opioids and cocaine in utero
MATERNAL RISK FACTORS
Teenage mother
Cigarette smoking during pregnancy
Anemia during pregnancy
Late or no prenatal care
Multiple births

increased capillary permeability with pulmonary edema. Histopathologic changes include microatelectasis, pulmonary capillary congestion, endothelial cell swelling, increased fluid leak, and hyaline membrane formation. This leads to pulmonary hypertension, V/Q mismatch, altered surfactant activity, hypoxemia, and decreased lung compliance.

Etiology

Table 4–14 lists antecedent events that may precipitate ARDS.

Clinical Presentation

Symptoms present a few hours to several days after the acute injury or antecedent event.

Physical Examination. Tachypnea is the initial symptom; work of breathing increases (retractions, nasal flaring, grunting) as lung compliance decreases.

Arterial Blood Gas Analysis. ABG determination reveals hypoxemia refractory to oxygen. The $Paco_2$ levels

TABLE 4–14 Lung Injury in Adult Respiratory Distress Syndrome

PRIMARY INJURY	SECONDARY INJURY
Aspiration	Shock
Near-drowning	Sepsis
Oxygen toxicity	Multiple trauma
Pulmonary infection	Long bone fracture
Pulmonary contusion	Massive blood transfusion
Toxic gas inhalation	Increased intracranial pressure
Smoke inhalation	Heroin overdose

are decreased initially in response to tachypnea; hypercarbia and respiratory acidosis develop as pulmonary disease worsens.

Management

The ultimate goals of management are to (1) provide adequate oxygenation, (2) treat the underlying disease, and (3) avoid complications.

Oxygen Therapy. Hypoxemia in ARDS is refractory to oxygen therapy, and greater than 60% oxygen is associated with lung parenchyma toxicity.

Mechanical Ventilation. Positive pressure ventilation is necessary to increase oxygenation and treat respiratory failure. PEEP is used to improve oxygenation in the hope of decreasing the high F_{IO_2} levels and increasing the functional residual capacity. Excess PEEP may overdistend the lung, reduce cardiac output, cause barotrauma, and worsen compliance. The lowest PEEP that can achieve the desired oxygenation level should be used. Inverse ratio ventilation may result in improved oxygenation with lower pressure levels. High-frequency oscillatory ventilation may be beneficial in some situations.

Extracorporeal Membrane Oxygenation. Patients who continue to deteriorate may be candidates for extracorporeal membrane oxygenation (ECMO), depending on the underlying disorder.

Aerosol Therapy. Bronchodilating agents may be administered through the mechanical ventilator for treatment of bronchospasm.

CPT. CPT may be indicated in patients with retained or excessive secretions. Suctioning of the airway should be kept to a minimum, because the negative pressure required for suctioning may lead to pulmonary edema, as well as reduce PEEP levels.

Stabilization of Circulation. Volume resuscitation may be needed with crystalloid, colloid, or hypertonic solutions. Optimal fluid balance may be difficult and requires careful attention to fluid status, nutritional support, and prevention of secondary infection.

Pharmacologic Support. Furosemide may be given for diuresis; dopamine or dobutamine may be needed to support cardiac output.

Complications

Mortality remains high. Most survivors recover normal lung mechanics; however, some maintain a reduced forced vital capacity. Nosocomial infections, air leak syndromes, and multiple organ system failure may lead to death.

NEAR-DROWNING

Near-drowning describes any victim who survives a minimum of 24 hours. Submersion results in lack of oxygen. If aspiration also occurs, pulmonary surfactant may be altered, with atelectasis and severe hypoxemia developing. Overall sequelae are the result of anoxia, pulmonary injury from aspiration, and hypothermia.

Incidence

Drowning is the second leading cause of injury in children older than 9 months of age. The incidence of drowning peaks in (1) children less than 4 years of age and (2) children 15 to 19 years of age. Risk factors are listed in Table 4–15.

Clinical Presentation

Neurologic Examination. Anoxic insult to the brain may lead to cerebral edema, which is manifested by increased intracranial pressure (ICP). The severity of the central nervous system (CNS) injury determines the neurologic abnormalities present. Findings range from alert and awake to comatose and flaccid.

TABLE 4–15 Risk Factors Associated With Near-Drowning

Absence of barriers
Drugs or alcohol use
Exhaustion
Hypothermia
Inadequate supervision
Inexperience in swimming
Mental retardation
Myocardial infarction
Seizure disorder
Trauma

Chest X-ray Findings. X-rays are consistent with pulmonary edema and aspiration.

Arterial Blood Gas Analysis. ABG determination reveals hypoxemia that is often refractory to oxygen therapy.

Management

Oxygen Therapy. Oxygen via cannula, hood, mask, or mechanical ventilation is indicated.

Resuscitation. Hypoxemia should be reduced as quickly as possible. Intubation with supplemental oxygen, positive pressure ventilation, and cardiac massage may be necessary. In cases of hypothermia, the patient must be warmed; methods include warmed IV fluids, warm blankets, heating of supplemental oxygen, and bladder and peritoneal irrigation with warm fluids.

Neurologic Management. The goal is to decrease the ICP, decrease cerebral metabolic needs, and maintain cerebral perfusion pressure at 35 to 45 mm Hg. The position of the head should be kept at midline. Attempts should be made to keep the ICP at a minimum.

Mechanical Ventilation. Volume ventilation is often needed in patients who experience severe hypoxemia, respiratory failure, or ARDS. The positive pressure is used to treat atelectasis and pulmonary edema. High rates may be instituted to reduce $Paco_2$ levels and ICP. Sedation and paralysis are often necessary to ventilate efficiently and maintain a low ICP.

TABLE 4–16 Prognostic Factors in Near-Drowning

FAVORABLE FACTORS	UNFAVORABLE FACTORS
Age <3 years	Submersion (warm water) >9 minutes
Submersion (warm water) <3 minutes	CPR duration >25 minutes
Ice in water	CPR needed on admission to emergency department
Core temperature <33° C	pH <6.85
Conscious on arrival	Fixed and dilated pupils >6 hours after admission
Presence of a pulse in the emergency department	Seizures persisting >24 hours

From Holbrook PR, Fields AI: Drowning and near-drowning. *In* Holbrook PR: Textbook of Pediatric Critical Care. Philadelphia, WB Saunders, 1993, pp 91–93.
CPR, cardiopulmonary resuscitation.

Complications

Poor neurologic outcome is not uncommon among survivors. The prognostic factors in near-drowning are listed in Table 4–16.

FOREIGN BODY ASPIRATION

Aspiration of foreign material into the trachea or bronchi may result in complete occlusion of the airway (e.g., from hot dogs, balloons) with strangulation and rapid death or in partial obstruction (e.g., from peanuts, popcorn) with wheezing.

Incidence

Foreign body aspiration occurs most often in infants and toddlers.

Clinical Presentation

Symptoms vary depending on the location of impaction and whether airway obstruction is complete or partial.

Physical Examination. Sudden onset of wheezing (usually unilateral), coughing, gagging, or stridor should raise suspicion. Severe respiratory distress, decreased breath sounds, cyanosis, and collapse usually indicate complete obstruction.

Chest X-ray Findings. Recurrent pneumonia in the same lobe is suspicious. More apparent on an expiratory film, asymmetric lung hyperinflation may be seen as a result of the ball-valve effect caused by a foreign body localized in a major bronchus. Some objects may be revealed on an x-ray film (safety pin, bolts), whereas others will not (peanut, apple skin).

Management

The Heimlich maneuver may be necessary in life-threatening situations. Removal of the foreign body by rigid bronchoscopy under general anesthesia may be indicated. Following removal of the foreign body, CPT may be needed to aid in secretion removal. A second bronchoscopy may be required because of reaccumulation of secretions.

Complications

Resolution of symptoms may be delayed following removal of the object. Reactive granulation tissue with infection may occur at the site of obstruction.

Bibliography

American Academy of Pediatrics—Task Force on Infant Positioning and SIDS—Kattwinkel J, Brooks J, Myerberg D: Positioning and SIDS. Pediatrics 1992; 89:1120.

Avery ME, First LR: Pediatric Medicine. Baltimore, Williams & Wilkins, 1989.

Blumer J: A Practical Guide to Pediatric Intensive Care, 3rd ed. St. Louis, CV Mosby, 1990.

Bokulic RE, Hilman BC: Interstitial lung disease in children. Pediatr Clin North Am 1994; 41:543.

Burg FD, Ingelfinger JR, Wald ER: Current Pediatric Therapy, vol 14. Philadelphia, WB Saunders, 1993.

Chernick V: Kendig's Disorders of the Respiratory Tract in Children, 5th ed. Philadelphia, WB Saunders, 1990.

Clochesy JM, Breu C, Cardin S, et al: Critical Care Nursing. Philadelphia, WB Saunders, 1993.

Committee on Infectious Diseases: Screening for tuberculosis in infants and children. Pediatrics 1994; 93:131.

Cooke JC, Currie DC, Morgan AD, et al: Role of computed tomography in diagnosis of bronchiectasis. Thorax 1987; 42:272.

Cressman WR, Myer CM III: Diagnosis and management of croup and epiglottitis. Pediatr Clin North Am 1994; 41:265.

Culbertson JL, Krous HF, Bendell DR: Sudden Infant Death Syndrome: Medical Aspects and Psychological Management. Baltimore, Johns Hopkins University Press, 1988.

Custer JR: Croup and related disorders. Pediatr Rev 1993; 14:19.

Dantzker DR: Cardiopulmonary Critical Care. Philadelphia, WB Saunders, 1991.

Evans DA, Wilmott RW: Pulmonary embolism in children. Pediatr Clin North Am 1994; 41:569.

Fanconi S, Kraemer R, Weber J, et al: Long-term sequelae in children surviving adult respiratory distress syndrome. J Pediatr 1985; 106:218.

Fandel I, Bancalari E: Near-drowning in children. Pediatrics 1976; 58:573.

Fiser DH: Adult respiratory distress syndrome. Pediatr Rev 1993; 14:163.

Freij BJ, Kusmiesz H, Nelson JD, McCracken GH: Parapneumonic effusions and empyema in hospitalized children: A retrospective review of 227 cases. Pediatr Infect Dis 1984; 3:578.

Griscom NT: Diseases of the trachea, bronchi, and smaller airways. Radiol Clin North Am 1993; 31:605.

Hilman B: Pediatric Respiratory Disease: Diagnosis and Treatment. Philadelphia, WB Saunders, 1993.

Hoffman HJ, Hillman HS: Epidemiology of the sudden infant death syndrome: Maternal, neonatal, and postneonatal risk factors. Clin Perinatol 1992; 19:717.

Holbrook PR: Textbook of Pediatric Critical Care. Philadelphia, WB Saunders, 1993.

Kamei RK: Chronic cough in children. Pediatr Clin North Am 1991; 38:593.

Katz R: Adult respiratory distress syndrome in children. Clin Chest Med 1987; 8:635.

Kilham H, Gillis J, Benjamin B: Severe upper airway obstruction. Pediatr Clin North Am 1987; 34:1.

Levin DL, Moriss FC, Toro LO, et al: Drowning and near-drowning. Pediatr Clin North Am 1993; 40:321.

Lyrene RK, Troug WE: Adult respiratory distress syndrome in a pediatric intensive care unit: Predisposing conditions, clinical course, and outcome. Pediatrics 1981; 67:790.

Marks MI: Pediatric Infectious Diseases for the Practitioner. New York, Springer-Verlag, 1985.

Mauro RD, Poole SR, Lockhart CH: Differentiation of epiglottitis from laryngotracheitis in the child with stridor. Am J Dis Child 1988; 142:679.

Mazzocco MC, Owens GR, Kirilloff LH, Rogers RM: Chest percussion and postural drainage in patients with bronchiectasis. Chest 1985; 88:360.

McLaughlin FJ, Goldmann DA, Rosenbaum DM, et al: Empyema in children: Clinical course and long-term follow up. Pediatrics 1984; 73:587.

National Asthma Education Program Expert Panel Report: Guidelines for the Diagnosis and Management of Asthma. Washington, DC, National Heart, Lung, and Blood Institute, National Institutes of Health, Publication No. 91-3042, 1991.

Orenstein DM, Bowen A: Cystic fibrosis: Clinical update for radiologists. Radiol Clin North Am 1993; 31:617.

Provisional Committee on Quality Improvement: Practice parameter: The office management of acute exacerbations of asthma in children. Pediatrics 1994; 93:119.

Quan L, Wentz KR, Gore EJ, Copass MK: Outcome and predictors of outcome in pediatric submersion victims receiving prehospital care in King County, Washington. Pediatrics 1990; 86:586.

Royall J, Levin DL: Adult respiratory distress syndrome in pediatric patients. I. Clinical aspects, pathophysiology, pathology and mechanisms of lung injury. J Pediatr 1988; 112:169.

Royall J, Levin DL: Adult respiratory distress syndrome in pediatric patients. II. Management. J Pediatr 1988; 112:335.

Sarnaik AP, Lieh-Lai M: Adult respiratory distress syndrome in children. Pediatr Clin North Am 1994; 41:337.

Snider DE Jr, Rieder HL, Combs D, et al: Tuberculosis in children. Pediatr Infect Dis J 1988; 7:271.

Starke JR, Jacobs RF, Joreb J: Resurgence of tuberculosis in children. J Pediatr 1992; 120:839.

Stempel DA, Szefler SJ: Management of chronic asthma. Pediatr Clin North Am 1992; 39: 1293–1310.

Taylor RW, Shoemaker WC: Critical Care: State of the Art, vol 12. Fullerton, CA, Society of Critical Care Medicine, 1991.

Weinberger M: Antiasthmatic therapy in children. Pediatr Clin North Am 1989; 36:1251.

Wilmott RW, Fiedler MA: Recent advances in the treatment of cystic fibrosis. Pediatr Clin North Am 1994; 41:431.

SECTION 5

Cardio-vascular Disorders

I. Circulation

A. Fetal circulation
B. Transitional changes

II. Congenital Heart Disease

A. Acyanotic heart disease
   1. Patent ductus arteriosus
   2. Atrial septal defect
   3. Ventricular septal defect
   4. Atrioventricular canal or endocardial cushion defect
   5. Aortic stenosis
   6. Coarctation of the aorta
   7. Hypoplastic left heart syndrome

B. Cyanotic heart disease
   1. Total anomalous pulmonary venous return
   2. Tetralogy of Fallot
   3. Complete transposition of the great arteries
   4. Pulmonary atresia, intact ventricular septum
   5. Tricuspid atresia
   6. Truncus arteriosus

III. Congestive Heart Failure

IV. Shock

A. True volume loss (hypovolemic shock)
B. Decreased peripheral vascular resistance (neurogenic shock)
C. Decreased myocardial performance (cardiogenic shock)
D. Septic shock

V. Respiratory Care Following Cardiovascular Surgery

A. Equipment needed at bedside
B. Mechanical ventilation
C. Airway management
D. Monitoring
E. Extubation
F. Postextubation care
G. Respiratory complications following cardiovascular surgery

Abbreviations

AS–aortic stenosis
ASD–atrial septal defect

AV–atrioventricular
CHD–congenital heart disease
CHF–congestive heart failure
CoA–coarctation of the aorta
HLHS–hypoplastic left heart syndrome
IVC–inferior vena cava
LA–left atrium
LV–left ventricle
MAST–military antishock trousers
PA–pulmonary artery
PDA–patent ductus arteriosus
PEEP–positive end-expiratory pressure
PS–pulmonary stenosis
PVR–pulmonary vascular resistance
RA–right atrium
RV–right ventricle
SVC–superior vena cava
TA–tricuspid atresia
TAPVR–total anomalous pulmonary venous return
TGA–transposition of the great arteries
TOF–tetralogy of Fallot
UV–umbilical vein
VSD–ventricular septal defect

CIRCULATION

Fetal Circulation

During fetal life, the exchange of oxygen and carbon dioxide occurs in the placenta and not in the lungs. Oxygenated blood diffuses from the maternal placental circulation to the fetal placental circulation, where it leaves the placenta via the umbilical vein (UV). Nearly 50% of the blood in the UV is shunted (bypassing the liver) through the ductus venosus to the inferior vena cava (IVC) and on to the right atrium (RA). This is the more highly oxygenated blood. The remainder of the oxygenated blood flows through the hepatic-portal venous system, where it mixes with blood from the liver and lower body and then returns to the IVC and RA. The blood flowing from the IVC into the RA tends to be shunted through the patent foramen ovale into the left atrium (LA) and then to the left ventricle (LV), where it is pumped out to the ascending aorta toward the head.

Less-oxygenated blood from the upper body returns to the heart via the superior vena cava (SVC). Normally this blood flows into the RA and on to the right ventricle (RV), where it is pumped to the pulmonary artery (PA). Most of this blood bypasses the high-resistance pulmonary vasculature and is shunted through the ductus arteriosus to the descending aorta, from which it will return to the placenta. About 8% of the total fetal cardiac output flows through the fluid-filled lungs and into the LA and LV, where it is then pumped to the descending aorta (Fig. 5–1).

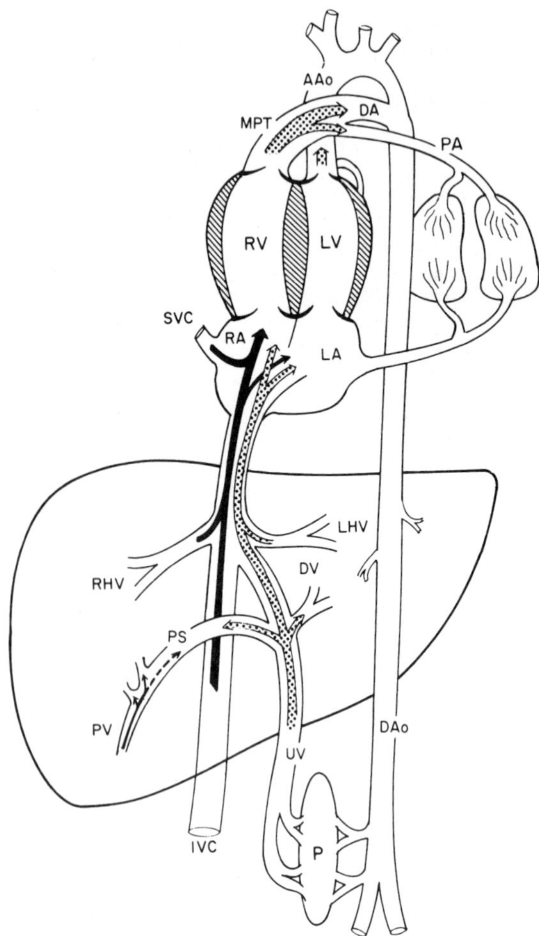

Figure 5–1 Normal fetal circulation and fetal flow patterns. AAo, ascending aorta; DA, ductus arteriosus; DAo, descending aorta; DV, ductus venosus; IVC, inferior vena cava; LA, left atrium; LHV, left hepatic vein; LV, left ventricle; MPT, main pulmonary trunk; P, placenta; PA, pulmonary arteries; PS, portal sinus; PV, portal vein; RA, right atrium; RHV, right hepatic vein; RV, right ventricle; SVC, superior vena cava; UV, umbilical vein. (From Creasy RK, Resnick R: Maternal and Fetal Medicine: Principles and Practice. Philadelphia, WB Saunders, 1984.)

Transitional Changes

Circulatory changes occurring at birth include the following:

1. The lungs expand after the infant's first breath. The increase in oxygenation causes pulmonary vascular resistance (PVR) to rapidly decrease, resulting in increased pulmonary blood flow.

2. The umbilical cord is cut, which removes the low-resistance placenta from the circulation. Systemic pressure rises, and gas exchange now occurs in the lungs.
3. The three fetal shunts close. *Foramen ovale:* Increased blood flow through the lungs and into the LA causes left atrial pressure to be greater than right atrial pressure. The foreman ovale functionally closes within minutes or hours in response to this reversal in pressure. *Ductus arteriosus:* Increased systemic pressure reverses blood flow through the ductus arteriosus; oxygenated blood from the aorta now flows through the ductus arteriosus into the PA. The increased oxygen concentration causes constriction of the ductus, usually in 24 to 72 hours. *Ductus venosus:* Within a few days after birth, the ductus venosus constricts and later becomes a ligament (Fig. 5–2; Table 5–1).

CONGENITAL HEART DISEASE

Congenital heart defects occur in approximately 1% of live births. Survival has improved considerably owing to earlier and improved diagnosis, improved surgical procedures (Table 5–2), technologic and pharmacologic developments, and continued progress in heart transplantation. The defects discussed in the following paragraphs are classified accordingly as acyanotic or cyanotic disorders.

Acyanotic Heart Disease

Patent Ductus Arteriosus

Failure of the ductus arteriosus to close results in persistent patency. As PVR falls after birth, the patent ductus arteriosus (PDA) allows a left-to-right shunt from the aorta to the PA. This results in increased pulmonary blood flow, which is associated with pulmonary hypertension and increased pressure load on the RV.

Incidence. There is a high incidence of PDA in low birth weight preterm infants (20%–60%) and in infants who have recovered or are recovering from respiratory distress syndrome. PDA also occurs in about 60% of term infants with congenital rubella syndrome. It is more common in females than in males (2:1). There may be an increased incidence at higher altitudes.

Clinical Presentation. Clinical features depend on the size of the defect, the magnitude of the left-to-right shunt, and the patient's ability to handle the extra volume load. If the defect is small, the patient may be asymptomatic, with only a short systolic murmur. Older children may have the classic continuous machinery murmur. Pulse pressure is wid-

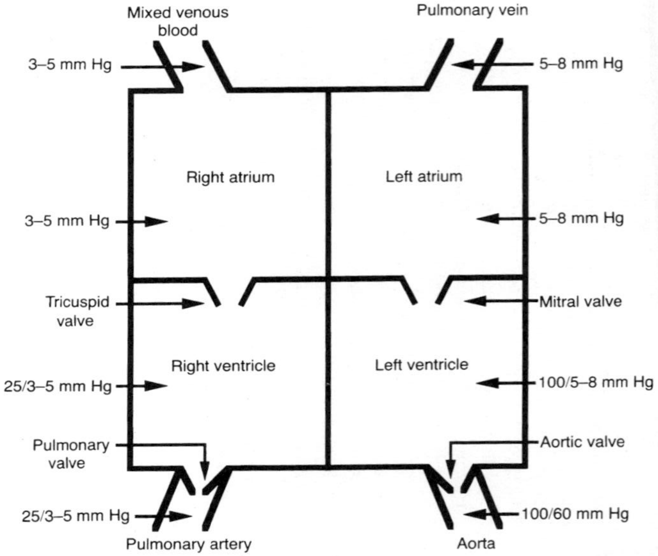

Figure 5–2 Pressures of the normal heart and great vessels of the older child.

TABLE 5–1 Blood Flow in Normal Circulation

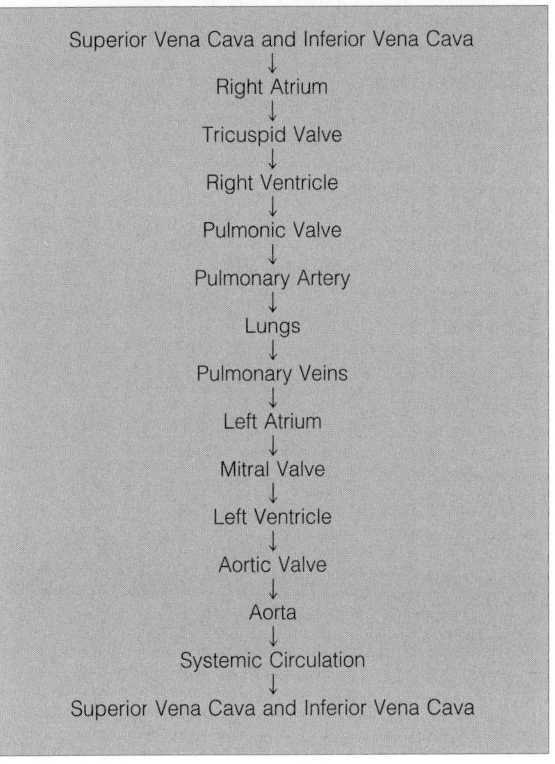

Superior Vena Cava and Inferior Vena Cava
↓
Right Atrium
↓
Tricuspid Valve
↓
Right Ventricle
↓
Pulmonic Valve
↓
Pulmonary Artery
↓
Lungs
↓
Pulmonary Veins
↓
Left Atrium
↓
Mitral Valve
↓
Left Ventricle
↓
Aortic Valve
↓
Aorta
↓
Systemic Circulation
↓
Superior Vena Cava and Inferior Vena Cava

ened, producing bounding peripheral pulses. The child may present with poor feeding, tachypnea, slow weight gain, fatigue, excessive sweating, and irritability, if the defect is large or progresses to left ventricular failure, or both.

Management. Indomethacin may be given orally or intravenously to constrict the ductus in premature infants. It has a high success rate; however, if the neonate has not responded to the drug after 48 to 72 hours of treatment, surgery is recommended. Surgical repair consists of ligation of the ductus arteriosus through a thoracotomy incision (Fig. 5–3).

Atrial Septal Defect

An atrial septal defect (ASD) is an opening in the septum between the right and left atria. The size and position of the defect vary considerably among patients. The three types of ASDs include ostium secundum, ostium primum, and sinus venosus. Since the left atrial pressure is greater than the

TABLE 5–2 Surgical Procedures Used for Management of Congenital Heart Disease

PROCEDURE	DESCRIPTION
	Palliative Procedures
Atrial septectomy	Surgical removal of part of the interatrial septum
Blalock-Taussig shunt	A shunt attaching the subclavian artery to the PA to increase pulmonary blood flow
Glenn shunt	A shunt attaching the right PA to the SVC to increase pulmonary blood flow
Norwood procedure	Performed in HLHS and consists of (1) the main PA connected to the aorta (an artificial PDA), (2) atrial septectomy to relieve pulmonary venous obstruction to the RA, and (3) a systemic-PA shunt to allow blood flow to the lungs
PA banding	A band is placed around the pulmonary artery to decrease the diameter and increase resistance to flow through the artery; this procedure does not correct the defect but serves to reduce pulmonary blood flow
Potts shunt	A shunt attaching the descending aorta to the PA to increase pulmonary blood flow

Rashkind balloon atrial septostomy	During cardiac catheterization, a catheter is advanced into the LA, the balloon is inflated, and then with a short tug the catheter is rapidly withdrawn across the atrial septum
Waterston-Cooley shunt	A shunt attaching the ascending aorta to the PA to increase pulmonary blood flow
	Corrective Procedures
Fontan procedure	The right systemic venous blood is routed directly from the vena cava or the RA to the PA through a fenestrated conduit
Mustard procedure	A patch is used to create an interatrial baffle to direct blood flow from the IVC and SVC to the LV and the pulmonary venous flow to the RV; used in cases of TGA
Rastelli procedure	Flow from the LV is directed to the aorta by an intraventricular patch-tunnel, and a conduit from the RV to the main PA is used to redirect the pulmonary and systemic blood; used in cases of TGA
Senning procedure	Part of the atrial wall is used to create an interatrial baffle to direct blood flow from the IVC and SVC to the LV and the pulmonary venous flow to the RV; used in cases of TGA

PA, pulmonary artery; SVC, superior vena cava; HLHS, hypoplastic left heart syndrome; PDA, patent ductus arteriosus; RA, right atrium; LA, left atrium; IVC, inferior vena cava; LV, left ventricle; RV, right ventricle; TGA, transposition of the great arteries.

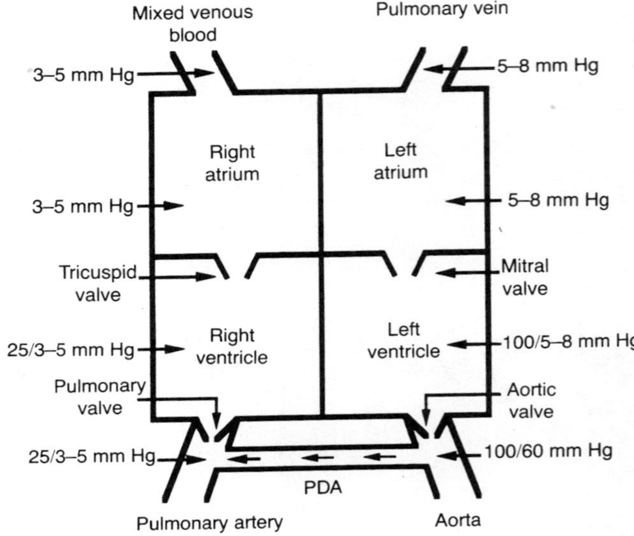

Figure 5–3 Patent ductus arteriosus—communication between the pulmonary artery and the aorta.

right during most of the cardiac cycle, the blood is shunted left to right, resulting in an increase in pulmonary blood flow. Pulmonary hypertension and congestive failure are rare.

Incidence. ASD occurs in approximately 7% of all cardiac defects. It is more common in females than in males (2:1).

Clinical Presentation. Most patients are asymptomatic until childhood or adolescence, when a murmur may be heard. If the shunt is large, the child may easily become fatigued and complain of dyspnea. Infants may have poor growth and lower respiratory tract infections. The chest x-ray film may or may not demonstrate cardiomegaly and may show increased pulmonary vascular markings.

Management. Spontaneous closure may occur. Elective surgical repair is the treatment for all ASDs clinically diagnosed. It is usually deferred until the child is near 5 years of age, except in those patients who have evidence of cardiac failure or pulmonary hypertension. Repair is usually via simple suture closure; however, a pericardial or polytetrafluorethylene (Teflon) patch may be needed in larger defects. Complications following surgery are rare, although pulmonary hypertension and cardiac failure have been noted, as have dysrhythmias, including bradycardia and atrial flutter (Fig. 5–4).

Ventricular Septal Defect

A ventricular septal defect (VSD) is an opening in the septum between the right and left ventricles. The size and location of the defects are variable, and they may occur as single or multiple lesions. Because of the relatively low resistance of the pulmonary vascular bed, most of the blood flow through a VSD is from left to right. The size of the defect determines the amount of shunting. The shunt can often be large, with the increased pulmonary blood flow resulting in pulmonary hypertension and congestive heart failure (CHF). Increased pulmonary blood flow causes increased return of blood to the left side of the heart, with a marked volume overload of the LV. If PVR increases and exceeds that of the systemic circulation, the shunt may become predominantly right to left.

Incidence. VSD is the most common congenital heart disease (CHD) in all age groups, occurring in approximately 20% of all patients with congenital heart anomalies.

Clinical Presentation. Clinical features are dependent on the size of the defect. Patients with small defects may be asymptomatic, with only a loud murmur that is commonly

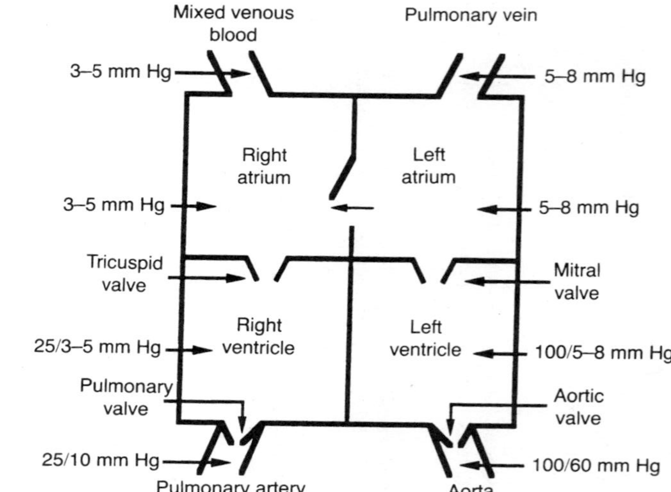

Figure 5–4 Atrial septal defect—communication between the right and left atria through the septum.

detected after 2 weeks of age. Larger defects present with symptoms primarily due to the left-to-right shunt and left ventricular failure. Symptoms include failure to thrive, tachypnea and increased work of breathing, excessive sweating and fatigue during feeding, and an increased anteroposterior diameter of the chest. Patients with a right-to-left shunt may exhibit cyanosis. Chest radiography may reveal cardiomegaly and increased pulmonary vascular markings.

Management. Small defects usually close spontaneously and are managed with only observation and prophylactic antibiotics to prevent endocarditis (e.g., during dental and surgical procedures). Larger defects are managed medically with digoxin and diuretics; surgical repair is considered when there is evidence of growth failure, repeated pulmonary infections, and further CHF. The defect is closed during surgery, usually by suturing; however, a large defect may require that a patch be sewn to the septum. In some patients it is not possible to repair multiple defects, and PA banding is performed (Fig. 5–5).

Atrioventricular Canal or Endocardial Cushion Defect

Embryologic development of the endocardial cushions results in the atrioventricular (AV) septa and the septal leaflets of both the mitral and tricuspid valves. Faulty development of the endocardial cushions and the AV septa results in varying degrees of cardiac defects that have a ‘‘scooped out’’ appearance; hence the term canal. The anomaly may be a partial-canal or complete-canal defect in which there is a large AV septal defect and a common AV valve. Left-to-right shunting at the atria or ventricles, or both, occurs, resulting in increased pulmonary blood flow and associated pulmonary hypertension and CHF. Mitral valve regurgitation may occur if the mitral valve is deformed.

Incidence. This condition is often associated with Down's syndrome, and males and females are affected equally.

Clinical Presentation. Symptoms seen early in life include dyspnea, fatigue, recurrent respiratory infections, and growth failure. Severe cardiac failure with cyanosis and respiratory failure may develop. The chest x-ray film may demonstrate cardiomegaly and a dilated PA. A systolic murmur is usually heard.

Management. Medical management of the CHF consists of digoxin and diuretic administration. Surgery is indicated when cardiac failure or growth failure continues and should be performed prior to 2 years of age, as the risk of pulmonary

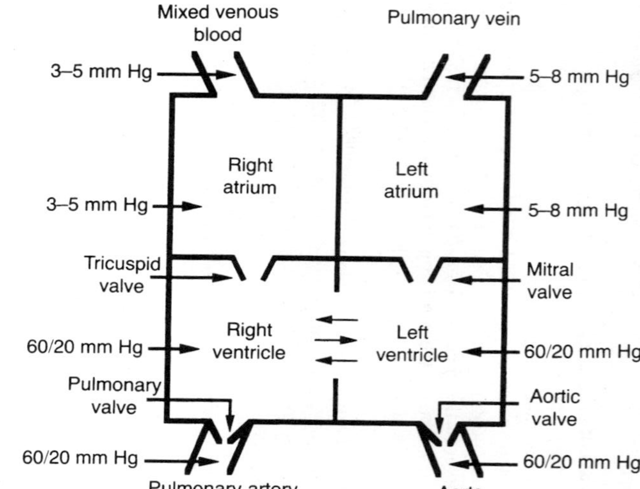

Figure 5–5 Ventricular septal defect—communication between the right and left ventricles through the septum.

vascular obstructive disease (irreversible pulmonary vascular disease) increases after 2 years. PA banding to decrease pulmonary blood flow is a palliative procedure and may be performed in patients younger than 6 months of age, who are at greater risk of surgical complications following complete repair. Complete repair includes closure of the AV septa and reconstruction of the AV valves to the new septum. Varying degrees of AV valve problems occur after surgery, including mitral regurgitation. Postoperative arrhythmias occur in some patients. Permanent pacemakers may be used in patients with persistent heart block or sinus node dysfunction. Prophylactic antibiotics are given to prevent bacterial endocarditis. There does not seem to be any difference in surgical mortality in patients with Down's syndrome when compared with those without it (Fig. 5–6).

Aortic Stenosis

Obstruction of blood from the LV may occur above, below, or at the level of the aortic valve. Supravalvar stenosis is a narrowing of the ascending aorta (described as a supravalvar coarctation) beginning right above the aortic valve, valvar stenosis is a narrowing of the aortic valve itself, and subaortic stenosis consists of a membranous diaphragm or fibrous ring encircling the left ventricular outflow tract just below the aortic valve. The obstruction to left ventricular outlet flow results in left ventricular hypertrophy. The more the obstruction, the greater the left ventricular pressure needed to provide systemic output. If left ventricular pressures are great enough, CHF results.

Incidence. Supravalvar stenosis is associated with Wiliams' syndrome (elfin facies and hypercalcemia of infancy). Valvar stenosis occurs in 3% to 6% of patients with CHD, often with PDA and coarctation of the aorta (CoA). It is the second most common congenital heart defect in young adults and occurs more often in males than in females (4 : 1). Subaortic stenosis occurs more often in males than in females (2 : 1).

Clinical Presentation. Most children are asymptomatic, with a murmur often detected during routine examinations. Fatigue, exertional dyspnea and anginal pain, syncope, and endocarditis may occur. Patients in cardiac failure may be irritable, pale or cyanotic, and hypotensive and present with tachycardia, tachypnea, retractions, and pulmonary congestion. Surprisingly the chest film usually demonstrates a normal heart; however, the child with CHF may have a massively enlarged heart.

Management. The malformed aortic valve is at high risk for infection; therefore, prophylactic antibiotics are given. Strenuous physical activity is avoided. Surgical management

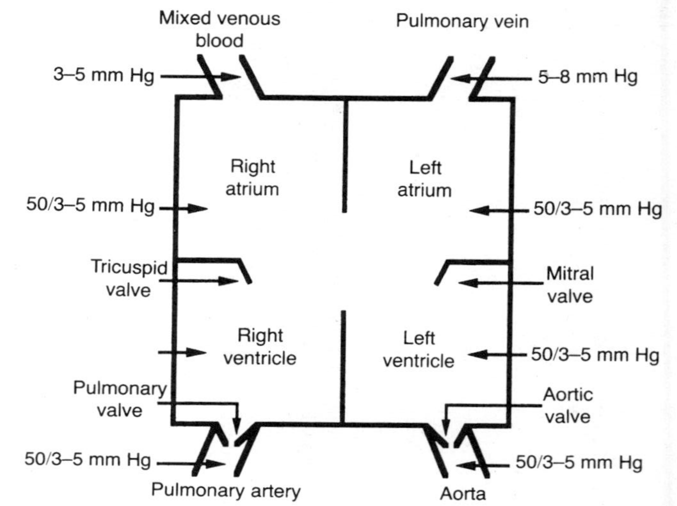

Figure 5–6 Atrioventricular canal defect—incomplete development of the atrial and ventricular septa, which allows complete cardiac mixing of blood.

consists of balloon valvuloplasty, valvotomy, or valve replacement. Calcification of valve leaflets may occur later in life and require valve replacement. Repair of supravalvar stenosis may include widening the lumen of the aorta or replacing the entire narrowed area with a prosthesis. Endocarditis remains a possible complication following surgery, and sudden death may occur even in asymptomatic patients (Fig. 5–7).

Coarctation of the Aorta

CoA occurs as a constriction or narrowing of the aortic lumen, usually located at the junction of the ductus arteriosus and the aortic arch (aortic isthmus). Obstruction may be a discrete narrowing or a long segment. Obstruction to left ventricular outflow may result in left ventricular failure with pulmonary edema, low output, and circulatory collapse (often associated with closure of the ductus arteriosus).

Incidence. CoA is the fifth or sixth most common CHD and is more common in males than in females (1.7 : 1). It is frequently associated with PDA, VSD, aortic stenosis (AS), and mitral valve abnormalities. It is commonly seen in patients with Turner's syndrome.

Clinical Presentation. Weak or absent femoral and pedal pulses are common. Upper limbs may demonstrate hypertension, with decreased pressure in the lower limbs. Infants frequently present with tachycardia, tachypnea, pallor, cyanosis, failure to thrive, and a weak cry. Murmurs may be present or absent. Chest x-ray film often reveals an enlarged heart with pulmonary vasculature congestion.

Management. Neonates may be treated with digitalis (for cardiac failure), diuretics (to limit vascular engorgement), and prostaglandins (to minimize ductus arteriosus constriction) prior to surgery. Surgical repair consists of relieving the obstruction via (1) an end-to-end anastomosis, (2) a patch aortoplasty, or (3) a subclavian flap procedure. Complications after surgery include residual obstruction, recoarctation, endocarditis, and persistent hypertension (Fig. 5–8).

Hypoplastic Left Heart Syndrome

Hypoplastic left heart syndrome (HLHS) is characterized by underdevelopment of the structures of the left side of the heart, the aortic valve, and the aorta. To survive, blood must be shunted from the small LA through the foramen ovale into the RA. A PDA supplies the entire systemic output at first, with output decreasing when the ductus closes. The RV becomes hypertrophied because of the increased blood flow. HLHS is fatal without surgery.

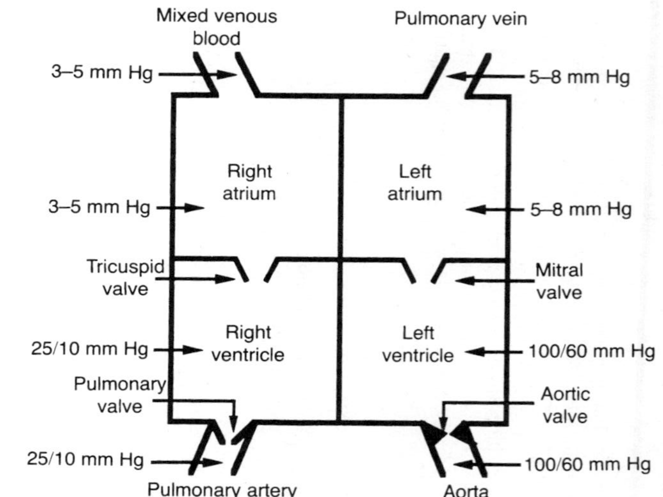

Figure 5–7 Aortic stenosis—outflow obstruction of the aorta, impeding blood flow from the left ventricle.

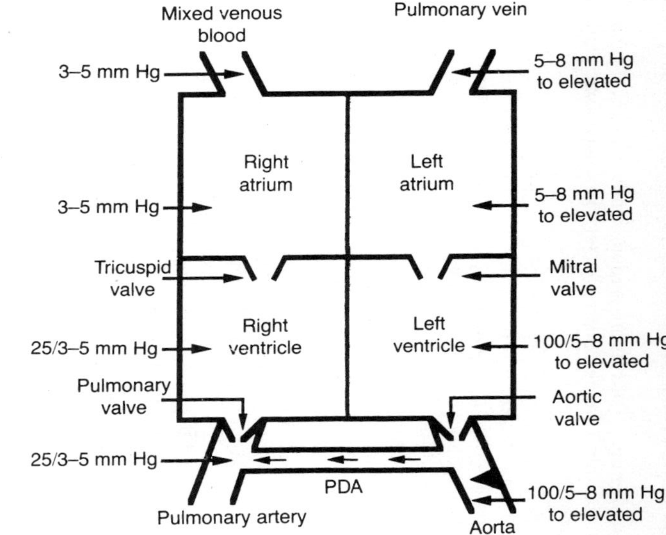

Figure 5–8 Coarctation of the aorta—severe narrowing of the aortic lumen, which decreases blood flow through the aorta. A PDA is often present to allow pulmonary blood flow when the coarctation is severe. PDA, patent ductus arteriosus.

Incidence. Patients are predominantly male (67%) and of normal birth weight; approximately 10% have extracardiac anomalies.

Clinical Presentation. Nearly all infants become symptomatic within 13 days of being born. Diminished peripheral pulses, pallor, tachycardia, tachypnea, dyspnea, and metabolic acidosis are present as the ductus begins to close. Cardiac failure is inevitable. The chest radiograph often reveals an enlarged, globular heart with right atrial enlargement.

Management. Immediate treatment includes prostaglandin E_1 given to maintain a PDA, digoxin and diuretics for cardiac failure, and mechanical ventilation. Some patients are not candidates for surgery and will die within days or weeks. Surgical management is accomplished in phases, with initial palliation using the Norwood procedure and a Fontan procedure performed approximately 6 months to 4 years later. The PA is the main outlet to systemic circulation, and the heart is operational as a single ventricle pump. Heart transplantation is another management approach (Fig. 5–9).

Cyanotic Heart Disease

Total Anomalous Pulmonary Venous Return

In total anomalous pulmonary venous return (TAPVR), the pulmonary veins have no connection with the LA and drain (directly or indirectly) into the RA. Connection may be at (1) the supracardiac level, (2) the cardiac level, (3) the infracardiac level, or (4) two or more of these levels. This results in the mixing of pulmonary and systemic blood returning to the RA, as well as in increased pressures and volume in the right side of the heart. Without pulmonary venous obstruction, there is increased pulmonary blood flow. In contrast, obstructed pulmonary veins result in low oxygen saturation and often a right-to-left shunt through a PDA.

Incidence. TAPVR is the abnormality in 2% of critically ill infants with cardiac problems. There is a male preponderance in TAPVR with connection to the portal vein (3 : 1), whereas other TAPVR anomalies occur equally in males and females.

Clinical Presentation. Clinical features often depend on the degree of pulmonary venous obstruction, with severe obstruction mimicking pulmonary disease and presenting with cyanosis and pulmonary edema in the infant's first days of life. Infants with unobstructed TAPVR are usually asymptomatic at birth, with tachypnea and feeding problems

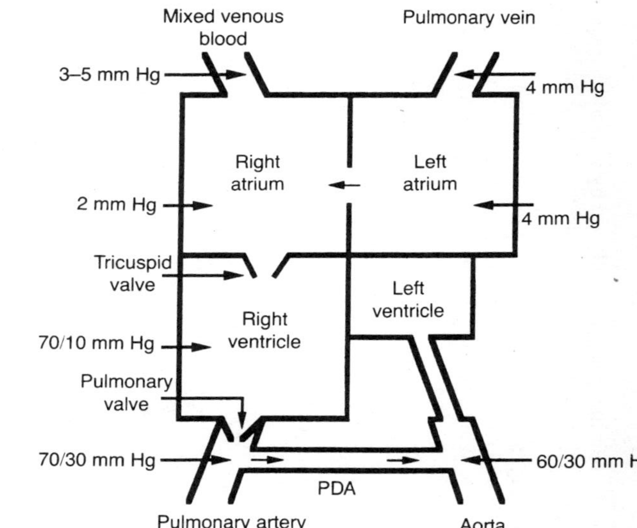

Figure 5–9 Hypoplastic left ventricle—underdeveloped left ventricle and severe narrowing of the ascending aorta. It may include mitral atresia (pictured here), lack of the mitral valve, aortic atresia, or lack of the aorta, or a combination. A PDA is necessary for systemic blood flow. PDA, patent ductus arteriosus.

being their first problems, followed by irritability, dyspnea, tachycardia, respiratory infections, and cardiac failure.

Management. Surgical correction varies according to the type of TAPVR, with the goal of redirecting blood flow to the LA. Without surgery, the prognosis is grim. Most patients are asymptomatic and healthy following surgery, although pulmonary venous obstruction develops in some (Fig. 5–10).

Tetralogy of Fallot

Tetralogy of Fallot (TOF) consists of (1) VSD, (2) pulmonary stenosis (PS), (3) overriding aorta, and (4) RV hypertrophy. Flow through the VSD depends on the degree of pulmonary stenosis. Mild PS causes a left-to-right shunt with increased pulmonary blood flow; more severe PS may result in bidirectional flow; and a right-to-left shunt develops, in the presence of severe right ventricular outflow obstruction, resulting in decreased pulmonary blood flow and desaturation of blood.

Incidence. TOF is the most common CHD among children surviving beyond the first year of life without surgery. It occurs in 10% to 15% of all children with CHD. There is a slight male preponderance.

Clinical Presentation. Clinical features vary from asymptomatic patients to those who are severely cyanotic at birth. Clubbing of the nails is present in patients with desaturation. Most have a systolic murmur. Chest x-ray film reveals a normal or small "boot-shaped" heart. Hypercyanotic spells ("Tet" spells) are believed to be due to an infundibular spasm that leads to an increased right-to-left shunt. They occur mostly in infants and consist of cyanosis, tachycardia, and tachypnea and may result in unconsciousness or a cerebrovascular accident.

Management. Palliative surgery is performed to increase pulmonary blood flow in patients who are not candidates for repair. Various systemic-pulmonary shunts may be used including Blalock-Taussig's, Potts', and Waterston's shunts. The Blalock-Taussig shunt is preferred by most. Surgical repair consists of (1) patching or suturing the VSD and (2) relief of the pulmonary stenosis. Following surgical repair, cyanosis disappears and nails return to a normal shape. Complications seen postoperatively are rare and include endocarditis, brain abscess, and cerebrovascular accident (Fig. 5–11).

Complete Transposition of the Great Arteries

In complete transposition of the great arteries (TGA), the aorta arises from the RV, and the PA arises from the LV.

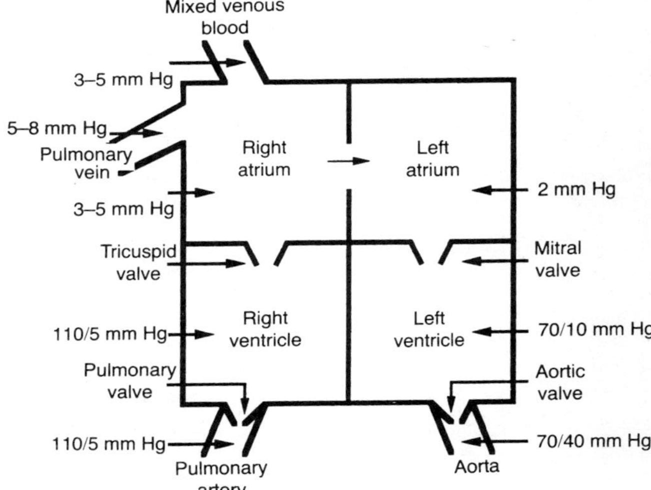

Figure 5–10 Total anomalous pulmonary venous return—pulmonary venous return is routed to the right atrium instead of the left atrium. Pulmonary drainage can be routed (1) above the heart (supracardiac), as pictured here; (2) through the heart (cardiac); (3) through the portal vein, ductus venosus, hepatic vein, or inferior vena cava (infracardiac); or (4) through the diaphragm or esophageal hiatus (subdiaphragmatic).

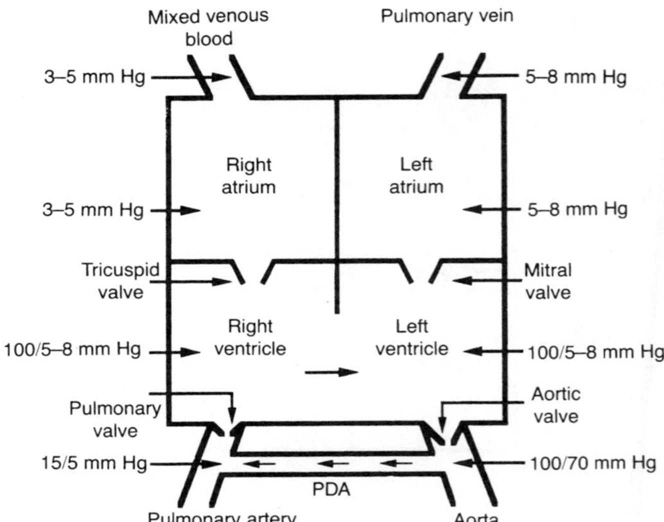

Figure 5–11 Tetralogy of Fallot—overriding aorta, pulmonary artery stenosis, right atrial hypertrophy, and a VSD. A PDA is often present to allow pulmonary blood flow if pulmonary stenosis is severe. PDA, patent ductus arteriosus.

This creates two parallel circuits of blood: (1) unoxygenated blood from the body flows from the RV to the aorta, then returns to the right side of the heart (systemic blood returns to the systemic circulation without being oxygenated) and (2) oxygenated blood from the lungs flows from the LV to the PA, then it returns to the lungs (oxygenated pulmonary blood returns to the pulmonary circulation without taking part in gas exchange). This defect is incompatible with life unless mixing between the two circulations takes place. Shunting through a PDA and the foramen ovale is usually sufficient immediately after birth. A VSD frequently exists and serves to mix the two circulations.

Incidence. TGA accounts for 5% to 7% of all congenital heart defects. Males are affected more often than females (2 : 1).

Clinical Presentation. Clinical features depend on the extent of mixing between the two circulations. Infants usually present with cyanosis, hypoxemia, and cardiac failure.

Management. Prostaglandin E_1 is given immediately after diagnosis to maintain the PDA. Prior to corrective surgery, a balloon atrial septostomy may be performed to create a large ASD and ensure adequate mixing between the two atria. Surgical repair consists mainly of an atrial switch procedure (Mustard or Senning). A Rastelli procedure, in which circulation is redirected at the ventricle level, is selected if the infant has a VSD and left ventricular outflow obstruction. Although a Rastelli procedure is relatively new, some are favoring an arterial switch (a Jatene procedure) (Fig. 5–12).

Pulmonary Atresia, Intact Ventricular Septum

In pulmonary atresia, the pulmonary valve does not develop and the RV is small, hypertrophied, or normal. There is complete obstruction to normal outflow from the RV. The LA receives blood from the right side of the heart through an ASD, and there is considerable volume overload on the LV. Since there is no blood flow from the RV to the pulmonary system, a PDA must be present to support life.

Incidence. This condition occurs in 1% to 3% of all congenital cardiac defects, with a slight male predominance.

Clinical Presentation. Cyanosis presents within hours of birth, with progressive hypoxemia and metabolic acidosis developing. The chest x-ray film may be normal or may reveal cardiomegaly.

Management. Prostaglandins are given to maintain the PDA, and a Blalock-Taussig shunt is established. To enhance

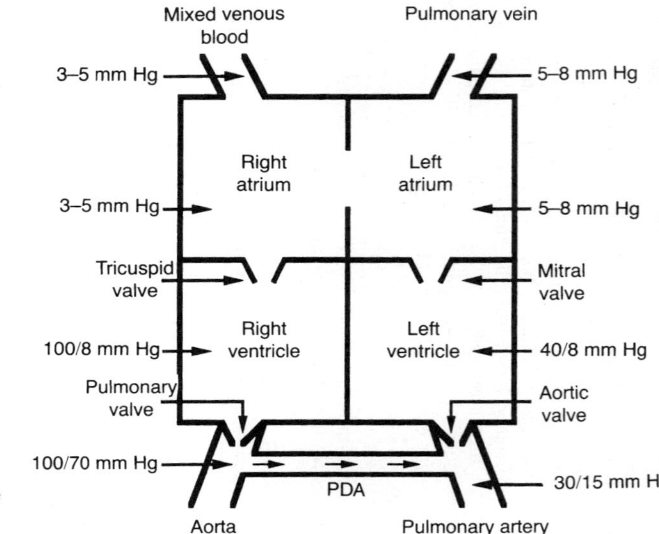

Figure 5–12 Transposition of the great arteries—the aorta arises from the right ventricle and the pulmonary artery arises from the left ventricle. A PDA is necessary to allow pulmonary blood flow. PDA, patent ductus arteriosus.

pulmonary blood flow, a Glenn procedure may be performed. Pulmonary valvotomy may be performed if the RV is large enough. If the RV is extremely small, the shunt may be removed and a Fontan procedure performed at a later date. Infant mortality remains high, even with surgery.

Tricuspid Atresia

In tricuspid atresia (TA), the tricuspid valve has not developed and there is no direct communication between the RA and the RV. An ASD is needed for blood to leave the RA, and a VSD is needed for blood to flow back into the RV. The RV is often hypoplastic. If the VSD is large and there is no pulmonary stenosis or atresia, pulmonary blood flow is increased and may result in pulmonary hypertension and CHF.

Incidence. TA is the 14th or 15th most common CHD in infants, occurring in 2% of all cases of CHD. There is a male preponderance (55%).

Clinical Presentation. Cyanosis or murmur occurs in the majority of infants within 24 hours of birth. CHF is common in patients with increased pulmonary blood flow.

Management. Palliative surgery is performed to increase pulmonary blood flow and improve oxygenation. Shunts may include the Blalock-Taussig, Waterston, or Glenn shunt. A Fontan procedure is performed when the child is older. Complications include endocarditis, brain abscess, pulmonary vascular obstructive disease, and life-threatening arrhythmias (Fig. 5–13).

Truncus Arteriosus

In truncus arteriosus, one large vessel (arterial trunk) rises from both ventricles via a single semilunar valve. The vessel gives rise to the pulmonary arteries, aorta, and coronary arteries. There is a VSD, and the truncal valve may be stenotic or incompetent. CHF occurs when PVR decreases and the left-to-right shunt becomes the predominant shunt.

Incidence. TA accounts for about 0.7% of heart defects. There is equal occurrence among males and females.

Clinical Presentation. CHF develops within the first days and weeks of life. Loud murmurs are present.

Management. Surgical repair consists of separating the pulmonary arteries from the truncus, closing the VSD, and providing a conduit between the RV and the PA. The RV-PA conduits are often replaced at a later age because of stenosis and calcification (Fig. 5–14).

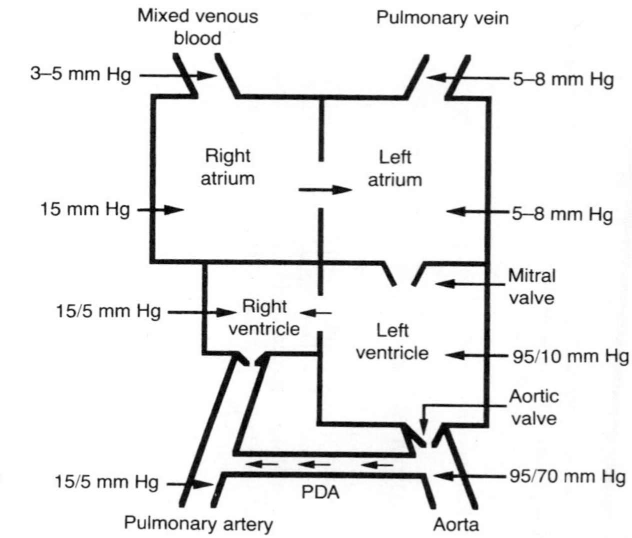

Figure 5–13 Hypoplastic right ventricle—due to either lack of a tricuspid valve, as pictured here, or pulmonary atresia. An ASD or patent foramen ovale is necessary for right atrial outflow of blood. A PDA is necessary to allow pulmonary blood flow. PDA, patent ductus arteriosus.

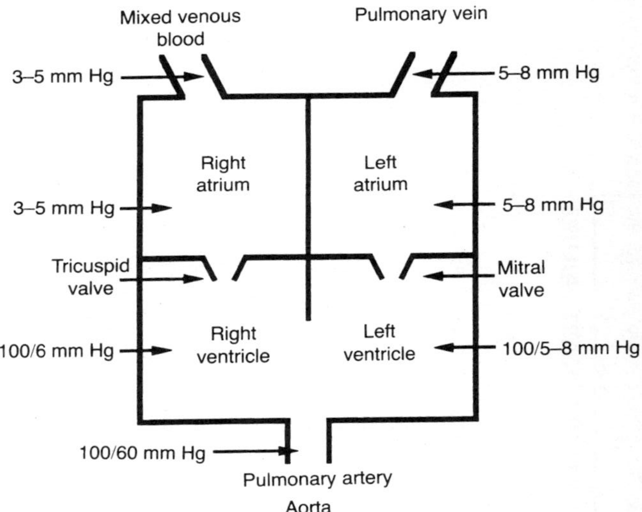

Figure 5–14 Truncus arteriosus—a single great artery arises from the ventricles carrying both pulmonary and systemic blood flow.

CONGESTIVE HEART FAILURE

CHF is a syndrome that occurs when the heart cannot supply the cardiac output that is demanded by the tissues. Failure is brought about by numerous factors (Table 5–3).

Clinical Presentation. Clinical findings vary and may include tachypnea, dyspnea, tachycardia, pallor, weak pulses, failure to thrive, diaphoresis, peripheral edema, and hepatomegaly. The systemic and pulmonary vascular resistance often determines the onset and severity of symptoms.

Management. Treatment includes (1) diuretics (furosemide) to decrease preload and reduce pulmonary edema; (2) oxygen to treat hypoxemia and reduce reactive pulmonary vasoconstriction; (3) inotropic agents (digoxin, dopamine) to improve myocardial contractility, increase cardiac output, and produce diuresis; (4) sedation (morphine sulfate, meperidine) for restlessness; (5) afterload reducers (captopril) to decrease systemic vascular resistance and increase cardiac output; and (6) antibiotics for infection.

SHOCK

Shock is a state of circulatory dysfunction resulting in inadequate delivery of oxygen and other nutrients; therefore, the body's metabolic demands are not met. Cellular metabolism is disrupted; if not improved, shock will be irreversible and death will occur even if the initiating problem is resolved. Shock is divided into three categories: true loss of intravascular volume, decreased peripheral vascular resistance, and decreased myocardial performance. Septic shock can encompass all three perturbations.

True Volume Loss (Hypovolemic Shock)

True volume loss occurs with acute fluid loss (hypovolemia) of water, electrolytes, and blood. Causes include diarrhea and vomiting; diabetes insipidus; hemorrhage from trauma, gastrointestinal bleeding, or surgery; burns; sepsis; and peritonitis. Clinical features are tachypnea, tachycardia, decreased peripheral perfusion, oliguria, cool extremities, and progressive hypotension. Treatment is aimed at replacing the lost volume and preventing further loss. Intravenous fluid infusion is given for dehydration and hemorrhagic shock. Patients should be given blood and placed in the Trendelenberg position.

TABLE 5–3 Causes of Congestive Heart Failure

CARDIAC	NONCARDIAC
Congenital	**Systemic**
Left-sided obstructive defects	Asphyxia
Hypoplastic left-sided heart syndrome	Hypoglycemia
Interrupted aortic arch	Hypocalcemia
Coarctation of the aorta	Hypomagnesemia
Aortic stenosis	Sepsis
Total anomalous pulmonary venous return (obstructed)	Kawasaki's disease
Cor triatriatum	Diffuse vasculitis
Left-to-right shunting defects	Neuromuscular degenerative disorders
Patent ductus arteriosus	**Pulmonary**
Ventricular septal defect	Upper airway obstruction (tonsillar hypertrophy, subglottic stenosis)
Atrioventricular septal defect	Bronchopulmonary dysplasia
Aortopulmonary window	Persistent primary pulmonary hypertension
Atrial septal defect	Cystic fibrosis
Total anomalous pulmonary venous return	**Hematologic**
Complex congenital defects	Anemia
Truncus arteriosus	Polycythemia
d-transposition of the great arteries with ventricular septal defect	**Renal**
Tricuspid atresia	Failure
Single ventricle	Intravascular volume overload
Other	Hypertension (renovascular)
Anomalous origin of left coronary artery	**Endocrine**
Pulmonary insufficiency	Hyperthyroidism
Tricuspid insufficiency	Hypothyroidism
Pulmonary stenosis	Adrenal insufficiency
Tetralogy of Fallot, absent pulmonary valve variant	**Vascular**
	Systemic arteriovenous fistula

Table continued on following page

TABLE 5-3 Causes of Congestive Heart Failure *Continued*

CARDIAC	NONCARDIAC
Congenital	**Vascular**
Postoperative	Multiple cutaneous hemangiomas
Myocardial ischemia	Large vascular tumor
Inadequate repair	
Ventricular dysfunction	
Acquired	
Dysrhythmia	
Complete heart block	
Supraventricular tachycardia	
Chronic tachycardia	
Other tachyarrhythmia	
Cardiomyopathy	
Myocarditis	
Endocardial fibroelastosis	
Anthracycline-induced	
Human immunodeficiency virus	
Hypertrophic	
Hypertensive	
Familial	
Storage disease	
Idiopathic	
Valvular dysfunction	
Rheumatic	
Acute bacterial endocarditis	

Decreased Peripheral Vascular Resistance (Neurogenic Shock)

Decreased peripheral vascular resistance results in the peripheral pooling of blood in arterioles and venous capacitance vessels and in the development of a relative hypovolemia. Causes include fever, anaphylaxis, central nervous system injury (high level of spinal cord, brainstem), vasodilating drugs, and sepsis. Clinical features are tachypnea, progressive hypotension with orthostatic changes, tachycardia, and warm extremities. The underlying problem should be treated and vasopressors given. Fluid therapy should be provided cautiously when head trauma has occurred.

Decreased Myocardial Performance (Cardiogenic Shock)

Causes of decreased myocardial performance include impaired cardiac function following CHD repair, CHD with impaired ventricular outflow, arrhythmias, cardiomyopathy, myocarditis, cardiac tamponade, anoxia, hypoglycemia, and hypothermia. Clinical features are similar to those in hypovolemia, with normal to decreased blood pressure, pulmonary edema, and hepatic enlargement possible. Treatment includes positive inotropic drugs to improve myocardial contractility (e.g., dopamine, dobutamine, epinephrine), oxygen, and antiarrhythmic agents (e.g., atropine, isoproterenol, lidocaine).

Septic Shock

Septic shock is the most common type of shock and encompasses many characteristics of the three types of shock described earlier. It occurs when sepsis becomes overwhelming, toxins produce peripheral vascular collapse, and cellular metabolism is directly impaired. Pathogens include bacteria, viruses, rickettsiae, and fungi. Clinical features range from a ''warm'' shock (with tachycardia, tachypnea, wide pulse pressure with normal blood pressure, warm and dry skin, and restlessness) to ''cold'' shock (with hypotension, narrow pulse pressure, shallow and rapid respirations, thready pulses, cold and clammy skin, cyanosis, oliguria, metabolic acidosis, and hypoxemia). Treatment includes immediate volume resuscitation to improve cardiac output, inotropic agents (dopamine, dobutamine), oxygen, respiratory and hemodynamic stabilization, and antimicrobial therapy, including rapid bacterial eradication if indicated. Military antishock (MAST) trousers are available in pediatric sizes.

RESPIRATORY CARE FOLLOWING CARDIOVASCULAR SURGERY

If possible, it is helpful to review the patient history and cardiovascular disorder before the patient is returned from surgery. Familiarity with the patient's preoperative status is often helpful in recognizing postoperative complications. The cardiovascular unit is usually notified of the patient's status and the approximate time he or she will arrive from surgery. The respiratory care equipment that will be needed should be at the bedside, ready to be placed on the patient immediately on arrival.

Equipment Needed at Bedside

A resuscitation bag and mask with tubing attached to the oxygen flowmeter or blender should be at the bedside along with an oxygen device (if ordered), a mechanical ventilator (if patient is intubated), suction equipment with appropriate-sized catheters, and sterile saline for lavage. All equipment should be tested and functioning properly before the patient returns from surgery.

Mechanical Ventilation

The surgical unit will usually notify the cardiovascular unit if the patient will return intubated and require mechanical ventilation. Ventilator settings should be established and the ventilator set up at the bedside for immediate use when the patient arrives. After the child is placed on the ventilator, breath sounds, chest expansion, color, heart rate, respiratory rate, and pulse oximetry values should be monitored. A complete ventilator check should be performed at this time.

Settings vary and are dependent on each patient's cardiorespiratory status. Settings are usually adjusted in an attempt to provide adequate oxygenation and normal $Pa{CO_2}$ levels. Postive end-expiratory pressure (PEEP) levels of 2 to 4 cm H_2O are usually set, except in patients with low cardiac output. Since positive pressure ventilation may decrease venous return and cardiac output, PEEP may not be used in the attempt to decrease mean airway pressure and reduce its effect on the cardiac output. This situation is often encountered in patients who have undergone the Fontan procedure and in those who experience cardiac tamponade.

Airway Management

Proper positioning of the endotracheal tube can be assessed by auscultation and chest radiography. Breath sounds should be equal bilaterally, and the chest x-ray film should show the tube positioned above the carina. Movement of the tube occurs easily in infants and children and may result in main stem intubation, which if not corrected can lead to atelectasis, hypoxemia, and barotrauma. If one suspects that the tube has migrated into a main stem bronchus, it may be pulled back very slowly and breath sounds assessed for improvement. If the tube requires retaping, at least two clinicians should be involved; one should stabilize the tube throughout the procedure while the other prepares and applies the tape. If repositioning the tube does not improve breath sounds, a chest x-ray film may be needed to confirm the tube position and to rule out complications such as atelectasis or pneumothorax. The intubated patient should be manually ventilated prior to suctioning, after each suction attempt, and prior to being placed back on the ventilator. Saline lavage may be used prior to suctioning if secretions are thick.

Monitoring

Oxygenation and ventilation may be assessed using blood gas values, pulse oximetry, and transcutaneous oxygen and carbon dioxide monitors. An arterial line is often in place postoperatively and is used to obtain blood gas samples. Continuous monitoring of oxygenation via pulse oximetry or transcutaneous monitors is a necessity in the immediate postoperative period.

Extubation

Prior to extubation, the oxygen device the patient will use should be assembled and ready for immediate use. Racemic epinephrine and aerosol therapy equipment should also be readily available to use following extubation in case the patient experiences subglottic edema. Equipment needed for reintubation should also be at the bedside in case the patient "fails" extubation. Respiratory effort, breath sounds, and color should be assessed immediately following extubation and frequently afterward. Signs of respiratory distress include tachypnea, retractions, grunting, gasping, stridor, and nasal flaring. The patient with stridor most likely has upper airway obstruction due to subglottic edema, and aerosol treatment with racemic epinephrine is indicated. If distress is not relieved, the patient may need to be reintubated.

Postextubation Care

Oxygen is usually delivered via hood, Venturi mask, or cannula. Incentive spirometry is administered in patients old enough to perform the maneuvers effectively. Chest physical therapy may be ordered for patients who have excessive secretions or in whom atelectasis has developed.

Respiratory Complications Following Cardiovascular Surgery

Complications causing respiratory impairment may develop following cardiovascular surgery.

1. *Atelectasis* is the most common complication in infants and children postoperatively and is usually a result of mucus plugging or main stem intubation. Treatment includes chest physical therapy and adequate suctioning for patients being mechanically ventilated; incentive spirometry may also be given if the patient has been extubated.
2. *Pneumothorax* may develop spontaneously from barotrauma caused by mechanical ventilation, during surgery

if the pleural space has been entered, or while the chest tube is being removed. Treatment varies and may include thoracentesis, chest tube placement, or simply frequent monitoring while the air is absorbed.

3. Injury to the thoracic duct during surgery may result in a *chylothorax*. This occurs most often during repairs near the aortic arch, such as CoA and AS. Treatment includes thoracentesis or chest tube drainage.
4. *Hemothorax* may develop and is considered a possibility if blood appears in a chest tube, the patient's lung compliance decreases (mean airway and peak pressures may increase depending on the type of ventilator used), breath sounds decrease, or hypotension develops. Treatment includes thoracentesis or chest tube placement and possibly blood replacement.
5. *Chronic respiratory failure* may develop in some patients postoperatively, and mechanical ventilatory support may be prolonged. Weaning may be a long process and the patient may experience numerous complications, including respiratory infections, barotrauma, and atelectasis.
6. Cardiovascular surgery patients may experience *pleural effusions* following CHF. Treatment includes thoracentesis or chest tube placement.

Bibliography

Adams FH, Emmanouilides GC, Riemenschneider TA: Moss' Heart Disease in Infants, Children, and Adolescents, 4th ed. Baltimore, Williams & Wilkins, 1989.

Fyler DC, Nadas AS: Cardiology. *In* Avery ME, First LR (eds): Pediatric Medicine. Baltimore, Williams & Wilkins, 1989.

Fyler DC, Buckley LP, Hellenbrand WE, et al: Reports of the New England Regional Infant Cardiac Program. Pediatrics 1980; 65(Suppl):376–460.

Hurst JW, Schlant RC: The Heart: Arteries and Veins, 7th ed. Philadelphia, JB Lippincott, 1990.

Ilbawi MN: Current status of surgery for congenital heart disease. Clin Perinatol 1989; 16:157–176.

Long WA: Fetal and Neonatal Cardiology. Philadelphia, WB Saunders, 1990.

Root RK, Sande MA: Septic Shock. New York, Churchill Livingstone, 1985.

Saez-Llorens X, McCracken G: Sepsis syndrome and septic shock in pediatrics: Current concepts of terminology, pathophysiology, and management. J Pediatr 1993; 123:497–508.

Santulli TV: An approach to the newborn with heart disease. *In* Pomerance JJ, Richardson CJ (eds): Neonatology for the Clinician. Norwalk, Appleton & Lange, 1993.

Zimmerman JL, Dietrich KA: Current perspectives on septic shock. Pediatr Clin North Am 1987; 34:131–163.

SECTION 6

Congenital, Neurologic, and Neuromuscular Disorders

I. Congenital Structural Disorders
   A. Bronchogenic cysts
   B. Choanal atresia
   C. Congenital diaphragmatic hernia
   D. Cystic adenomatoid malformation
   E. Esophageal atresia and tracheoesophageal fistula
   F. Gastroschisis
   G. Lobar emphysema
   H. Macroglossia
   I. Mandibular hypoplasia
   J. Omphalocele
   K. Pectus carinatum
   L. Pectus excavatum
   M. Pulmonary sequestration
   N. Tracheomalacia
   O. Vascular ring

II. Neurologic Disorders
   A. Increased intracranial pressure
   B. Intracranial pressure monitoring
   C. Medical management of increased intracranial pressure
   D. Reye's syndrome

III. Neuromuscular Disorders
   A. Guillain-Barré syndrome
   B. Myasthenia gravis

Abbreviations

ABG–arterial blood gas
AP–anteroposterior
CAM–cystic adenomatoid malformations
CDH–congenital diaphragmatic hernia
CPT–chest physical therapy
CT–computed tomography
EA–esophageal atresia
ECMO–extracorporeal membrane oxygenation
ETT–endotracheal tube
FTT–failure to thrive
GBS–Guillain-Barré syndrome
GE–gastroesophageal
ICP—intracranial pressure
LDH–lactate dehydrogenase
MG–myasthenia gravis
PDA–patent ductus arteriosus

PEEP–positive end-expiratory pressure
PT–prothrombin time
PTT–partial thromboplastin time
PVR–pulmonary vascular resistance
SGOT–serum glutamic-oxaloacetic transaminase
SGPT–serum glutamic-pyruvic transaminase
TEF–tracheoesophageal fistula
TOF–tetralogy of Fallot
VSD–ventricular septal defect

CONGENITAL STRUCTURAL DISORDERS

Bronchogenic Cysts

Abnormal embryologic development results in nonfunctional cystic lesions called bronchogenic cysts. The cysts can develop in the bronchial wall, pleura, mediastinum, or lung itself; most are located near the carina. Cysts located near the carina may compress the major bronchi.

Diagnosis. The chest x-ray film reveals a circular or ovoid mass with smooth borders.

Clinical Presentation. The patient may be asymptomatic or may present with respiratory distress, stridor, wheezing, hemoptysis, or recurrent pulmonary infections.

Management. Treatment consists of surgical resection.

Complications. Complications include rupture, hemorrhage, infection, and compression of other structures.

Choanal Atresia

Bony or membranous blockage of the posterior nares constitutes choanal atresia; the blockage may be unilateral or bilateral. Because an infant is an obligate nose breather, bilateral atresia results in severe respiratory distress and possibly death by asphyxia.

Incidence. Choanal atresia occurs in 1 in 700 live births, and is seen more often in girls than in boys (2 : 1). Unilateral atresia occurs twice as often as does bilateral atresia. Fifty percent of patients with choanal atresia have congenital anomalies known as CHARGE (*c*olobomas, congenital *h*eart defects, choanal *a*tresia, *r*etarded development, *g*enital hyperplasia, *e*ar anomalies).

Diagnosis. The diagnosis is suspected if a catheter cannot be passed into the nasopharynx. Diagnosis is confirmed by a facial computed tomography (CT) scan and possibly endoscopy.

Clinical Presentation. The patient may present with respiratory distress (severe if there is bilateral atresia), cyanosis (may occur only during feeding), and no movement of the alae nasi.

Management. Until surgery is undertaken, an oral airway or endotracheal tube (ETT) should be inserted and gavage feedings instituted. Making the infant cry and breathe through the mouth may relieve distress also. Surgical correction consists of excision of the obstruction; ETTs are placed in the nares to stent the choanae and prevent postoperative obstruction from swelling. Prophylactic antibiotics are given.

Complications. Problems include restenosis of the choanae. Tracheostomy or long-term intubation may be necessary in severe cases associated with other craniofacial abnormalities.

Congenital Diaphragmatic Hernia

Congenital diaphragmatic hernia (CDH) results from failure of the posterolateral pleuroperitoneal canals of the diaphragm to fuse during fetal development, causing herniation of the viscera into the pleural cavity. Compression of the lung during intrauterine development results in varying degrees of pulmonary hypoplasia, which is most notable on the side of the hernia but may involve both lungs. Increased muscularization around the pulmonary arteries is also present. A cycle of worsening hypoxia and pulmonary hypertension occurs (Fig. 6–1). Eighty-five percent of CDH cases occur on the left side and 15% occur on the right side; bilateral defects are rare.

Incidence. The incidence of CDH is 1 in 2000 to 5000 births. Table 6–1 lists associated anomalies.

Diagnosis. Prenatal diagnosis may be made via ultrasonography. The diagnosis may be confirmed with amniography. The chest x-ray film at birth reveals gas-filled loops of bowel in the chest, a displaced mediastinum, and pulmonary hypoplasia.

Clinical Presentation

Physical Examination. Classic symptoms include a flat or scaphoid abdomen with absent or decreased breath sounds over the involved side and bowel sounds heard in the thorax. The severity of respiratory distress depends on the volume of herniated bowel and the degree of pulmonary hypoplasia.

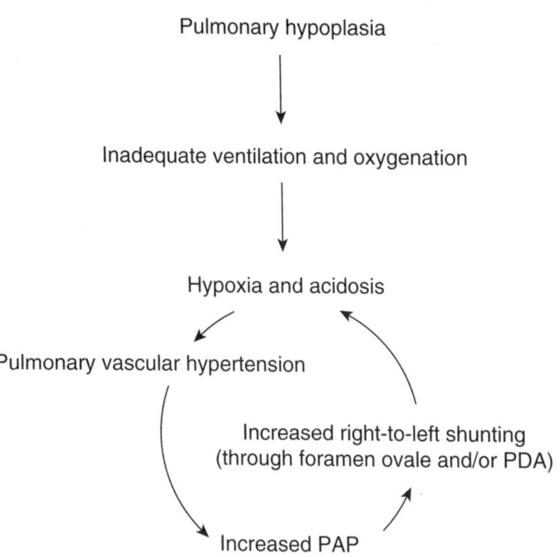

Figure 6–1 Cycle of worsening hypoxia seen with congenital diaphragmatic hernia, beginning with the hypoplastic lungs being unable to adequately ventilate and oxygenate and leading to hypoxia and acidosis. PDA, patent ductus arteriosus; PAP, pulmonary artery pressure.

TABLE 6–1 Anomalies Associated With Congenital Diaphragmatic Hernia
Beckwith-Wiedemann's syndrome
DiGeorge's sequence
Cornelia deLange's syndrome
Trisomy 13
Trisomy 18
Atrial septal defect
Ventricular septal defect
Tetralogy of Fallot
Marfan's syndrome
Hiatal hernia
Club foot
Hydrocephaly

Tachypnea, cyanosis, retractions (subcostal and intercostal), and a barrel-shaped chest are common.

Arterial Blood Gas Analysis. The arterial blood gas (ABG) analysis reveals severe hypoxemia, hypercarbia, and mixed metabolic and respiratory acidosis. Table 6–2 lists factors that affect pulmonary vascular resistance (PVR).

Management. In cases of prenatal diagnosis, the mother should have delivery performed at a center with extracorporeal membrane oxygenation (ECMO) facilities.

Preoperative Management. The goal is to avoid acidosis, barotrauma, and pulmonary hypertension. Resuscitation with ventilation via an ETT is preferred over mask ventilation (less gaseous distention of the stomach and intestines in the chest). A nasogastric tube is inserted to decrease gastric distention in the chest. A chest tube is inserted if a pneumothorax is present. Arterial access with an umbilical artery catheter is necessary for frequent ABG analysis. Unnecessary stimulation should be avoided because the pulmonary vasculature is hyperreactive; a proper environment includes low lights and minimal noise around the infant's bed.

Oxygen Therapy. Oxygen therapy is given to reduce hypoxia and PVR.

Nitric Oxide. Nitric oxide may be given endotracheally to reduce PVR.

Mechanical Ventilation. High-frequency oscillator ventilation or ventilation management that includes low volumes,

TABLE 6–2 Factors That Affect Pulmonary Vascular Resistance in Patients With Congenital Diaphragmatic Hernia

INCREASE RESISTANCE	DECREASE RESISTANCE
Hypoxemia	Oxygenation
Hypercarbia	Hyperventilation
Acidosis	Alkalosis
Hypothermia	Tolazoline
Lights	Nitric oxide
Loud noises	Prostaglandin E_1
Suctioning	
Pain	

high rates, short inspiratory times, and low peak pressures may be used. PVR may be reduced by inducing alkalosis with $Paco_2$ levels less than 35 mm Hg.

Pharmacologic Support. Bicarbonate infusions may be given to induce alkalosis. Vasodilator therapy with tolazoline may be efficacious in decreasing PVR. Sedation is used to decrease the risk of triggering pulmonary vasoconstriction.

Surgical Repair. Surgery consists of reducing the viscera from the chest, repairing the diaphragmatic defect, and stabilizing the mediastinum. Delaying surgery for hours to days may improve survival by allowing time for the pulmonary vessels to dilate, for reactivity of the pulmonary vasculature to diminish, and for PVR to decrease.

Postoperative Management. Intubation and ventilation are maintained. Efforts to reduce PVR are maintained.

Extracorporeal Membrane Oxygenation. ECMO may be used before or after surgical repair in patients who demonstrate pulmonary hypertension, clinical deterioration, and worsening hypoxemia in spite of pharmacologic support, volume resuscitation, and abnormally high ventilator settings, including peak inspiratory pressures greater than 35 cm H_2O. ECMO is used to stabilize pulmonary hypertension and to treat or prevent barotrauma—it is not used to treat the pulmonary hypoplasia (it cannot be used long enough to allow pulmonary growth). The patient is weaned from ECMO as PVR decreases.

Complications. The lung continues to grow, with alveoli increasing in number and airways increasing in diameter. In CDH, however, the total number of airways is decreased; therefore, the number of alveoli is reduced. Pneumothorax, increased PVR, right ventricular failure (cor pulmonale), recurrent hernia, gastroesophageal (GE) reflux, hemorrhage (including intracranial), and restrictive airway disease may also occur after repair.

Cystic Adenomatoid Malformation

A hamartoma or overgrowth of embryonal pulmonary tissue in a disorganized fashion in the region of end bronchioles is termed a cystic adenomatoid malformation (CAM). Alveolar growth is suppressed. The lesion may be a single large cavitary or solid cyst or may be multiple small cysts.

Incidence. CAM is frequently associated with hydramnios, prematurity, and anasarca.

Clinical Presentation. Symptoms depend on the amount of lung involved, but respiratory distress (tachypnea, retractions, cyanosis, nasal flaring) soon after birth is common. Shift of the mediastinum toward the opposite side may occur. The chest radiography reveals multiple densities and air bubbles, occasionally with air-fluid levels. The chest x-ray film may appear similar to that seen in CDH.

Management. Early surgical excision is performed, usually with lobectomy or pneumonectomy.

Complications. The prognosis is usually excellent. Large lesions may result in pulmonary hypoplasia and pulmonary hypertension, which may have a worse outcome.

Esophageal Atresia and Tracheoesophageal Fistula

Failure of the esophagus and trachea to separate during fetal development results in a communication between the trachea and the esophagus or the esophagus' ending in a blind pouch. Esophageal atresia (EA) results in obstruction of passage of saliva or food, whereas tracheoesophageal fistula (TEF) causes aspiration of salivary contents or gastric secretions. Figure 6–2 illustrates the defects, with EA and a distal TEF being the most common (85%). Proximal and distal EA without TEF is the second most common (5%). The H-type fistula is the third most common (3%). Proximal and distal TEF occurs in 2% of cases; a proximal fistula with a distal atresia is rarest (1%).

Incidence. These conditions are often associated with other anomalies known by the acronym VACTRL: *v*ertebral, *a*nal (atresia), *c*ardiac (ventricular septal defect [VSD], patent ductus arteriosus [PDA], tetralogy of Fallot [TOF]), *t*racheoesophageal (fistulas, atresia), *r*enal, *l*imb (polydactyly).

Diagnosis. TEF and EA may be diagnosed prenatally via ultrasonography. It is suspected in cases of polyhydramnios. In cases of EA, resistance will be met when an attempt is made to pass a nasogastric tube. Chest radiography will reveal the tube ending or coiling in the pouch. Air in the bowel is seen with a distal TEF, whereas absence of gas in the bowel suggests EA without TEF. A barium swallow is indicated for the diagnosis of TEF. Endoscopy may be needed for confirmation.

Clinical Presentation. Symptoms depend on the defect and the size of the fistula. They include drooling, with excessive oral secretions; coughing; choking; cyanosis; and vary-

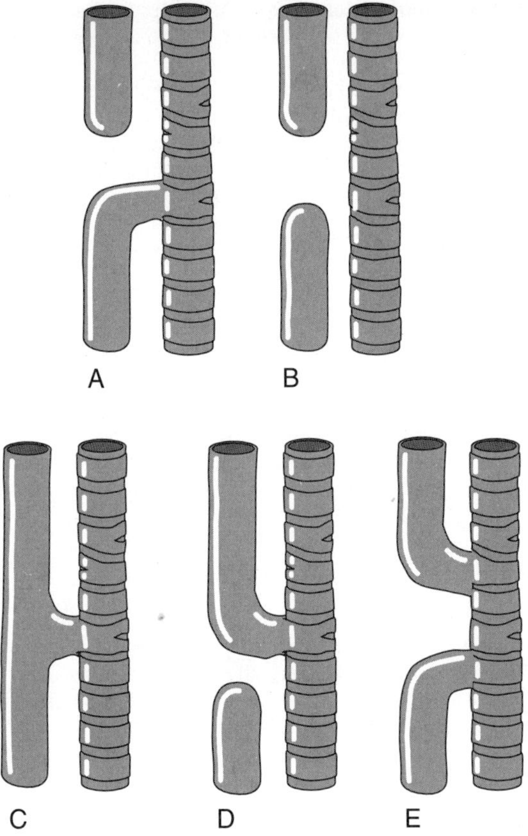

Figure 6–2 Five anatomic classifications describing tracheoesophageal fistula and esophageal atresia. *A,* Esophageal atresia with a distal tracheoesophageal fistula. *B,* Esophageal atresia with a "long gap" of missing esophagus between a proximal blind-ending pouch and a distal esophageal pouch. *C,* Tracheoesophageal fistula without esophageal atresia, "H-type." *D,* Esophageal atresia with a proximal fistula, similar to the H-type fistula, and a small distal esophageal pouch with no tracheoesophageal fistula. *E,* Esophageal atresia with a proximal and distal tracheoesophageal fistula.

ing degrees of respiratory distress. Symptoms may be pronounced during feedings.

Management

Preoperative Management. Head-up positioning and securing of a sump tube for continuous suctioning of the pouch are carried out to decrease the chance of aspiration. Chest physical therapy (CPT) is indicated to remove secretions. Antibiotics are given because of the risk of aspiration pneumonia. Gastrostomy may be necessary until definitive repair is performed. Infants with severe respiratory distress and low birth weight often require mechanical ventilation.

Surgical Repair. Repair of the esophagus with division of the fistula is performed in stable patients. End-to-end anastomosis of the esophagus is the repair of choice for atresia. Repair may be delayed in infants with associated anomalies, pulmonary disease, or prematurity and low birth weight. GE fundoplication may be performed in infants who have GE reflux and recurrent pneumonias.

Postoperative Management. Mechanical ventilation may be indicated. CPT is often necessary because of recurrent pneumonias.

Complications. Complications include pneumonia, infection, recurrent fistula formation, esophageal strictures, tracheomalacia, aspiration, bradycardia, apnea, and respiratory arrest. Pulmonary problems are often due to GE reflux.

Gastroschisis

A full-thickness defect of the abdominal wall lateral to the umbilical opening with herniation of abdominal contents constitutes gastroschisis. Herniation of bowel loops occurs most often; the liver may also herniate. Herniation usually occurs on the right side of a normal, intact umbilical cord. The abdominal contents are not covered by a sac or membrane. The bowel loops may be matted together from chemical peritonitis.

Incidence. Gastroschisis occurs in 1 in 20,000 births. Other associated anomalies are rare. It is often associated with prematurity and intrauterine growth retardation.

Diagnosis. Gastroschisis is suspected prenatally with elevation of maternal alpha-fetoprotein levels. Prenatal ultrasonography may reveal the defect. Diagnosis is confirmed at birth on examination of the abdomen.

Management. A prenatal diagnosis prompts the mother to have delivery at a tertiary center. On delivery, the infant is placed in a bowel bag (feet first to the armpits) to minimize dehydration and hypothermia. Antibiotics are given and fluids administered intravenously.

Surgical Repair. Closure of the defect is desired; however, the viscera may not fit back into the peritoneal cavity because of the diminished size secondary to the absence of abdominal contents in utero. In this case, a staged reduction is performed to gradually reduce the viscera into the abdominal cavity (this may take 5 to 14 days). A prosthetic silo is constructed, with the protruding viscera wrapped to maintain moisture and prevent infection. This wrapping is suspended from a support hanging over the abdomen, and the silo is gradually reduced in size until the contents are within the cavity and closure can be performed.

Mechanical Ventilation. Ventilation is usually required, with sedation and paralysis until after the silo is removed and closure is performed.

Nutritional Support. Central venous hyperalimentation is necessary following repair.

Complications. Complications include the need for long-term hyperalimentation as well as hyperalimentation-induced hepatic dysfunction and short-gut syndrome.

Lobar Emphysema

Overdistention of one lobe of the lung, usually an upper lobe, results in lobar emphysema, which is often due to obstruction in a segmental or lobar bronchus. A cartilaginous defect may cause the bronchus to collapse during expiration, resulting in airway obstruction and air trapping. Obstruction may be so severe that no air enters the trachea or main bronchus, and venous return to the right heart is blocked.

Diagnosis. The diagnosis is confirmed by chest radiography, which reveals a hyperlucent lobe with a surrounding zone of atelectasis. Diagnosis is critical; ventilation of the child in respiratory distress may lead to rapid distention of the affected lobe and circulatory collapse.

Clinical Presentation. The child presents with progressive respiratory distress with tachypnea, retractions, cough, wheezing, stridor, and cyanosis. Symptoms often worsen during feeding.

Management. The condition may resolve spontaneously or bronchoscopy or surgical resection of the lobe may be required.

Complications. The postoperative course is good. Tension emphysema and pulmonary infection may occur.

Macroglossia

Macroglossia is a greatly enlarged tongue that causes respiratory distress by pharyngeal obstruction. Relative macroglossia occurs with a normal-sized tongue in an undersized oral cavity.

Incidence. It is often associated with other disorders, including hypothyroidism, acromegaly, the Beckwith-Wiedemann syndrome, Down's syndrome, lymphangioma, and hemangioma.

Diagnosis. The diagnosis is made on physical examination.

Management. Mild cases may be treated with prone positioning. In severe cases, surgical correction should be performed by 1 year of age (before speech development).

Complications. Complications include hypoxia and carbon dioxide retention.

Mandibular Hypoplasia

Bilateral hypoplasia of the mandible constitutes mandibular hypoplasia. Micrognathia, glossoptosis, and posterior displacement of the tongue associated with a cleft palate are known as the Pierre Robin syndrome. Posterior displacement of the relatively large tongue often produces airway obstruction.

Diagnosis. The diagnosis is made on physical examination.

Clinical Presentation. Symptoms of upper airway obstruction are common, for example, stridor, retractions (suprasternal, subcostal), tachypnea, and cyanosis. Symptoms may worsen during feeding or sleeping or when the infant is placed in the supine position.

Management. Mild cases are treated by placing the patient in the prone position and administering oxygen. Feedings are carefully monitored and performed with special nipples. Intraoral and nasopharyngeal tubes or prostheses are used in mild to moderate cases. Severe cases may require surgery to keep the tongue in an anterior position. Tracheostomy is required in the most severe cases. Many cases resolve by 1 year of age with adequate nutrition and growth of the mandible.

Complications. Pulmonary edema, pulmonary hypertension, and cor pulmonale may develop from chronic obstruction. Failure to thrive (FTT), malnutrition, and pneumonia are also seen.

Omphalocele

An omphalocele is a defect of the abdominal wall at and just superior to the umbilical opening, with herniation of the abdominal contents into the base of the umbilical cord. The abdominal contents are covered with amniotic membrane and peritoneum, which protect the intestine from exposure to amniotic fluid.

Incidence. Omphalocele occurs in 1 in 3000 to 10,000 births. It is associated with other anomalies in 50% of cases, including trisomy 13, trisomy 18, and trisomy 21; the Beckwith-Wiedemann syndrome; and congenital heart disease (tetralogy of Fallot being most common).

Diagnosis. Omphalocele is suspected prenatally with elevation of maternal alpha-fetoprotein levels. Prenatal ultrasonography may reveal the defect. Diagnosis is confirmed at birth on examination of the abdomen.

Management. Treatment follows the same course as that for gastroschisis.

Complications. Problems include a prolonged need for hyperalimentation as well as bowel obstruction, sepsis, a perforated viscus, and complications resulting from other anomalies (Table 6–3).

Pectus Carinatum

Anterior protrusion of the sternum constitutes pectus carinatum, which is also known as pigeon breast.

TABLE 6–3 Comparison of Gastroschisis and Omphalocele

GASTROSCHISIS	OMPHALOCELE
Normal umbilical cord insertion	Base of umbilical cord insertion is into the hernia
Intestines are not covered by membrane or sac	Intestines are covered by protective amnion and peritoneum
Usually an isolated lesion; rarely occurs with other congenital anomalies	Often occurs with other significant congenital anomalies
Often occurs in premature births	Not associated with prematurity

Incidence. This condition is not as common as pectus excavatum. Males are affected more often than females.

Management. Surgical repair is performed most often for cosmetic purposes and consists of sternal osteotomies and chondrectomy of cartilages.

Pectus Excavatum

Pectus excavatum consists of altered growth of the cartilaginous ends of the ribs as they meet the sternum, resulting in varying degrees of depression of the lower sternum. The decreased anteroposterior (AP) diameter of the chest leads to decreased lung expansion, altered airflow due to distortion of the bronchi, and decreased air exchange and secretion clearance.

Incidence. This is the most common chest wall deformity. It is much more common than pectus carinatum and is associated with Marfan's syndrome and congenital heart disease.

Diagnosis. The diagnosis is made on physical examination.

Clinical Presentation. Decreased exercise tolerance, dyspnea, chest pain, stridor, wheezing, cough, and repeated upper respiratory tract infections may occur.

Management. Surgical repair is indicated for symptomatic patients. Most clinicians opt to delay repair until the patient is 4 to 7 years of age. Repair in the older adolescent and young adult may involve major chest wall reconstruction.

Complications. Complications include pneumonia, a reduced capacity for exercise, kyphoscoliosis, breast asymmetry, and a psychologic impact including withdrawal from social contact (resulting from peer ridicule and embarrassment caused by the cosmetic defect). Most children recover well, although postoperative complications may include infection, dislodged prostheses, cardiac tamponade, and pneumothorax.

Pulmonary Sequestration

Separation of potentially mature lung tissue from the rest of the tracheobronchial tree, resulting in separation of the pulmonary and systemic circulations, is called pulmonary sequestration. Areas are either nonaerated or aerated via collateral airways (pores of Kohn). Intrapulmonary sequestrations occur most often in the left lower lobe and may harbor recurrent infections. Extrapulmonary sequestrations are frequently associated with CDH.

Diagnosis. The diagnosis may be elusive. An arteriogram is diagnostic.

Clinical Presentation. Chronic cough, wheezing, tachypnea, recurrent pneumonias, hemoptysis, a large shunt, a heart murmur, and cardiac failure may be seen.

Management. Surgical excision with careful attention to the vasculature is performed.

Tracheomalacia

In tracheomalacia, the tracheal lumen lacks the support of the cartilaginous rings, which may be absent, malformed, or too pliable. This leads to tracheal stenosis and obstruction, with the tracheal lumen narrowing during inspiration and expiration. It may be a congenital defect or may be due to compression of the trachea from a vascular ring or tumor.

Diagnosis. A contrast tracheogram, laryngoscopy, or bronchoscopy, or a combination of these modalities, may be performed. The diagnosis may be established by exclusion of other disorders (vascular ring, tumor, tracheal web, foreign body).

Clinical Presentation. Infants may present with wheezing, stridor, cough, respiratory distress, prolonged expiration, and cyanosis. Infection with increased pulmonary secretions may be seen.

Management. Antibiotics are given to treat infection. CPT may be indicated for secretion removal. Tracheostomy is rarely needed. Surgical repair usually is not necessary because the tracheal cartilage becomes stiffer, usually by 1 year of age.

Vascular Ring

Various types of vascular anomalies that compromise the esophagus or trachea, or both, are encompassed in the term vascular ring. The types of anomalies are listed according to location: right aortic arch, double aortic arch, anomalous innominate or left carotid artery, aberrant right subclavian artery, and pulmonary artery ''sling.'' Compression and narrowing of the tracheoesophageal area lead to airway narrowing and obstruction.

Diagnosis. Clinical symptoms raise suspicion. Children are often mistakenly treated for asthma. The diagnosis is confirmed by angiocardiography.

Clinical Presentation. Symptoms may begin in the newborn period or later in development, usually depending on the type of ring. Stridor, wheezing, apnea, retractions (subcostal, suprasternal, and intercostal), tachypnea, and cyanosis are common. Symptoms may worsen during feeding or crying.

Management. Surgical repair is necessary for patients with severe respiratory distress, recurrent infections, and FTT. Antibiotics, oxygen therapy, and CPT to treat secretions and pneumonia may be indicated.

Complications. Tracheomalacia or malacia of a main stem bronchus are rare complications.

NEUROLOGIC DISORDERS

Increased Intracranial Pressure

Normal intracranial pressure (ICP) is 0 to 15 mm Hg. ICP greater than 15 mm Hg is considered increased. Causes of increased ICP are listed in Table 6–4. Symptoms of increased ICP are listed in Table 6–5. Levels of consciousness are often monitored using the Glasgow Coma Scale (Table 6–6). The Children's Coma Scale (Table 6–7) was developed to assess infants and toddlers who are unable to speak or follow commands.

Intracranial Pressure Monitoring

Monitoring is most frequently performed through insertion of a subarachnoid screw or bolt or intraventricular catheter that is connected to a transducer system for pressure measurement.

Cerebral perfusion pressure (CPP) is a means of assessing cerebral blood flow. Normal pressure = 60 to 80 mm Hg. The formula for obtaining CPP is:

$$\text{CPP} = \text{Mean arterial pressure} - \text{ICP}$$

In cases of increased ICP, the goal is to maintain a CPP greater than 50 mm Hg and an ICP less than 15 mm Hg.

Medical Management of Increased Intracranial Pressure

Head Positioning. The head and body should be aligned with the head kept midline and the head of the bed elevated 30 to 40 degrees.

TABLE 6–4 Causes of Increased Intracranial Pressure

CEREBRAL EDEMA	INCREASED CEREBRAL BLOOD VOLUME
Hypoxia	Hypoxia
Ischemia	Hypercarbia
Poisons	Arteriovenous malformations
Hypoglycemia	Intracranial hemorrhage
Trauma	Trauma
Reye's syndrome	Prematurity and anoxia
Irritation	Prematurity and positive pressure ventilation
INCREASED CEREBROSPINAL FLUID VOLUME	Reduced cerebral venous return
Congenital hydrocephalus	High intrathoracic pressure
Birth trauma	Valsalva's maneuver
Meningitis	Hematomas
Brain tumors	**MASS LESIONS**
Cerebrospinal fluid tumors	Intracranial tumors
Obstructed shunts	Intracranial abscess

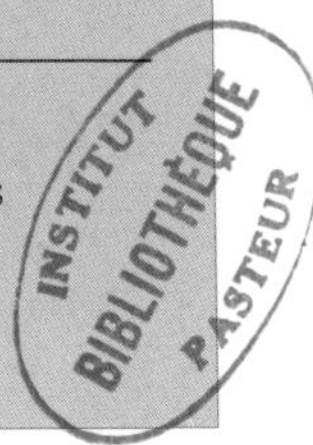

Oxygenation. The Pa_{O_2} is maintained at greater than or equal to 100 mm Hg. One must be aware that the use of positive end-expiratory pressure (PEEP) may increase intrathoracic pressure and result in increased ICP.

Hyperventilation. Decreasing the Pa_{CO_2} levels leads to cerebral vessel constriction and decreased cerebral blood volume, resulting in a reduction in the ICP. Pa_{CO_2} levels should not be maintained at less than 25 mm Hg.

Diuretics. Mannitol and glycerol are osmotic diuretics that reduce ICP by decreasing the blood viscosity and decreasing cerebral blood volume.

Glucocorticosteroids. Steroids such as dexamethasone are most useful in reducing edema surrounding mass lesions. They are not beneficial in the edema seen after hypoxic-ischemic injuries.

Analgesia. Pain may cause hypoventilation and Valsalva's maneuver, which increase ICP. Analgesics, sedatives, and paralyzing agents may be given.

TABLE 6–5 Signs and Symptoms of Increased Intracranial Pressure

Irritability
Lethargy
Decreased eye contact in infants
Confusion
Mood swings
Fixed, dilated, oval-shaped pupils
Decreased or absent pupil constriction response to light
Blurred vision
Diplopia
Strabismus
Papilledema (edema of the optic disc)
Unilateral papilledema, indicating a lesion behind affected eye
Systolic hypertension with bradycardia (Cushing's reflex)
Headache
Vomiting in the absence of nausea
Tachycardia with fluctuations in arterial blood pressure
Hypotension
Cheyne-Stokes respirations (alternating hyperpnea-bradypnea)
Central neurogenic hyperventilation
Apneustic breathing (prolonged inspiration and expiration)
Cluster breathing (irregular breathing with apnea)
Ataxic breathing (extremely irregular breathing)
Neurogenic pulmonary edema
Decreased motor function
Decorticate rigidity
Decerebrate posturing
Babinski's reflex
Decreased response to painful stimuli
Separation of cranial sutures
Increased head circumference in infants
Full or bulging anterior fontanelle in infants
High-pitched cry in infants

TABLE 6-6 Glasgow Coma Scale

I. Best Motor Response	
Obeys	6
Localizes	5
Withdraws (flexion)	4
Abnormal flexion	3
Extensor response	2
Nil	1
II. Verbal Response	
Oriented	5
Confused conversation	4
Inappropriate words	3
Incomprehensible sounds	2
Nil	1
III. Eye Opening	
Spontaneous	4
To speech	3
To pain	2
Nil	1
COMA SCORE = I + II + III	

From Ghajar J, Hariri RJ: Management of pediatric head injury. Pediatr Clin North Am 1992; 39:1093–1126.

TABLE 6-7 Children's Coma Scale

Ocular response: maximum score = 4
- 4 Pursuit
- 3 Extraocular movement intact, reactive pupils
- 2 Fixed pupils or extraocular movement impaired
- 1 Fixed pupil and extraocular movement paralyzed

Verbal response: maximum score = 3
- 3 Cries
- 2 Spontaneous respirations
- 1 Apneic

Motor response: maximum score = 4
- 4 Flexes and extends
- 3 Withdraws from painful stimuli
- 2 Hypertonic
- 1 Flaccid

TOTAL MAXIMUM SCORE = 11

TOTAL MINIMUM SCORE = 3

From Ghajar J, Hariri RJ: Management of pediatric head injury. Pediatr Clin North Am 1992; 39:1093–1126.

Pentobarbital Coma. Barbiturates are given to induce a coma, resulting in reduced cerebral blood flow, decreased edema formation, and a lowered metabolic rate of the brain. It is useful in the treatment of Reye's syndrome. Weaning from the coma is begun when the ICP no longer rises during barbiturate dosage reductions. Seizures may occur during weaning from pentobarbital.

Hypothermia. Cerebral blood volume is decreased by hypothermia. It is frequently used concurrently with pentobarbital coma. Body temperature is usually kept at 27° to 31° C. Rewarming is performed slowly.

Anticonvulsants. These are given to prevent or control seizures, or both.

Avoiding Increased ICP. Hyperoxygenation and hyperventilation should be performed prior to, during, and after any activity that may cause an increase in the ICP, such as ETT suctioning or patient transport. Suctioning should be limited to less than 10 seconds in total duration. The ICP should be allowed to stabilize between patient activities. Mechanical ventilation increases intrathoracic pressure and may increase ICP; therefore, ventilation should be instituted using the lowest peak and mean airway pressures possible for adequate ventilation and oxygenation. CPT should be used with caution as it may aggravate the ICP. Valsalva maneuvers and coughing should be avoided. A quiet environment around the patient's bed, including low lights and minimal noise, may help maintain reduced ICP levels.

Reye's Syndrome

Acute, progressive encephalopathy with fatty degeneration and infiltration into the internal organs, especially notable in the liver, characterizes Reye's syndrome. Serum ammonia levels rise, liver dysfunction occurs, and cerebral edema develops without evidence of inflammation.

Etiology. The cause is unknown. It is associated with influenza, varicella, and salicylate (aspirin) use.

Incidence. Reye's syndrome occurs most often in children 4 to 16 years old. There is an increased occurrence during viral illness epidemics. It affects males and females equally.

Diagnosis. The diagnosis is made if the patient has a characteristic history (viral prodrome) and elevated serum ammonia and liver enzyme levels, and other disorders are ruled out. A liver biopsy may be performed when the diagnosis is in question. The syndrome should be highly suspected in children presenting with symptoms of encephalopathy, especially when vomiting occurs following a viral-like illness.

Clinical Presentation

History. Symptoms are preceded by a viral illness such as influenza, varicella (chickenpox), or gastroenteritis.

Physical Examination. Symptoms usually appear within 1 week after the onset of the viral illness and may begin with the sudden onset of mild nausea and vomiting, with the child recovering fully. Other children may progress to confusion, combativeness, unresponsiveness, and coma. Staging of the symptoms is used to determine treatment and prognosis (Table 6–8). The faster a child progresses through the stages, the poorer the prognosis.

Laboratory Values. Elevated levels of serum glutamic-oxaloacetic transaminase (SGOT), serum glutamic-pyruvic transaminase (SGPT), lactate dehydrogenase (LDH), and serum ammonia are hallmarks of Reye's syndrome. Serum ammonia levels greater than 300 mg/dl are associated with poor outcome. Other laboratory findings may include hypoglycemia, metabolic acidosis, respiratory alkalosis, and a prolonged prothrombin time (PT) and partial thromboplastin time (PTT).

Management. Treatment is related to individual symptoms. Monitoring in an ICU should include a neurologic assessment, ammonia and liver enzyme levels, and an ICP determination in severe cases. Patients in Stages III through V require intensive treatment to reduce the high ICP levels (see Medical Management of Increased Intracranial Pressure). Seizures are treated with phenytoin (Dilantin).

Complications. Complete neurologic recovery and normal liver function occur in many patients. Neurologic sequelae often occur in patients who progressed beyond Stage II or who were not diagnosed and treated early. Death occurs in patients with uncontrollable increased ICP.

NEUROMUSCULAR DISORDERS

Guillain-Barré Syndrome

Guillain-Barré Syndrome (GBS) is an acute demyelinating polyneuropathy in which destruction of the myelin sheath results in impaired nerve impulse conduction. Nerve degeneration may occur. Progressive motor weakness may lead to respiratory failure.

TABLE 6–8 Clinical Stages of Reye's Syndrome

	CONSCIOUSNESS	MOTOR	SEIZURES	OTHER
Stage I	Lethargy, responds to pain	None	None	Vomiting, rash, hepatic dysfunction, hyperventilation
Stage II	Delirium, combative	Hyperactive reflexes, sluggish pupils	None	Hepatic dysfunction, hyperventilation
Stage III	Coma	Decorticate rigidity, sluggish pupils, doll's eyes	None	Hepatic dysfunction, hyperventilation
Stage IV	Coma	Decerebrate rigidity, sluggish large pupils, no oculocephalic reflex	None	Minimal hepatic dysfunction
Stage V	Coma	No reflexes, flaccid, fixed pupils	Present	Respiratory arrest, serum ammonia >300 mg/ml

Etiology. The cause is unknown but may result from an abnormal immune response to infection. Certain triggering events often occur within 30 days of the symptoms, including immunosuppressive states (from chemotherapy, organ transplantation) and viral infections (upper respiratory tract infection, varicella, cytomegalovirus, viral immunization).

Diagnosis. Features are so characteristic that the diagnosis is often made without laboratory confirmation. Lumbar puncture with elevated concentrations of protein in cerebrospinal fluid confirms the diagnosis.

Clinical Presentation. Onset is usually sudden. Muscle weakness progresses rapidly and affects the legs or arms first and is relatively symmetric. Table 6–9 lists common signs and symptoms.

Management. Management of GBS is largely symptomatic.

Bedside Pulmonary Function Testing. The vital capacity and negative inspiratory force should be monitored every 2 to 4 hours.

TABLE 6–9 Symptoms Often Found in Guillain-Barré Syndrome

Limb paresthesia (numbness, tingling, burning sensations)
Hyperesthesia (lightest touch is painful)
Muscle aches and cramps
Muscle weakness (progressive, ascending, symmetric)
Paralysis (including respiratory muscles)
Lack of tendon reflexes in weak muscles
Bilateral facial weakness
Dysphagia
Impaired gag and swallow reflexes
Pupil dilatation and constriction
Inability to talk or blink
Facial flushing
Diaphoresis
Orthostatic hypotension
Bradycardia
Heart block
Bowel and bladder dysfunction

Pulmonary Toilet. Deep breathing techniques are necessary to prevent atelectasis. CPT may be indicated if secretions pool.

Physical Therapy. Passive and active range-of-motion exercises are necessary to prevent contractures.

Mechanical Ventilation. Table 6–10 lists factors that indicate the need for intubation and mechanical ventilation. Ventilation may be necessary for several weeks. Weaning is started with recovery of muscle strength.

Complications. Aspiration, atelectasis, pneumonia, and respiratory failure may occur. Complete recovery can be expected if the child is well ventilated during the time of profound paralysis.

Myasthenia Gravis

Myasthenia gravis (MG) encompasses disorders of the neuromuscular junction characterized by muscle weakness and fatigue.

Etiology. MG may occur as three syndromes.

Congenital Myasthenia Gravis and Familial Infantile Myasthenia Gravis. Caused by genetic defects, familial infantile MG has respiratory failure as a prominent feature. Congenital MG symptoms are milder, and the mother does not have MG.

Juvenile Myasthenia Gravis. This is an immune-mediated form of MG that is encountered from late infancy through adulthood. Two forms are recognized: ocular MG (eye muscles are affected) and generalized MG (moderate to severe weakness of bulbar and limb muscles).

TABLE 6–10 Clinical Factors Indicating the Need for Mechanical Ventilation in the Patient With Guillain-Barré Syndrome

Vital capacity ≤30% of predicted value or <15 ml/kg body weight
Negative inspiratory force ≤−20 cm H_2O
Inability to cough, swallow, or clear oral secretions
Pharyngeal paralysis

Transitory Neonatal Myasthenia Gravis. This is observed in offspring of mothers with MG and is believed to be due to the transfer of antibody from the mother to the normal fetus.

Diagnosis. The response to anticholinesterase is used for the diagnosis, which is established if weakness and respiratory distress are reversed after the administration of edrophonium chloride (Tensilon). Elevated concentrations of the antibodies against the acetylcholine receptor are found in patients with the generalized form of juvenile MG and in infants with transitory neonatal MG.

Clinical Presentation. The onset of symptoms varies with the different types of MG and are listed in Table 6–11.

Management

Congenital and Familial Myasthenia Gravis. Long-term treatment with neostigmine or pyridostigmine is needed to prevent sudden apneic episodes. Intubation and mechanical ventilation may be needed in cases of severe respiratory failure.

Juvenile Myasthenia Gravis. Anticholinesterase drugs are given to children with ocular involvement. Thymectomy is performed, followed by plasma exchange if weakness is extreme. Corticosteroids should be started immediately after surgery.

Transitory Neonatal Myasthenia Gravis. Exchange transfusion should be performed in newborns with severe weak-

TABLE 6–11 Symptoms Often Found in Myasthenia Gravis

Muscle weakness (progressive, descending)
Tendon reflexes are present
Ptosis
Diplopia
Difficulty feeding
Inability to suck in infants
Weak cry and facial expressions in infants
Tachypnea
Fatigability with exercise
Arthrogryposis
Paralysis (including respiratory muscles)
Thyroiditis
Collagen vascular disease

ness and respiratory distress. Administration of neostigmine before feeding improves sucking and swallowing; the dose is reduced as symptoms resolve.

Complications. Aspiration, pneumonia, upper airway obstruction from the inability to handle secretions, and apnea are complications seen with MG. Respiratory failure resulting in death may occur if monitoring and treatment are inadequate.

Cholinergic Versus Myasthenic Crisis. Overmedication with anticholinesterase drugs may result in muscle weakness. This is referred to as a cholinergic crisis. Administration of edrophonium chloride is termed a Tensilon test and will distinguish between a cholinergic crisis and a myasthenic crisis. If the patient's symptoms worsen after edrophonium administration, the patient is experiencing a cholinergic crisis. If symptoms improve, the patient is experiencing a myasthenic crisis. Because acute respiratory failure may occur with the test, resuscitation and airway management equipment (laryngoscope and ETT) should be immediately available.

Bibliography

Avery GB, Fletcher MA, MacDonald MG: Neonatology. Pathophysiology and Management of the Newborn, 4th ed. Philadelphia, JB Lippincott, 1994.

Avery ME, First LR: Pediatric Medicine. Baltimore, Williams & Wilkins, 1989.

Bailey PV, Connors RH, Tracy TF, et al: A vital analysis of extracorporeal membrane oxygenation for congenital diaphragmatic hernia. Surgery 1989; 106:611.

Burg FD, Ingelfinger JR, Wald ER: Current Pediatric Therapy, vol 14. Philadelphia, WB Saunders, 1993.

Caplan MS, MacGregor SN: Perinatal management of congenital diaphragmatic hernia and anterior abdominal wall defects. Clin Perinatol 1989; 16:917.

Chernick V: Kendig's Disorders of the Respiratory Tract in Children, 5th ed. Philadelphia, WB Saunders, 1990.

Dillon PW, Cilley RE: Newborn surgical emergencies: Gastrointestinal anomalies, abdominal wall defects. Pediatr Clin North Am 1993; 40:1289.

Fanaroff AA, Martin RJ: Neonatal-Perinatal Medicine. St. Louis, Mosby-Year Book, 1992.

Fenichel GM: Clinical Pediatric Neurology: A Sign and Symptoms Approach, 2nd ed. Philadelphia, WB Saunders, 1993.

Ghajar J, Hariri RJ: Management of pediatric head injury. Pediatr Clin North Am 1992; 39:1093.

Graef JW: Manual of Pediatric Therapeutics, 5th ed. Boston, Little, Brown, 1994.

Haller JA Jr, Turner CS: Diagnosis and operative management of chest wall deformities in children. Surg Clin North Am 1981; 61:1199.

LeRoux PD, Jardine DS, Loeser JD: Pediatric intracranial pressure monitoring in hypoxic and nonhypoxic brain injury. Child Nervous System 1991; 7:34.

Misulis KE, Fenichel GM: Genetic forms of myasthenia gravis. Pediatr Neurol 1989; 5:205.

Nakayama DK, Motoyama ED, Tagge EM: Effect of preoperative stabilization on respiratory system compliance and outcome in newborn infants with congenital diaphragmatic hernia. J Pediatr 1991; 118:793.

Pomerance JJ, Richardson CJ: Neonatology for the Clinician. Norwalk, CT, Appleton & Lange, 1993.

Sabiston DC, Spencer FC: Gibbon's Surgery of the Chest, 4th ed. Philadelphia, WB Saunders, 1983.

Surgeon General's advisory on the use of salicylate in Reye's syndrome, 1981: Reye's syndrome and salicylate usage. MMWR 1982; 31:51.

Weinstein S, Stolar CJH: Newborn surgical emergencies: Congenital diaphragmatic hernia and extracorporeal membrane oxygenation. Pediatr Clin North Am 1993; 40:1315.

SECTION 7

Neonatal Disorders

Abbreviations

ALTE–apparent life-threatening event
AP–anteroposterior
BPD–bronchopulmonary dysplasia
bpm–beats per minute
CBC–complete blood count
CPAP–continuous positive airway pressure
CPR–cardiopulmonary resuscitation
CPT–chest physical therapy
CSF–cerebrospinal fluid
ECMO–extracorporeal membrane oxygenation
EEG–electroencephalogram
FTT–failure to thrive
GER–gastroesophageal reflux
IMV–intermittent mandatory ventilation
IPPB–intermittent positive pressure breathing
IVH–intraventricular hemorrhage
MAS–meconium aspiration syndrome
NEC–necrotizing enterocolitis
PAP–pulmonary artery pressure
PDA–patent ductus arteriosus
PIE–pulmonary interstitial emphysema
PPHN–persistent pulmonary hypertension of the newborn
PROM–premature rupture of membranes
PVR–pulmonary vascular resistance
RDS–respiratory distress syndrome
ROP–retinopathy of prematurity
SIDS–sudden infant death syndrome
TTN–transient tachypnea of the newborn
WBC–white blood cell

APNEA

Apnea is the cessation of respiratory airflow for greater than or equal to 20 seconds with or without bradycardia or cyanosis. Types include *central* (no respiratory effort), *obstructive* (respiratory effort without airflow), *mixed* (combination of central and obstructive apnea), and *apnea of prematurity* (apnea in an infant less than 37 weeks of gestation). *Periodic breathing* is three or more apneic periods lasting greater than or equal to 3 seconds within a 20-second period. Physiologic effects of apnea include hypoxia, hypercarbia, bradycardia, hypotension, and depressed cardiac function.

Etiology. Causes of apnea are listed in Table 7–1.

Diagnosis. Screening tests should include chest and abdominal x-ray films (for pulmonary changes, necrotizing enterocolitis [NEC]); head ultrasound (for intraventricular hemorrhage [IVH]); arterial blood gas (ABG) (for hypoxia); complete blood count (CBC) (for sepsis); blood, urine, and cerebrospinal fluid (CSF) cultures (for sepsis); and electrolytes, calcium, and glucose levels (for metabolic disturbances). Other tests that may be needed for accurate diagnosis include an electroencephalogram (EEG), pneumogram (monitors heart rate and chest wall movement; 3-channel pneumogram includes a nasal thermistor to detect airflow), and polysomnogram (monitors EEG and muscle movement during sleep).

Clinical Presentation. Symptoms associated with apnea may include bradycardia, cyanosis, snoring, choking, mouth breathing, and changes in respiratory pattern. Apnea of prematurity usually presents after 3 days of life and is not associated with any other abnormality. Apnea within the first 24 hours of life is often associated with infection.

An *apparent life-threatening event* (ALTE) refers to a frightening episode characterized by a combination of apnea, a color change, a marked change in muscle tone, and choking or gagging. It can occur at any age, usually at 2 to 3 months of age.

Management. The goal of management is to treat the underlying cause of apnea and prevent further apneic episodes.

Underlying Causes. Treatment may include blood transfusions (anemia); prone, upright positioning and frequent small feedings with thickened formula (gastroesophageal reflux [GER]); glucose administration (hypoglycemia); and surgical repair.

Monitoring. Monitoring includes heart rate and pulse oximetry. When alarms sound, the infant should be checked for airway obstruction, bradycardia, and cyanosis.

Tactile Stimulation. Gentle shaking or tapping of the infant's feet may resolve spells. An oscillating water bed or "bump" bed may stimulate respiration. Bump beds are

TABLE 7–1 Causes of Apnea in the Newborn

- Abnormal coordination of swallowing
- Acidosis
- Airway obstruction
- Airway stimulation
  - Fluid in the airway
  - Suctioning
- Anemia
- BPD
- Cardiovascular abnormalities
- Choanal atresia
- Central hypoventilation syndromes
- Craniofacial abnormalities
  - Beckwith-Weidemann's syndrome
  - Down's syndrome
  - Macroglossia
  - Micrognathia
  - Pierre Robin syndrome
- Gastroesophageal reflux
- Hypocarbia
- Hypoglycemia
- Hypothermia
- Hypoxia
  - Hypovolemia
  - Pulmonary disorders (RDS, TTN, atelectasis)
- Immaturity of respiratory control (apnea of prematurity)
- Infection
  - Group B streptococci
  - Meningitis
  - Pertussis
  - Pneumonia
  - Respiratory syncytial virus
  - Sepsis
- Maternal drug addiction
- Metabolic abnormalities
  - Hyperammonemia
  - Hypocalcemia
  - Hypoglycemia
  - Hyponatremia
- Drug depression
  - Analgesics
  - Narcotics
  - Prostaglandins
  - Sedatives

TABLE 7–1 Causes of Apnea in the Newborn
Continued

NEC
Prolonged Valsalva maneuvers
Coughing
Crying
Defecation
Seizures
Temperature changes

BPD, bronchopulmonary dysplasia; RDS, respiratory distress syndrome; TTN, transient tachypnea of the newborn; NEC, necrotizing enterocolitis.

constructed by connecting a rubber glove (placed under the infant's mattress pad) to a pressure ventilator or intermittent positive pressure breathing (IPPB) machine with a set respiratory rate and inspiratory pressure.

Oxygen Therapy. Low F_{IO_2} settings (.23 to .25) often resolve episodes.

Resuscitation. Bag and mask for ventilation should be kept at the bedside. Intubation, ventilation, and cardiac compressions are indicated if the infant does not respond to tactile stimulation and bag-mask ventilation.

Pharmacologic Therapy. Drugs used to treat apnea include theophylline, caffeine, and doxapram. Mechanisms of action are unclear. Methylxanthines (theophylline, caffeine) may worsen GER.

Continuous Positive Airway Pressure. CPAP is commonly used after pharmacologic therapy has failed to relieve spells. It is usually delivered by nasal prongs at 2 to 5 cm H_2O.

Mechanical Ventilation. This is indicated if the preceding interventions fail or if apnea is associated with severe hypoxia and bradycardia.

Home Care. Home apnea-bradycardia monitors are used with infants who have abnormal apnea or bradycardia at the time of hospital discharge or those who experience a severe ALTE. Monitors are also used in siblings (including identical twins) of sudden infant death syndrome (SIDS) victims, infants with tracheostomies, and infants with central hypoventilation syndrome. Alarm settings for monitors may include a 15- to 20-second time delay for the respiratory signal, low heart rate alarm of 70 to 80 beats per minute (bpm), and high heart rate alarm greater than 220 bpm. The low heart rate alarm is adjusted downward every 2 months in increments of 10 bpm. If oxygen saturation (Sao_2) is monitored, the low alarm is set at less than 85%. Parents should be trained in how to respond to the alarms and in cardiopulmonary resuscitation (CPR). Monitors may be discontinued when there is no recurrence of apnea or the infant is no longer felt to be at increased risk of cardiopulmonary arrest or death. Theophylline and caffeine may be continued at home.

Complications. Complications include pulmonary hypertension, hypoxic-ischemic brain damage, and SIDS.

BRONCHOPULMONARY DYSPLASIA

Bronchopulmonary dysplasia (BPD) is chronic lung disease that occurs in premature infants in whom increased levels of oxygen and mechanical ventilation were required in the first week of life and who continue to have oxygen dependence, radiographic abnormalities, and respiratory symptoms after 28 days of life. Pulmonary changes may include increased alveolar-capillary permeability, airway inflammation, pulmonary fibrosis, destruction of alveolar septa, absence of cilia resulting in mucus retention, atelectasis, hyperinflation, and a decreased number of alveoli and small pulmonary arteries. This leads to decreased pulmonary compliance and increased resistance, airflow obstruction, air trapping, bronchial hyperreactivity, and increased work of breathing and caloric expenditure.

Etiology. Table 7–2 lists factors associated with the development of BPD.

TABLE 7–2 Factors Associated With the Development of Bronchopulmonary Dysplasia

Prematurity	Aspiration
Low birth weight	Surfactant deficiency
Cardiac failure	Respiratory distress syndrome (RDS)
Pulmonary barotrauma	Sepsis
Apnea of prematurity	Genetic predisposal
Mechanical ventilation	Endotracheal intubation
Pulmonary hypoplasia	Pulmonary dysmaturity
Prolonged exposure to high Fio_2 levels	

Diagnosis. The history, clinical picture, and radiographic findings lead to the diagnosis of BPD.

Clinical Presentation

Physical Examination. Tachycardia, tachypnea, dyspnea, retractions, grunting, nasal flaring, cough, paradoxical ("see-saw") respirations, wheezing, prolonged expiration, and rhonchi are found. The child is often pale or cyanotic, irritable, and exhibits poor weight gain and failure to thrive (FTT).

Arterial Blood Gas Analysis. Hypoxemia (often 50 to 70 mm Hg) and hypercarbia (often 50 to 90 mm Hg) may be seen; pH may be normal.

Chest X-ray Findings. The radiograph is variable according to the stage of disease. It ranges from increased lung densities and diffuse atelectasis with fluid accumulation to the chronic picture of atelectasis, hyperinflation, cystic changes, fibrosis, and cardiomegaly.

Management

Oxygen Therapy. Oxygen is given to treat chronic hypoxia, reduce pulmonary hypertension (prevent cor pulmonale), and reduce caloric expenditures (improve weight gain). Clinical goals often include maintaining Pa_{O_2} levels at greater than 55 mm Hg or Sa_{O_2} levels at greater than 90%.

Mechanical Ventilation. Various ventilator strategies may be used. The goal is to provide adequate oxygenation and ventilation while minimizing barotrauma. Pressure ventilators are used in the early stages of BPD; volume ventilators are needed to treat the increased airway resistance and decreased compliance present in the later stages. Tracheostomy is indicated in some infants who require long-term ventilatory support. Weaning is a slow process often taking weeks to months. Volume ventilation with slow weaning modes such as pressure support are often used.

Monitoring. Pulse oximetry is used to monitor oxygenation; capillary or ABG analysis is used to monitor pH and P_{CO_2} levels.

Drug Therapy. Table 7–3 lists medications used in the treatment of BPD.

Aerosol Therapy and Chest Physical Therapy. Bronchodilators may be delivered via small-volume nebulizer, metered dose inhaler, and dry powder inhalation. Chest physical therapy (CPT) is indicated in infants with increased mucus production. Treatment frequency varies depending on active infections and the ability to remove secretions.

TABLE 7-3 Pharmacologic Agents Used in the Management of Bronchopulmonary Dysplasia

BRONCHODILATORS	PULMONARY VASODILATORS
Methylxanthines	Hydralazine
Theophylline	Diltiazem
Caffeine	Nifedipine
Beta-adrenergics	**DIURETICS**
Albuterol	Furosemide
Terbutaline	Spironolactone
Metaproterenol	Chlorothiazide
Anticholinergics	Hydrochlorothiazide
Atropine	**ANTIOXIDANTS**
ANTIINFLAMMATORY AGENTS	Vitamin E
Cromolyn sodium	Vitamin A
Nedocromil sodium	Superoxide dismutase
CORTICOSTEROIDS	
Dexamethasone	

Home Care. Oxygen therapy and mechanical ventilation are often required on discharge. Home apnea-bradycardia monitoring may be indicated. Parents should be instructed in equipment care and CPR.

Complications. Infection is the greatest risk in chronic stages of disease. Airway injuries sustained during intubations, suctioning, and mechanical ventilation may result in stenosis (tracheal, subglottic, bronchial), polyps, granulomas, tracheomalacia, and bronchomalacia. Other complications include pulmonary hypertension, reactive airway disease, abnormal pulmonary function (air trapping, decreased airflow), growth failure, neurologic and developmental abnormalities (speech delay, learning disabilities, attention deficit, cerebral palsy), and death (resulting from respiratory failure, tracheal obstruction, sepsis, pulmonary hypertension, congestive heart failure).

MECONIUM ASPIRATION SYNDROME

Meconium is the first bowel discharge of an infant, usually passed within 48 hours after delivery. If the meconium is passed into the amniotic fluid in utero, it may be aspirated by the fetus and result in airway obstruction and atelectasis (physical obstruction of the glottis, trachea, or airways), air trapping (ball-valve effect with partial obstruction), airway inflammation (chemical pneumonitis), infection, and increased pulmonary vascular resistance (PVR) (due to profound hypoxia).

Etiology. Meconium passage in utero occurs most often in term or postterm infants who experience intrauterine stress or hypoxia. It is believed that in utero hypoxia results in intestinal peristalsis and sphincter relaxation, allowing the meconium to pass. Other theories of causes of meconium passage include vagal responses (compression of the umbilical cord or fetal head), breech delivery, fetal acidosis, and spontaneous passage by a mature fetus.

Diagnosis. Meconium aspiration syndrome (MAS) is suspected whenever there is meconium staining of amniotic fluid. The diagnosis is made whenever the infant has clinical signs of respiratory distress and meconium is present below the vocal cords.

Clinical Presentation

Labor and Delivery. Delivery is usually through meconium-stained fluid (''pea soup''). Labor may be prolonged and include significant intrauterine stress or hypoxia, breech delivery, and abnormal fetal heart rhythms. Skin, nails, and cord may be yellow-tinged; skin may be peeling; nails may be long; and the cord may lack or have little Wharton's jelly. Apgar scores may vary at 1 minute; however, signs of respiratory distress present quickly.

Physical Examination. Respiratory distress often depends on the viscosity of the meconium and may include tachypnea with gasping respirations, grunting, nasal flaring, and retractions. Breath sounds are decreased with crackles, the anteroposterior (AP) diameter of the chest may be increased, and cyanosis is present.

Arterial Blood Gas Analysis. Hypoxemia is present; hypercarbia occurs with moderate to severe MAS. Mixed respiratory and metabolic acidosis develops as obstruction and inflammation progress.

Chest X-ray Findings. The appearance of the radiograph varies; it may be similar to that seen in bacterial pneumonia. It usually reveals widespread involvement with areas of atelectasis and hyperexpansion. Pulmonary air leaks (pulmonary interstitial emphysema [PIE], pneumothorax, pneumomediastinum) may be present.

Management

Delivery Room Intervention. Pharyngeal suction with a bulb syringe should be performed when the infant's head is delivered. Intratracheal suctioning is indicated immediately after delivery if there are signs of in utero fetal distress, the neonate requires ventilation in the delivery room, the meconium is thick or particulate, or pharyngeal suctioning was not performed.

Oxygen Therapy. Mild cases may require only an oxygen hood.

Continuous Positive Airway Pressure. Nasal prongs at 3 to 6 cm H_2O may improve oxygenation; this increases the risk of barotrauma.

Mechanical Ventilation. Infants with severe hypoxemia and respiratory distress that do not respond to CPAP should be intubated and ventilated. Sedation and paralysis are often required. Since these infants are at high risk of barotrauma, the goal is to adequately ventilate and oxygenate with the lowest mean airway pressures possible. Hyperventilation is often necessary to treat the pulmonary hypertension. High-frequency ventilation is often used to provide lower pressures.

Extracorporeal Membrane Oxygenation. Infants with severe MAS and pulmonary hypertension may require extracorporeal membrane oxygenation (ECMO).

New Interventions. Surfactant replacement therapy (meconium may inhibit surfactant), nitric oxide inhalation (to reduce PVR), and liquid ventilation with perfluorochemicals (able to ventilate at lower pressures) may find a role in the future management of MAS.

Complications. Depending on the severity of disease, MAS may result in barotrauma, increased intracranial pressure with IVH, pulmonary hypertension, air leaks, infection, chronic obstructive pulmonary disease, exercise-induced bronchospasm, cerebral palsy, and death.

PERSISTENT PULMONARY HYPERTENSION OF THE NEWBORN

Persistent pulmonary hypertension of the newborn (PPHN) is a clinical syndrome consisting of pulmonary vasoconstriction with severely increased PVR and right-to-left shunting. The foramen ovale and ductus arteriosus remain open (resulting from increased PVR) and severe hypoxia and acidosis develop, worsening the pulmonary vasoconstriction.

Etiology. Pulmonary capillary bed hypoplasia, alveolar capillary dysplasia, pulmonary smooth muscle hypertrophy and hyperplasia, and abnormal levels of vasoactive agents (increased vasoconstrictors, decreased vasodilators) are primary causes of PPHN. Table 7–4 lists underlying disorders that frequently result in PPHN.

Diagnosis. Various tests may be used to assist in the diagnosis.

TABLE 7–4 Factors Associated With Persistent Pulmonary Hypertension of the Newborn

FETAL FACTORS

- Intrauterine stress
  - Hypoxia
  - Acidosis
- Placental vascular abnormalities

MATERNAL FACTORS

- Diabetes
- Hypoxia
- Cesarean section

PHARMACOLOGIC FACTORS

- Prostaglandins
- Indomethacin
- Salicylate
- Diphenylhydantoin

PULMONARY FACTORS

- Pneumonia
- Meconium aspiration
- Pulmonary hypoplasia
- Diaphragmatic hernia
- Respiratory distress syndrome
- Transient tachypnea of the newborn
- Lobar emphysema

HEMATOLOGIC FACTORS

- Increased hematocrit
- Septicemia
- Maternal-fetal blood loss
  - Abruptio placentae
  - Placenta previa
- Acute blood loss
- Neonatal hyperviscosity
- Polycythemia

CARDIOVASCULAR FACTORS

- Systemic hypotension
- Congenital heart disease
- Shock

OTHER FACTORS

- Central nervous system disorders
- Neuromuscular disease
- Hypoglycemia
- Hypocalcemia

Hyperoxia Test. Little or no increase in the Pa_{O_2} level after administration of 100% oxygen indicates a right-to-left shunt or congenital heart disease.

Preductal-Postductal P_{O_2} Comparison. Right-to-left shunting is indicated if a preductal Pa_{O_2} measurement is more than 20 mm Hg greater than a postductal Pa_{O_2} measurement. (A normal test result does not rule out PPHN.)

Hyperoxia-Hyperventilation Test. PPHN is confirmed if the Pa_{O_2} level is greater than 100 mm Hg after hyperventilation to maintain a Pa_{CO_2} of 20 to 25 mm Hg.

Doppler Flow–Cardiac Catheterization. Foramen ovale and patent ductus arteriosus (PDA) shunts can be observed; elevated pulmonary artery pressure (PAP) indicates PPHN.

Clinical Presentation. Infants are usually cyanotic and present within 12 hours of life with severe respiratory distress, including tachypnea, retractions, grunting, and nasal flaring.

Arterial Blood Gas Analysis. Severe hypoxemia (Pa_{O_2} often < 40 mm Hg) refractory to oxygen therapy is common. Hypercarbia and acidosis may develop.

Chest X-ray Findings. The radiograph varies depending on the associated disorder. Cardiomegaly may be present (due to increased right ventricular afterload).

Management

Oxygen Therapy. High F_{IO_2} levels are administered to produce pulmonary vasodilation and reduce the PVR.

Mechanical Ventilation. If the hypoxemia does not respond well to an F_{IO_2} of 1.0, intubation and ventilation are indicated. Hyperventilation (maintaining Pa_{CO_2} levels at 25 to 35 mm Hg [sometimes lower] and pH $\geq$ 7.5) is used to induce respiratory alkalosis, which, in turn, produces pulmonary vasodilation. Ventilatory rates greater than 100 breaths per minute and peak inspiratory pressures greater than 35 cm H_2O may be necessary. Sedation (phenobarbital, lorazepam) and paralysis (pancuronium) may be needed for infants who "fight" the ventilator. High-frequency ventilation has been used to treat some infants with PPHN.

Vasodilator Therapy. Tolazoline has been used extensively to reduce PVR, although the effect is inconsistent; nitroprusside and nitroglycerin have also been used. Since tolazoline may cause systemic hypotension, inotropic agents (dopamine, dobutamine) may be given with tolazoline to augment cardiac output and systemic blood pressure. Inhaled nitric oxide is a promising new therapy in producing pulmonary vasodilation and has been shown to improve oxygenation in infants with PPHN.

Extracorporeal Membrane Oxygenation. Infants who are not responsive to the preceding management approaches may be candidates for ECMO.

Complications. PPHN infants may experience hearing loss, seizures, cerebral infarction, IVH, and BPD. The mortality rate ranges from 20% to 40% (an increase in survival is seen when ECMO is used).

PNEUMONIA

Newborns with pneumonia often have hyaline membranes, alveolar capillary leakage, inflammation, interstitial pneumonitis, necrosis of the lung, and pulmonary hemorrhage.

Etiology

Transplacental. Infection is transmitted across the placenta to the fetus in utero, usually resulting from a maternal viral infection.

Perinatal. Infection is acquired during labor and delivery, most often through contaminated amniotic fluid or extended exposure to bacteria in the vaginal tract. Premature rupture of membranes (PROM) more than 12 to 24 hours prior to delivery increases the risk of pneumonia.

Postnatal. Nosocomial infection from equipment, procedures, visitors, or caregivers may result in pneumonia. Table 7–5 lists organisms often responsible for neonatal pneumonia.

Diagnosis. Throat, blood, urine, and cerebrospinal fluid (CSF) cultures should be performed when pneumonia is suspected. A white blood cell (WBC) count with tracheal or gastric aspirates may be necessary.

Clinical Presentation. Table 7–6 lists clinical signs and symptoms in the infant with neonatal pneumonia. The chest x-ray film may look similar to that in respiratory distress syndrome (RDS), transient tachypnea of the newborn (TTN), or BPD. It often reveals diffuse, bilateral densities and air-spaces with bronchograms.

Management

Oxygen Therapy. An oxygen hood is indicated to relieve hypoxemia.

TABLE 7–5 Pathogens Often Responsible for Pneumonia in Neonates

PNEUMONIA ACQUIRED TRANSPLACENTALLY
Listeria monocytogenes
Haemophilus influenzae
Mycobacterium tuberculosis
Treponema pallidum
Toxoplasma
Syphilis
Rubella
Varicella zoster
Cytomegalovirus
Herpes simplex virus
Human immunodeficiency virus
PNEUMONIA ACQUIRED DURING LABOR AND DELIVERY
Group B beta-hemolytic streptococcus
Klebsiella
Escherichia coli
Chlamydia trachomatis
NOSOCOMIAL PNEUMONIA ACQUIRED AFTER DELIVERY
Pseudomonas
Serratia marcescens
Staphylococcus aureus
Staphylococcus epidermidis
Klebsiella
Candida albicans
Respiratory syncytial virus
Cytomegalovirus
Herpes simplex virus

Mechanical Ventilation. Infants with respiratory failure and hypoxemia who do not respond to oxygen therapy should be intubated and ventilated. Some infants may require high rates, inspiratory pressures, and F_{IO_2} levels.

Extracorporeal Membrane Oxygenation. Infants who are not responsive to the preceding management approaches may be candidates for ECMO.

TABLE 7–6 Clinical Manifestations and Complications of Neonatal Pneumonia

Respiratory distress
Tachypnea
Cyanosis
Grunting
Nasal flaring
Retractions
Apnea
Poor peripheral perfusion
Tachycardia
Lethargy
Temperature instability
Abdominal distention
Excessive jaundice
Asphyxia
Septic shock
Persistent fetal circulation
Pulmonary hemorrhage
Pulmonary edema
Myocardial insufficiency
Pleural effusion
Hypotension
Disseminated intravascular coagulation
Hypoxemia
Hypercarbia
Respiratory acidosis
Metabolic acidosis
Barotrauma
Intraventricular hemorrhage
Bronchopulmonary dysplasia
Necrotizing enterocolitis

Monitoring. Pulse oximetry, transcutaneous monitors, and capillary or ABG values should be used to evaluate the adequacy of oxygenation and ventilation.

Drug Therapy. Antibiotics and antiviral agents should be administered, depending on results of cultures. Broad-spectrum antibiotics are often given for at least 72 hours or until definitive culture results are obtained.

Complications. Pneumonia in the newborn may result in IVH, barotrauma, NEC, BPD, neurologic damage, and developmental delay. Morbidity and mortality depend on the organism involved and the clinical course.

PULMONARY BAROTRAUMA

Lung overdistention created during manual or mechanical ventilation causes alveolar rupture, with air escaping into the interstitium. Air leaks may result in compression of small airways and pulmonary arterioles, increased PVR, atelectasis, decreased compliance, and increased intrathoracic pressure. Air leaks include PIE, pneumothorax, pneumomediastinum, pneumopericardium, and pneumoperitoneum.

Diagnosis. The chest x-ray film confirms the diagnosis.

Clinical Presentation. The clinical presentation varies with the size and location of the gas accumulation. Symptoms may include tachypnea, retractions, bradycardia, hypotension, restlessness and irritability, distended neck veins, cyanosis, wheezing, and decreased breath sounds.

Pulmonary Interstitial Emphysema

PIE consists of extrapulmonary gas within the interstitial space. The chest x-ray film may be similar to that seen in RDS, with white areas, small to large bubbles, and air bronchograms. There is often a mediastinal shift toward the unaffected side. PIE may resolve spontaneously, or the infant may need to be positioned with the affected side down.

Pneumothorax

Extrapulmonary gas in the intrapleural space may occur gradually or suddenly. It may be spontaneous or due to pulmonary disease or positive pressure ventilation. Infants may be asymptomatic or present with severe respiratory distress in cases of tension pneumothorax. The chest radiograph often reveals a shift of the trachea, heart, and mediastinum toward the unaffected side with the ribs separated and the diaphragm pushed downward. Treatment may include needle aspiration or chest tube insertion, or both.

Pneumomediastinum

Extrapulmonary gas in the mediastinal space may cause severe distress, or the infant may be asymptomatic. Most cases resolve spontaneously.

Pneumopericardium

Extrapulmonary gas tracked along the great vessels into the pericardial sac carries a high risk of morbidity and mortality. Treatment includes needle aspiration or chest tube insertion.

Complications. Bronchopleural fistulas, IVH, and BPD are associated with air leaks. Chest tube insertion may result in hemorrhage, lung puncture, infarction, and phrenic nerve injury with eventration of the diaphragm. The earlier the onset of air leaks after birth, the higher the mortality rate.

Transillumination of the Chest. A transilluminator may be used to diagnose a pneumothorax; it may be difficult to distinguish between a pneumomediastinum and a pneumopericardium. The room (area around the infant's bed) should be darkened. The infant is placed in the supine position and the light probe placed anteriorly on the chest and moved to different areas for comparison. In infants without air leaks, there should be a 2- to 3-cm lucent area surrounding the probe tip. The lucent area increases in size in the presence of intrathoracic air. False-positive results may occur if there is increased subcutaneous fat (infants of diabetic mothers) or chest wall edema. False-negative results may occur if the volume of free air is less than 20 ml. Transillumination of extremities may be performed for localization of vessels for puncture.

RESPIRATORY DISTRESS SYNDROME

Also called hyaline membrane disease, RDS usually affects premature infants and is believed to be the result of an insufficient amount of surfactant and immature pulmonary development. This condition, along with the preterm infant's overly compliant chest wall, leads to atelectasis. Hypoxia, hypercarbia, and acidosis cause pulmonary vasoconstriction and pulmonary hypertension, which may result in right-to-left shunting through the foramen ovale and PDA.

Diagnosis. The history, clinical presentation, laboratory values, and chest radiograph are diagnostic for RDS.

Clinical Presentation

History. Most infants are premature and have evidence of respiratory distress on delivery. Apgar scores are often less than 5.

Physical Examination. Tachypnea, retractions (intercostal, subcostal, "see-saw" appearance), grunting, nasal flaring, cyanosis, and increased work of breathing are evident.

Breath sounds are diminished. Very premature infants may be hypotonic and unresponsive.

Arterial Blood Gas Analysis. Moderate to severe hypoxemia, varying degrees of hypercarbia, and mixed respiratory and metabolic acidosis are present. The Pa_{CO_2} level is often low initially but rises as the work of breathing increases and the infant tires.

Chest X-ray Film. Chest films typically reveal diffuse, fine, granular densities (ground-glass appearance). Air bronchograms and a slightly enlarged heart may be seen.

Management

Surfactant Replacement. Surfactant may be given prophylactically (at delivery) or therapeutically (after signs of RDS are apparent). (See Section 9 for surfactant replacement therapy guidelines.)

Oxygen Therapy. An oxygen hood is provided to relieve the hypoxia with the goal being to maintain the Pa_{O_2} at greater than 50 mm Hg.

Continuous Positive Airway Pressure. Nasal prongs are used to provide a CPAP of 4 to 6 cm H_2O (7 to 8 cm H_2O in infants weighing >1500 g) in infants who cannot maintain oxygenation via hood.

Mechanical Ventilation. Intubation and ventilation are indicated if the infant requires greater than 80% oxygen with a CPAP of 10 cm H_2O. Some small infants with severe respiratory distress may require intubation and mechanical ventilation immediately after birth. Pressure ventilators are used with the initial setting listed in Table 7–7. High-frequency ventilation may be necessary in some infants in whom conventional ventilation continues to fail or in those who have severe air leaks.

Monitoring. Pulse oximetry, transcutaneous oxygen–carbon dioxide monitors, and capillary or ABG analysis are used for assessment of oxygenation and ventilation.

Chest Physical Therapy. Therapy is indicated in infants with persistent atelectasis.

Drug Therapy. Sedation (phenobarbital, lorazepam) and paralysis (pancuronium) may be necessary in infants who "fight" the ventilator.

Complications. BPD, reactive airway disease, air leaks, IVH, retinopathy of prematurity (ROP), infection, and NEC are complications often found in RDS survivors.

TABLE 7–7 Suggested Initial Settings for Time-Cycled, Pressure-Limited Ventilation

CONDITION	POSITIVE INSPIRATORY PRESSURE (cm H_2O)	POSITIVE END-EXPIRATORY PRESSURE (cm H_2O)	RATE (breaths per minute)	INSPIRATORY TIME (sec)	FLOW (L/min)
Normal compliance	10–12	2–4	10–20	0.3–0.7	5–8
RDS (IMV)	18–22	3–6	20–30	0.3–0.5	5–8
RDS (SIMV)	20–22	3–6	20–30	0.2–0.3	5–8
Meconium aspiration with atelectasis	30–60	3–6	20–40	0.5–1.0	8–12
Meconium aspiration with pulmonary hypertension	<20	2–3	40–60	0.3–0.5	5–8
Persistent pulmonary hypertension (hyperventilation)	20–25	2–4	60–100	0.3–0.5	6–10

RDS, respiratory distress syndrome; SIMV, synchronized intermittent mandatory ventilation; IMV, intermittent mandatory ventilation.

RETINOPATHY OF PREMATURITY

Once termed retrolental fibroplasia, ROP is a disorder of the newly forming retinal blood vessels that develops in premature infants weeks after birth. Vasoconstriction of the vessels results in ischemic injury and eruption of vessels into the vitreous. In the majority of patients, this process regresses spontaneously. In advanced stages, it may lead to retinal hemorrhage, fibrosis, retinal detachment, and blindness. The term retrolental fibroplasia best describes changes that occur in these late stages.

Etiology. Hyperoxia is believed to cause the vasoconstriction and obliteration of the vessels; however, other factors have been implicated in the development of ROP (Table 7–8).

Diagnosis. Diagnosis is confirmed by ophthalmoscopic examination.

Clinical Presentation. The location of damage to the retina is described in clock hours on the area of the eye. The extent and severity of ROP is identified by five stages: *Stage I:* A thin, flat, white demarcation line separates the avascular retina from the vascularized retina. *Stage II:* The line becomes a wider elevated ridge extending into the retina and vitreous. *Stage III:* Extraretinal fibrovascular proliferation is added to the ridge. *Stage IV:* Partial retinal detachment is present. *Stage V:* Total retinal detachment ensues. *Plus Disease:* A plus sign is added to the stage number of ROP to indicate that vessels posterior to the ridge have become dilated and tortuous. Although ROP in some infants regresses spontaneously, other times it suddenly and rapidly

TABLE 7–8 Risk Factors Associated With Retinopathy of Prematurity

Prematurity	Apnea
Low birth weight	Hypoxia
Oxygen therapy	Acidosis
Bradycardia	Hypercarbia
Heart disease	Infection
Blood transfusions	Respiratory distress syndrome (RDS)
Bronchopulmonary dysplasia (BPD)	Multiple births
Intraventricular hemorrhage (IVH)	Anemia

progresses to "plus disease." This is associated with a poorer outcome.

Management. Cryotherapy is used to treat Stage III or early Stage IV ROP. Complications of the procedure include apnea, bradycardia, and decreased oxygen saturation. Vitamin E (antioxidant) administration is controversial but has been reported to result in increased regression of plus disease. Side effects include sepsis, NEC, and IVH. Follow-up eye examinations by an ophthalmologist familiar with ROP are recommended.

Complications. Complications associated with ROP include myopia, strabismus, nystagmus, amblyopia, cataracts, glaucoma, retinal pigment changes, inflammation, vision in only one eye, corneal degeneration and late retinal detachment.

TRANSIENT TACHYPNEA OF THE NEWBORN

Also known as RDS, Type II and "wet lung" syndrome, TTN is a relatively benign disease characterized by tachypnea and respiratory distress that begin shortly after birth. It occurs most often in term infants who have been delivered via cesarean section.

Etiology. It is believed that TTN is the result of delayed resorption of fetal lung fluid. The fluid overload reduces lung compliance and tidal volume while increasing dead space.

Diagnosis. The diagnosis is usually made by exclusion of other causes of neonatal respiratory distress. It is similar in clinical presentation to RDS, group B streptococcal pneumonia, and PPHN.

Clinical Presentation

Physical Examination. Tachypnea (60 to 150 breaths/min) with shallow respirations is the distinguishing feature. Cyanosis, grunting, retractions, and nasal flaring may also be present.

Arterial Blood Gas Analysis. Mild to moderate hypoxemia, hypercapnia, and respiratory acidosis may occur.

Chest X-ray Findings. Chest films may reveal pulmonary vascular congestion, prominent perihilar streaking, fluid in the interlobular fissures, hyperexpansion, and flat diaphragms.

Management

Oxygen Therapy. An oxygen hood with an F_{IO_2} less than 0.4 may resolve the distress. Infants are often breathing room air within 48 hours.

Continuous Positive Airway Pressure. Nasal prongs with pressures of 3 to 5 cm H_2O may be indicated when higher FIO_2 levels are needed.

Mechanical Ventilation. Intubation and ventilation are occasionally indicated in the infant (often preterm) who is unable to clear the alveoli of fluid. Ventilator settings are usually low with peak inspiratory pressures of 18 to 22 cm H_2O, PEEP settings of 3 to 4 cm H_2O, and intermittent mandatory ventilation (IMV) rates of 15 to 20 breaths per minute. Weaning is fairly rapid, with ventilatory support rarely needed for more than 24 hours.

Complications. Although rare, air leaks occur in some infants who require mechanical ventilation.

Bibliography

Abman SH, Groothius JR: Pathophysiology and treatment of bronchopulmonary dysplasia: Current issues. Pediatr Clin North Am 1994; 41:277.

Aranda JV, Thurman T: Methylxanthines in apnea of prematurity. Clin Perinatol 1979; 6:87.

Avery GB, Glass P: Retinopathy of prematurity: What causes it. Clin Perinatol 1988; 15:917.

Avery GE, Fletcher MA, MacDonald MG: Neonatology, 4th ed. Philadelphia, JB Lippincott, 1994.

Bancalari E, Stocker JT: Bronchopulmonary Dysplasia. Washington, DC, Hemisphere Publishing Corp, 1988.

Cloutier MM: Nebulized steroid therapy in BPD. Pediatr Pulmonol 1993; 15:111.

Committee on Neonatal Ventilation/Meconium/Chest Compressions: Guidelines proposed at the Conference on Cardiopulmonary Resuscitation and Emergency Cardiac Care, Dallas, 1992. JAMA 1992; 268:2276.

Davis JM, Sinkin RA, Aranda JV: Drug therapy for BPD. Pediatr Pulmonol 1990; 8:117.

Dennehy PH: Respiratory infections in the newborn. Clin Perinatol 1987; 14:667.

Donn SM, Faix RG: Transillumination in neonatal diagnosis. Clin Perinatol 1985; 12:3.

Fanaroff AA, Martin RJ: Neonatal-Perinatal Medicine Diseases of the Fetus and Infant, 5th ed, vol II. St. Louis, Mosby-Year Book, 1992.

Farrell PM, Taussig LM: BPD and Related Chronic Respiratory Disorders: 90th Ross Conference on Pediatric Research. Columbus, OH, Ross Laboratories, 1986.

Goetzman BW: Meconium aspiration. Am J Dis Child 1992; 146:1282.

Greenough A: BPD: Early diagnosis, prophylaxis and treatment. Arch Dis Child 1990; 65:1082.

Hazinski TA: BPD. *In* Chernick V (ed): Kendig's Disorders of the Respiratory Tract in Children, 5th ed. Philadelphia, WB Saunders, 1990, pp 300–320.

Holtzman RB, Banzhaf WC, Silver RK, Hageman JR: Perinatal management of meconium staining of the amniotic fluid. Clin Perinatol 1989; 16:825.

Keens TG, Ward SLD: Apnea spells, sudden death, and the role of the apnea monitor. Pediatr Clin North Am 1993; 40:897.

Keith LG, Witter FR: Textbook of Prematurity. Boston, Little, Brown, 1993.

Kinsella JP, Abman SH: Inhalational nitric oxide therapy for persistent pulmonary hypertension of the newborn. Pediatrics 1993; 91:997.

Leistner HL: Apnea in infants and children. *In* Zimmerman S, Gildea J (eds): Critical Care Pediatrics. Philadelphia, WB Saunders, 1985.

Merritt TA, Northway WH, Boynton BR: Bronchopulmonary Dysplasia. Boston, Blackwell Scientific Publications, 1988.

Miller MJ, Martin RJ: Apnea of prematurity. Clin Perinatol 1992; 19:789.
National Institutes of Health Consensus Development Conference on Infantile Apnea and Home Monitoring. 1987. US Department of Health and Human Services. Bethesda, MD, NIH publication 87-2905.
Phelps DL: Retinopathy of prematurity. Pediatr Clin North Am 1993; 40:705.
Pomerance JJ, Richardson CJ: Neonatology for the Clinician. Norwalk, CT, Appleton & Lange, 1993.
Pramanik AK, Holtzman RB, Merritt TA: Surfactant replacement therapy for pulmonary diseases. Pediatr Clin North Am 1993; 40:913.
Roberts JD Jr, Shaul PW: Advances in the treatment of persistent pulmonary hypertension of the newborn. Pediatr Clin North Am 1993; 40:983.
Rush MC, Hazinski TA: Current therapy of BPD. Clin Perinatol 1992; 19:563.
Taeusch HW, Ballard RA, Avery ME: Schaffer and Avery's Diseases of the Newborn, 6th ed. Philadelphia, WB Saunders, 1991.
Toney SB: Apnea. *In* Fleischer GR, Ludwig S (eds): Textbook of Pediatric Emergency Medicine, 3rd ed. Baltimore, Williams & Wilkins, 1993.
Troug WE, Jackson JC: Alternative modes of ventilation in the prevention and treatment of BPD. Clin Perinatol 1992; 19:621.
Walsh-Sukys MC: Persistent pulmonary hypertension of the newborn: The black box revisited. Clin Perinatol 1993; 20:127.
Wiswell TE, Bent RC: Meconium staining and the meconium aspiration syndrome: Unresolved issues. Pediatr Clin North Am 1993; 40:955.
Yousefzadeh D, Hammerman C, Choi J, Bui K: Persistent pulmonary hypertension of the newborn: Managing the unmanageable? Clin Perinatol 1989; 16:137.

SECTION 8

Therapeutic Procedures

I. Oxygen Therapy
- A. Indications
- B. Complications
- C. Oxygen therapy delivery systems
- D. Hyperbaric oxygen therapy

II. Humidity Therapy
- A. Indications
- B. Humidity to patients on mechanical ventilation
  - 1. Heated pass-over humidifier
  - 2. Heat and moisture exchanger
  - 3. Heated wire circuits

III. Aerosol Therapy
- A. Indications
- B. Small-volume nebulizer
  - 1. Nonintubated patients
  - 2. Intubated or tracheostomized patients
- C. Metered dose inhaler
- D. Small-particle aerosol generator

IV. Incentive Spirometry
- A. Indications
- B. Contraindications
- C. Complications
- D. Procedure

V. Intermittent Positive Pressure Breathing
- A. Therapeutic goals
- B. Indications
- C. Contraindications
- D. Complications
- E. Procedure

VI. Chest Physical Therapy
- A. Indications
- B. Contraindications
- C. Complications
- D. Comparison of techniques
- E. Monitoring during therapy

VII. Surfactant Replacement Therapy
- A. History
- B. Function and composition of surfactant
- C. Types of exogenous surfactants

D. Indications
   1. Prophylaxis
   2. Rescue therapy
E. Contraindications
F. Administration
   1. Exosurf
   2. Survanta
G. Dosage frequency
H. Monitoring during therapy
I. Complications
J. Surfactant replacement therapy for other disorders

VIII. Extracorporeal Membrane Oxygenation

A. Neonatal extracorporeal membrane oxygenation
B. Pediatric extracorporeal membrane oxygenation
C. Blood flow during extracorporeal membrane oxygenation and the extracorporeal membrane oxygenation circuit
   1. Venoarterial extracorporeal membrane oxygenation
   2. Venovenous extracorporeal membrane oxygenation
D. Patient management during extracorporeal membrane oxygenation
E. Complications

Abbreviations

ACT–activated clotting times
AD–Autogenic drainage
CPAP–continuous positive airway pressure
CPT–chest physical therapy
DPPC–dipalmitoylphosphatidylcholine
ECLS–extracorporeal life support
ECMO–extracorporeal membrane oxygenation
ELSO–extracorporeal life support organization
ERV–expiratory reserve volume
ETT–endotracheal tube
FET–forced expiratory technique
HBO–hyperbaric oxygen
HFCC–high-frequency chest compression
HME–heat and moisture exchanger
IPPB–intermittent positive pressure breathing
MDI–metered dose inhaler
OI–oxygen index

PD–postural drainage
PEEP–positive end-expiratory pressure
PEP–positive expiratory pressure
PG–phosphatidylglycerol
RDS–respiratory distress syndrome
SPAG–small-particle aerosol generator
SVN–small-volume nebulizer
TLC–total lung capacity
VA–venoarterial
V_T–tidal volume
VV–venovenous

OXYGEN THERAPY

Indications

Oxygen therapy is used to prevent or relieve hypoxemia.

Complications

Table 8–1 lists complications of oxygen therapy in the neonatal and pediatric patient.

Oxygen Therapy Delivery Systems

Oxygen delivery devices are classified as either *low-flow* or *high-flow systems*. Low-flow systems may not meet the patient's inspiratory demand and the F_{IO_2} is inconsistent, depending on the patient's respiratory rate and tidal volume. High-flow systems can meet or exceed the patient's inspiratory demand and the F_{IO_2} does not change with variations in the patient's respiratory pattern (Fig. 8–1). Table 8–2 lists devices commonly used with neonatal and pediatric patients.

Hyperbaric Oxygen Therapy

Hyperbaric oxygen therapy (HBO) involves intermittent inhalation of 100% oxygen at increased atmospheric pressure. Table 8–3 lists indications for clinical use of HBO therapy and Table 8–4 lists complications of HBO administration.

HUMIDITY THERAPY

Indications

The goal of humidity therapy is to provide enough heat and humidification to the airway to approximate normal

TABLE 8–1 Complications of Oxygen Therapy in the Neonatal and Pediatric Patient

COMPLICATION	MECHANISM OF ACTION
Oxygen-induced hypoventilation	Occurs primarily in patients whose baseline Pa_{CO_2} is >50 mm Hg. Increasing Pa_{O_2} >60 mm Hg decreases stimulation of peripheral chemoreceptors, thus decreasing ventilation.
Absorption atelectasis	F_{IO_2} of 1.0 decreases N_2 partial pressures in alveoli, causing them to collapse. F_{IO_2} >0.55 creates shunt effect and worsens hypoxemia.
Retinopathy of prematurity	Increased Pa_{O_2} >100 mm Hg causes retinal vasoconstriction, which may damage endothelial cells and lead to fibrotic changes in eye tissue.
Chronic lung toxicity (BPD)	Resulting from both high F_{IO_2} and sustained high Pa_{O_2}. Biochemical products derived from oxygen reduction cause varying degrees of structural and metabolic changes within tissue cells.

N_2, nitrogen; BPD, bronchopulmonary dysplasia.

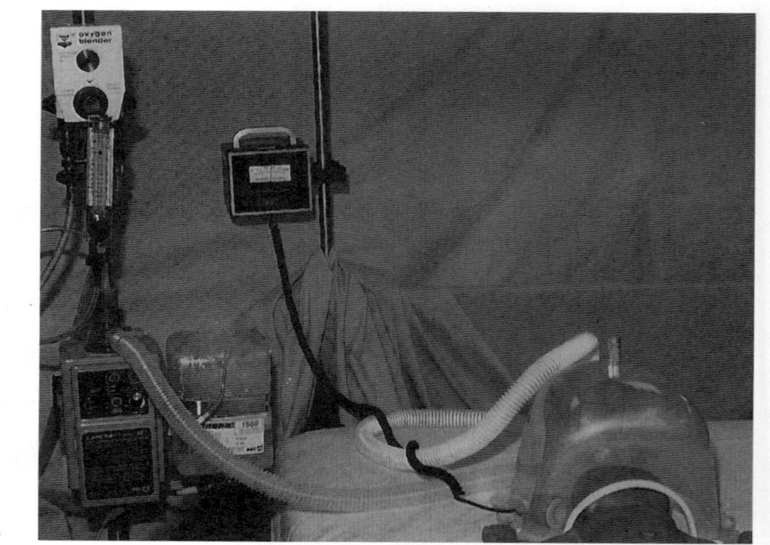

Figure 8–1 *See legend on opposite page*

inspiratory conditions. Indications for humidity therapy include:

- Humidity deficits
  - Delivery of medical gases
  - Upper airway bypassed (intubation, tracheostomy)
- Hypothermia (addition of heat to inspired air needed)
- Airways hyperreactive to inspired cold air
- Thick secretions

Humidity to Patients on Mechanical Ventilation

Patients who are being mechanically ventilated via an endotracheal tube (ETT) or tracheostomy require heated humidity therapy. Common mechanisms include (1) heated pass-over humidifiers and (2) heat and moisture exchangers.

Heated Pass-over Humidifier

Heated pass-over humidifiers direct gas over the surface of a water reservoir and collect humidity from the water that vaporizes over the surface of the reservoir chamber; some systems incorporate a wick that absorbs water from the reservoir. When using these systems on neonatal and pediatric patients, the following should be considered.

1. Temperature probes must be used in all circuits. The temperature of the gas may become excessive if the heater is left on while gas flow is stagnant in the ventilator circuit. If the temperature probe is positioned at the wye or on the expiratory limb of the ventilator circuit, heat from the exhaled gases is falsely interpreted as a higher temperature, and the servo-controlled heater reduces the temperature or turns off completely, resulting in delivery of dry gas to the patient.
2. Water supply to the humidifier may be a manual or continuous feed system. Open systems (which pour water from a bottle into the humidifier chamber) cause interruption of ventilation and may result in contamination of the humidifier or water. Continuous feed systems resupply water without opening the humidity reservoir; care must be taken not to overfill the humidifier chamber, which could lead to ventilator malfunction or patient lavage.

Figure 8–1 Infant oxygen hood with gas delivered through an oxygen blender system with heated humidification. The oxygen analyzer sensor is placed inside the hood close to the infant's head.

TABLE 8–2 Oxygen Delivery Devices and Considerations for Use in Neonatal and Pediatric Patients

DEVICE	DESCRIPTION	INDICATIONS	CONSIDERATIONS
Nasal cannula	Two soft prongs are sized to fit into the nares	Patients who require an F_{IO_2} of <0.5	F_{IO_2} is inconsistent; eating-talking does not change F_{IO_2}; blenders may be used to wean F_{IO_2} in neonates
Nasal catheter	Soft, plastic tube placed through nose into oropharynx	Patients who require an F_{IO_2} of <0.5	F_{IO_2} is inconsistent; secure to face with tape; change catheter daily
Simple mask	Mask fits over nose and mouth	Patients who require an F_{IO_2} of 0.35 to 0.6 for short times (postoperative transport)	F_{IO_2} is inconsistent; minimum flow of 6 L/min; elastic strap may cause skin irritation or uncomfortable fit
Partial rebreather	Mask with reservoir bag attached that fills with 100% oxygen and patient's exhaled gas	Patients who require an F_{IO_2} of 0.5 to 0.7	F_{IO_2} is inconsistent; set flow rate so that bag is partially inflated during inspiration; elastic strap may cause uncomfortable fit or skin irritation

Nonrebreather	Mask with reservoir bag and one-way valves to keep patient from rebreathing any exhaled gas	Patients who require an F_{IO_2} near 1.0; delivery of special gas mixes (helium-oxygen)	F_{IO_2} is inconsistent; tight fit of mask is needed to maintain high F_{IO_2}; set flow rate to keep bag partially inflated during inspiration; elastic strap may cause uncomfortable fit or skin irritation
Venturi mask	Mask with air entrained to provide high flow at a specific F_{IO_2}	Patients who require a controlled, low to moderate F_{IO_2} level	F_{IO_2} remains consistent with changes in ventilatory pattern; resistance to gas flow may cause lower gas flow and increased F_{IO_2} delivery to the patient; elastic strap may cause skin irritation and uncomfortable fit
Oxygen tent	Plastic tent that totally encloses patient's body	Patients who require cool, high humidity with an F_{IO_2} of <0.5	F_{IO_2} is inconsistent because of leaks when tent is opened for patient care; oxygen analyzer is necessary to monitor F_{IO_2}; do not allow electric toys, percussors, or vibrators in tent (fire risk from sparks); fog in tent may frighten child and also make it difficult to observe the child

Table continued on following page

TABLE 8–2 Oxygen Delivery Devices and Considerations for Use in Neonatal and Pediatric Patients *Continued*

DEVICE	DESCRIPTION	INDICATIONS	CONSIDERATIONS
Oxygen hood	Clear box or cylinder that covers the head; oxygen is delivered via blender or nebulizer	Neonates or infants requiring oxygen	Nebulizer set at 100% and oxygen or air bled in reduces noise levels in hood and makes F_{IO_2} regulation easier; blender is best for reducing noise and regulating F_{IO_2}; continuously analyze oxygen; heated humidity is necessary with neonates and infants; monitor temperature and maintain at or near body temperature; minimum flow of 7 L/minute; hoods may be placed on neonates inside an isolette

TABLE 8–3 Indications for Hyperbaric Oxygen Therapy

Decompression sickness
Iatrogenic air embolism
Carbon monoxide poisoning
Ischemic disorders
  Skin ulcers
  Crush injuries
  Clostridium myonecrosis
  Skin grafts
  Irradiated tissue

3. Tubing condensation is drained away from the patient; water traps are used when possible. Universal precautions are used and condensate is treated as infectious waste.

Heat and Moisture Exchanger

Also known as an artificial nose, a heat and moisture exchanger (HME) heats and humidifies the patient's inspired air by retaining heat and moisture from the exhaled breaths. Considerations for HME use in neonatal and small pediatric patients include the following:

1. A cuffless ETT allows heat and humidity to bypass the HME, decreasing the HME's efficiency.
2. The amount of dead space volume that an HME adds should be considered before use.
3. Circuit resistance may be increased with an HME, which may result in increased work of breathing.

TABLE 8–4 Complications Associated With Hyperbaric Oxygen Therapy

Pulmonary complications
  Oxygen toxicity
  Barotrauma (i.e., pneumothorax, embolism)
Central nervous system complications
  Seizures, convulsions
  Muscle fibrillations
Safety hazards
  Increased fire potential
Other
  Claustrophobia
  Ear or sinus barotrauma

4. An HME is removed during aerosol administration.
5. An HME is not used in patients with thick, copious, or bloody secretions.

Heated Wire Circuits

1. Heated wire circuits help to reduce tubing condensation, the amount of water wasted, and the risk of contamination (for both patient and clinician).
2. The temperature difference is set so that a few drops of condensate form near the patient connector.
3. Improper use of a heated wire circuit may result in overheating and meltdown of the circuit.
4. The circuit must not be covered with a blanket or crimped in the bedrail.

AEROSOL THERAPY

Indications

Aerosol therapy is used to

- Increase humidification
- Improve bronchial hygiene
- Deliver medication

Small-Volume Nebulizer

A small-volume nebulizer (SVN) is typically used to deliver small volumes of medication in an aerosol form. Table 8–5 lists the factors that may reduce particle deposition in the neonate and infant.

TABLE 8–5 Factors Reducing the Rate and Depth of Aerosol Particle Deposition in the Neonate and Infant

Large tongue in proportion to oral airway
Nose breathing
Narrow airway diameter
Faster respiratory rate
Small tidal volume
Inability to hold breath and coordinate inspiration
High inspiratory flow rate during respiratory distress and crying

Nonintubated Patients

The following should be considered when providing aerosol therapy to neonatal and pediatric patients who are not intubated.

1. Mouth breathing allows greater deposition. A mouthpiece is used instead of a mask in patients who can cooperate and tolerate it comfortably.
2. Laughing during a treatment encourages infants to breathe through their mouths.
3. A slow inspiratory flow rate with end-inspiration breath-holding (10 seconds optimal) improves deposition.
4. High inspiratory flow rates that occur during crying may greatly reduce aerosol deposition.
5. The strap on the mask is removed and the patient (or parent) is allowed to hold the nebulizer to his or her face (Fig. 8–2). (The strap is often uncomfortable and too "confining" for young patients.)
6. A pacifier or bottle must not be left in the patient's mouth during the therapy.

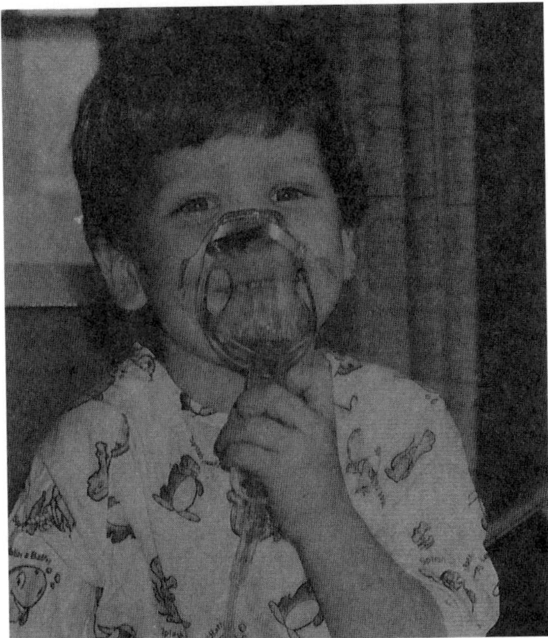

Figure 8–2 Three-year-old patient holding a nebulizer for aerosol therapy. Notice that the straps on the mask have been removed. The patient has been instructed to hold the mask firmly to his face.

Intubated or Tracheostomized Patients

The following should be considered when providing aerosol therapy to neonatal and pediatric patients who have an ETT or tracheostomy in place.

1. An ETT increases airway resistance and decreases aerosol deposition.
2. An SVN attached to an anesthesia (resuscitation) bag can deliver medication to the airways. Care must be taken to stabilize the ETT to prevent inadvertent extubation caused by the additional weight of the bag and SVN.
3. If a patient is on mechanical ventilation and SVN therapy is provided via an anesthesia bag, the same pressure, rate, and F_{IO_2} should be used.
4. An occasional sigh with a slight inspiratory hold may enhance the volume and depth of medication delivered.
5. When SVN therapy is provided in-line through a ventilator circuit, a large amount of aerosol deposits in the circuit and proximal airway. The nebulizer should be placed in the inspiratory limb of the circuit approximately 10 to 20 cm back from the wye.
6. Continuous nebulizer flow may increase the tidal volume (V_T), inspiratory pressure, and expiratory resistance during mechanical ventilation. It may also alter the performance of any mode of ventilation (e.g., pressure support).
7. When placing an SVN in-line with a time-cycled pressure-limited ventilator, the flow rate on the ventilator may need to be decreased to allow for the increased continuous flow from the nebulizer (check each ventilator's manual for specifics).

Metered Dose Inhaler

The correct use of a metered dose inhaler (MDI) is described in Table 8–6. Proper patient instruction is essential, and several repeated instruction sessions usually improve performance. Figure 8–3 illustrates how to estimate the contents of an MDI cannister. The use of a holding chamber or spacer should be encouraged in pediatric patients (Fig. 8–4).

Small-Particle Aerosol Generator

The small-particle aerosol generator (SPAG) (ICN Pharmaceuticals Inc., Costa Mesa, CA) is manufactured for the administration of the antiviral agent ribavirin. It consists of a nebulizer that produces an aerosol and a drying chamber that reduces particle size and transports the particles to the patient. The SPAG may be used with a mask, hood, tent, or ventilator. Ribavirin is administered continuously for 12

TABLE 8–6 The Seven-Step Technique for Using a Metered Dose Inhaler

Warm and shake the MDI vigorously
Hold MDI upright
Place mouthpiece 4 cm away from mouth
Exhale normally
Inhale slowly and deeply
Spray MDI as intubation begins
Hold breath 5 to 10 seconds
Exhale slowly
Note: Wait 1 minute between each spray of medication

MDI, metered dose inhaler.

to 18 hours each day and is repeated for 3 to 7 consecutive days. The following steps are taken to protect the clinician from exposure to the drug.

1. Therapy is provided in a negative pressure, single-patient room with six air exchanges per hour ventilated to the outside or with a local exhaust ventilation through a high-efficiency particulate air filter.
2. The aerosol is contained by
    - Using a canopy over the delivery device
    - Using a scavenging system for spontaneously breathing patients (Fig. 8–5)
    - Filtering the expiratory limb of the ventilator circuit when used with a mechanical ventilator
3. The ETT is fitted with a minimal amount of air leakage to limit environmental contamination with ribavirin.
4. The nebulizer is turned off 5 minutes prior to opening the tent or hood and 1 minute before disconnecting the ventilator.
5. Clinicians who have substantial contact with the drug are required to wear protective equipment (i.e., goggles, respiratory masks, gown, gloves).
6. Pregnant or lactating women are prevented from having contact with the drug.
7. Tandem filters are used at the end of the expiratory limb of the ventilator circuit before gas reenters the ventilator.
8. A water seal pop-off valve and one-way valve are used between the SPAG and the point of entry into the ventilator circuit immediately distal to the output of the humidifier. The level is set slightly greater than the positive end-expiratory pressure (PEEP) or continuous positive

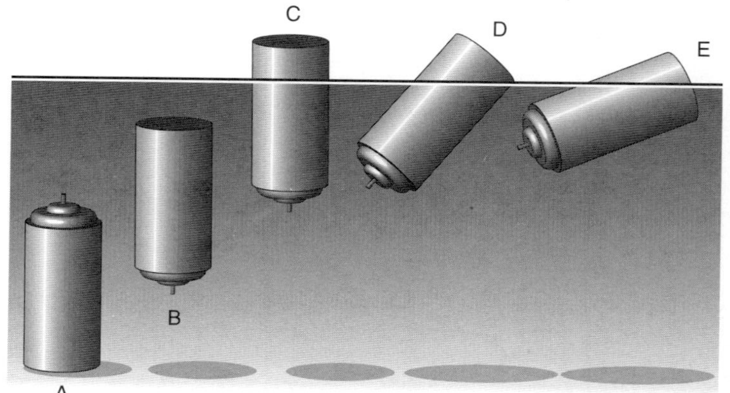

Figure 8–3 To determine the contents of an MDI canister, the canister is placed into a bowl of water. *A,* If it sinks to the bottom, it is full. *B,* If it floats under the surface, it is three-quarters full. *C,* If it floats upright on the surface, it is one-half full. *D,* If it floats sideways at a 45-degree angle on the surface, it is one-quarter full. *E,* If it floats sideways on the surface, it is empty.

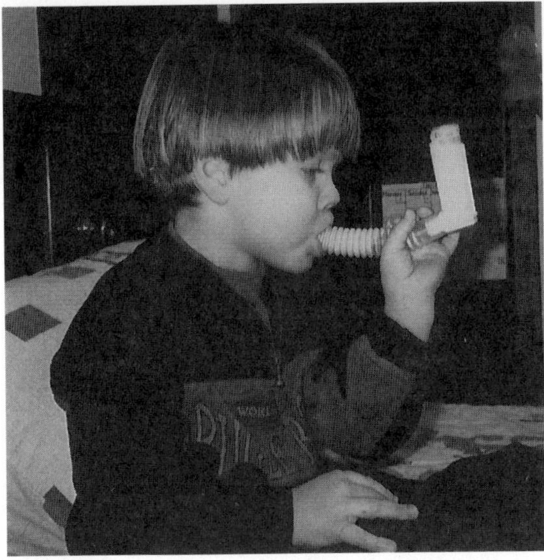

Figure 8–4 A 4-year-old patient using corrugated aerosol tubing as a spacer device with an MDI.

airway pressure (CPAP) level to prevent excessive V_T delivery during ventilator inflations.

9. A high-pressure alarm is provided on the inspiratory side of the ventilator circuit.
10. When using a time-cycled pressure-limited ventilator, the flow of the SPAG is added to the total flow of the patient. Flow of the ventilator and drying chamber must be adjusted to optimize ventilation.

INCENTIVE SPIROMETRY

Indications

Table 8–7 lists clinical conditions that may benefit from incentive spirometry. For incentive spirometry to be effective in the pediatric patient, he or she must be able to breathe volumes exceeding his or her normal V_T.

Contraindications

Incentive spirometry is contraindicated in patients who cannot cooperate or follow instructions concerning proper use of the device.

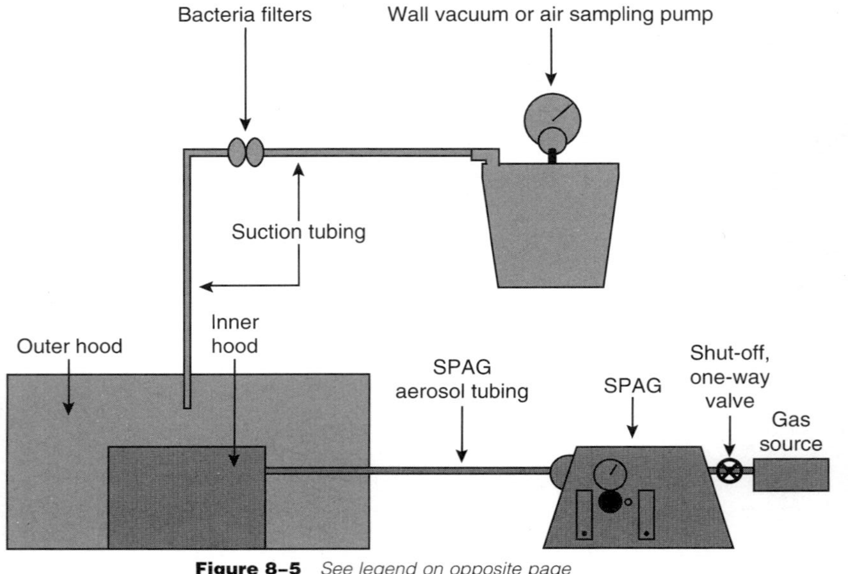

Figure 8–5 *See legend on opposite page*

TABLE 8–7 Indications for Incentive Spirometry

Abdominal surgery
Thoracic surgery
Surgery in patients with pulmonary disease
Atelectasis
Restrictive lung defects associated with quadriplegia
Restrictive lung defects associated with a dysfunctional diaphragm

Complications

- Hyperventilation
- Fatigue
- Pain
- Bronchospasm (if the patient exhales forcefully)
- Airway closure (if the patient exhales forcefully)
- Hypoxia (if oxygen therapy is interrupted during the procedure)

Procedure

1. The procedure and its purpose are thoroughly explained to the patient and parents. The teaching session is conducted preoperatively if possible.
2. The patient is positioned sitting upright if possible.
3. The chest is auscultated and the volume goal is set on the incentive device.
4. The patient is instructed to exhale normally, place his or her mouth tightly around the mouthpiece, inhale slowly and deeply, and hold the breath at end-inspiration for 3 to 5 seconds.
5. A short time to rest is allowed between maneuvers.
6. The patient is encouraged and assisted with coughing. A pillow or folded blanket is placed over the incision area to splint the area during coughs.
7. Breath sounds are reassessed after coughing, and the patient (and parents) are encouraged to perform the maneuvers independently between scheduled treatment sessions.

Figure 8–5 Double-containment system for safe administration of ribavirin. Two scavenger units with high-efficiency particulate air filters reduce the clinician's exposure to ribavirin by evacuating the space between the hood and the tent.

INTERMITTENT POSITIVE PRESSURE BREATHING

Therapeutic Goals

Intermittent positive pressure breathing (IPPB) is felt to be effective if the following goals are met:

- V_T during IPPB is greater than 25% of the spontaneous V_T
- Increased peak flow or FEV_1
- Effective cough
- Secretion clearance
- Improved breath sounds
- Improved chest radiograph

Indications

IPPB is indicated most often in the older patient who needs increased lung expansion but has failed to respond to other lung volume expansion therapies (e.g., these patients may have neuromuscular disease or chest wall deformity inhibiting inspiratory efforts).

Contraindications

Contraindications to IPPB therapy in infants and children are listed in Table 8–8.

Complications

Complications associated with IPPB therapy are listed in Table 8–9.

Procedure

1. The procedure and its purpose are explained to the patient and parents. The machine is manually cycled on and the patient is allowed to listen to the sound of the gas flow. The patient is also allowed to examine the mouthpiece (or mask) and circuit.
2. The patient is positioned in an upright position if possible.
3. Therapy is begun at a low pressure (10 cm H_2O) and is gradually increased to the desired level. The gas flow rate is set according to the individual patient's needs. Sensitivity may need to be increased for patients using a mask or mouthseal.
4. The patient's heart rate, respiratory rate, and breath sounds are monitored prior to, during, and after the treat-

TABLE 8–8 Contraindications to Intermittent Positive Pressure Breathing Therapy

ABSOLUTE
Tension pneumothorax
RELATIVE
Uncooperative patient with uncoordinated breathing
Intracranial pressure >15 mm Hg
Recent facial, oral, or skull surgery
Tracheoesophageal fistula
Recent esophageal surgery
Active hemoptysis
Active, untreated tuberculosis
Radiographic evidence of blebs
Hemodynamic instability
Nausea
Air swallowing
Inexperienced clinician

ment. The patient's spontaneous V_T is determined prior to therapy and the V_T is monitored several times during therapy (or continuously with a spirometer attached to the machine) to determine if lung volume is being augmented.

CHEST PHYSICAL THERAPY

Chest physical therapy (CPT) is used to prevent and clear pulmonary secretions that cannot be removed with normal clearance mechanisms. The goals of CPT also include the prevention of lung collapse due to mucus plugging. The severity of the patient's illness and his or her ability to tolerate the techniques determine the extent of the therapy required.

Indications

CPT is indicated when there is acute or chronic excessive secretion production or mucus plugging of large airways that does not clear with coughing or suctioning. Table 8–10 lists common clinical indications in the neonatal and pediatric population.

TABLE 8–9 Complications Associated With Intermittent Positive Pressure Breathing

Bronchospasm
Gastric distention and ileus
Nosocomial infection
Decreased venous return
Hyperventilation
Hypocarbia
Hypoventilation
Impaction of secretions
Fatigue
Air trapping
Barotrauma, pneumothorax
Increased airway resistance
Hemoptysis
Hyperoxia
Reduction of respiratory drive in patients with COPD
Increased ventilation-perfusion mismatch
Psychologic dependence

COPD, chronic obstructive pulmonary disease.

Contraindications

Disorders in which CPT may be contraindicated are listed in Table 8–11. Therapy modification may be required in some patients because of various medical or surgical factors.

Complications

Complications associated with CPT techniques are listed in Table 8–12.

Comparison of Techniques

CPT consists of techniques designed to remove secretions from the lungs (Table 8–13). The various techniques used are discussed.

Postural Drainage (PD). PD is a technique in which the patient is placed in various positions while gravity is used to move secretions from the peripheral airways to larger

TABLE 8–10 Indications for Chest Physical Therapy

Disorders resulting in hypersecretion and sputum retention
- Cystic fibrosis
- Bronchitis
- Bronchiectasis
- Asthma
- Pneumonia

Inability to cough effectively resulting in sputum retention
- Tracheostomy
- Endotracheal intubation
- Neuromuscular disease or injury

Before and after abdominal or chest surgery in patients with lung disorders

Acute lobar atelectasis due to mucus plugging

bronchi. Figures 8–6 and 8–7 illustrate the positions used during drainage in children and infants.

Percussion. With the patient in various drainage positions, the chest wall is percussed using a cupped hand or a mechanical device.

Vibration. With the patient in various drainage positions, both of the clinician's hands are placed (one on top of the other) over the patient's chest and vibrations are produced by tensing and contracting the shoulder and arm muscles.

Forced Expiratory Technique (FET). The patient forcibly exhales with an open glottis from a mid- to low-lung volume. (FET is also known as "huff coughing.") The maneuver is repeated several times, followed by coughs. It may be used alone or with other CPT techniques.

Positive Expiratory Pressure (PEP). An expiratory resistor device is used to generate positive airway pressure during active expiration. PEP may be used with or without postural drainage.

Autogenic Drainage (AD). AD is a series of breathing exercises: (1) beginning with slow, controlled breathing at the expiratory reserve volume (ERV) level, (2) the volume is increased with a normal V_T range and exhalation halfway into ERV, and (3) the depth of inspiration is increased to TLC while exhalation remains halfway into ERV.

High-Frequency Chest Compression (HFCC). Intermittent chest wall compressions at high frequencies are pro-

TABLE 8–11 Contraindications to Chest Physical Therapy

ABSOLUTE CONTRAINDICATIONS
Frank hemoptysis
Empyema
Foreign body aspiration
Untreated tension pneumothorax
Severe asthma exacerbation
Displaced fractured ribs
RELATIVE CONTRAINDICATIONS
Unstable cardiac status
Cardiac arrhythmias
Immediate postoperative period following tracheostomy
Immediate postoperative period following tracheobronchial reconstruction
Low platelet count (<50,000 cells/mm^3)
MODIFIED POSITIONING REQUIRED
Increased intracranial pressure
Hypertension
Abdominal distention
Compromised diaphragm movement
Continuous feedings
Chest tube or gastrostomy tube in place
Severe gastroesophageal reflux
Premature neonates at risk of intraventricular hemorrhage

duced via a snug-fitting inflatable vest connected to a high-performance air compressor.

Monitoring During Therapy

The following should be monitored in patients receiving CPT:

- Oxygen saturation (via pulse oximetry)
- Heart rate

TABLE 8–12 Complications Associated With Chest Physical Therapy

Hypoxemia
Tachypnea
Increasing dyspnea
Rib fractures
Positional hypotension or hypertension
V/Q alterations from postural changes
Atelectasis
Bronchospasm
Increased oxygen consumption
Increase in gastroesophageal reflux episodes
Vomiting
Aspiration
Increased intracranial pressure
Increase in intraventricular hemorrhage
Bruising
Cyanosis
Hemorrhage (high risk in patients with recent tracheostomy or prosthetic cardiac patch)
Inadvertent extubation or main stem intubation
Displaced tube (chest or gastrostomy)
Cardiac arrhythmias

- Respiratory rate
- Breathing pattern
- Skin color
- Breath sounds

Measures are taken to prevent heat loss while performing CPT on infants in a temperature-regulated environment (e.g., isolette).

SURFACTANT REPLACEMENT THERAPY

History

Surface tension abnormalities were recognized as factors in neonatal lung expansion in the 1940s. In the mid-1950s, the existence of lung surfactant was reported. This was followed in 1959 with Avery and Mead's reporting that respiratory distress syndrome (RDS) in infants resulted from a

Text continued on page 266

TABLE 8–13 Comparison of Chest Physical Therapy Techniques

Technique	Comments
Postural drainage	Maintain each position for 1–5 minutes if percussion or vibration is included; hold positions longer if drainage alone is provided; keep patient in bed (not on lap) during therapy if patient is mechanically ventilated or has multiple tubes or intravenous lines in place
Percussion	Do not percuss over the spine, sternum, bony prominences, last few ribs, abdomen, sutured areas, kidneys, liver, and below rib cage
Vibration	Perform while the patient exhales
Forced expiratory technique	May be more effective in older children who require less supervision; may be more effective if used with positive expiratory pressure therapy; cannot be used in infants and small children; interspersed with deep relaxed breathing; may prevent bronchospasm and promote a more effective cough
Positive expiratory pressure	Effective in mobilizing secretions in cystic fibrosis patients; cannot be used in infants and small children
Autogenic drainage	Cannot be used in infants and small children
High-frequency chest compression	Does not require patient to perform postural drainage; may decrease the risk of dynamic airway collapse in patients with cystic fibrosis or bronchiectasis; bears little resemblance to manual percussion; requires commercially made vest that must be snug-fitting; financial arrangements must be made before home use is possible

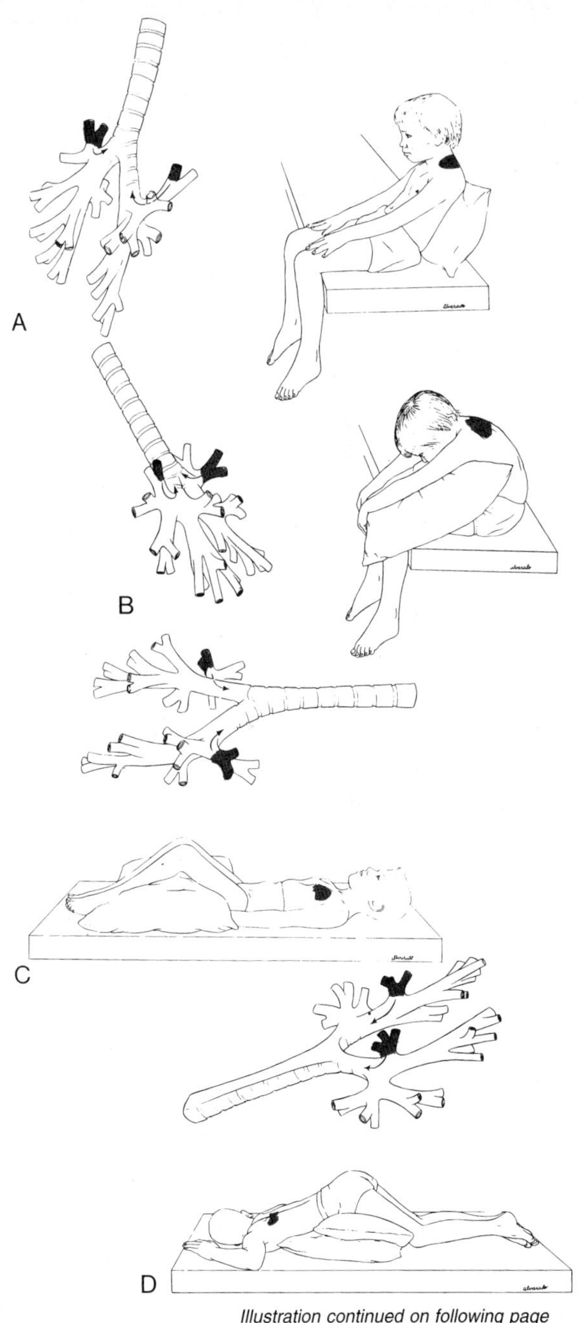

Illustration continued on following page

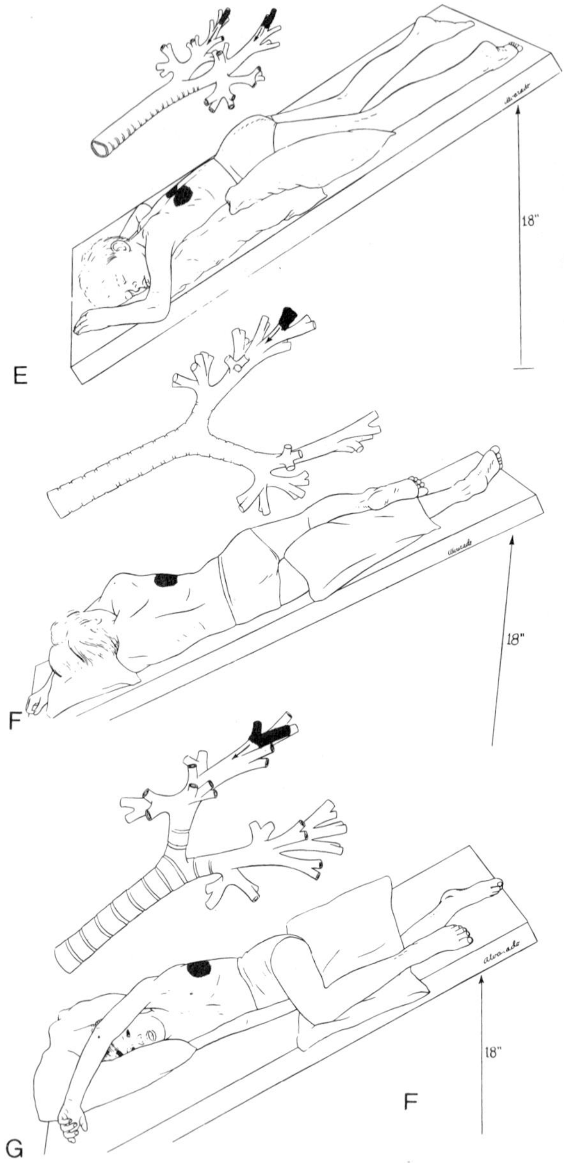

18"

E

18"

F

18"

F

G

Illustration continued on opposite page

Figure 8–6 Postural drainage positions for the child or adult. The model of the tracheobronchial tree above the child illustrates the segmental bronchi being drained. The stippled area over the child's

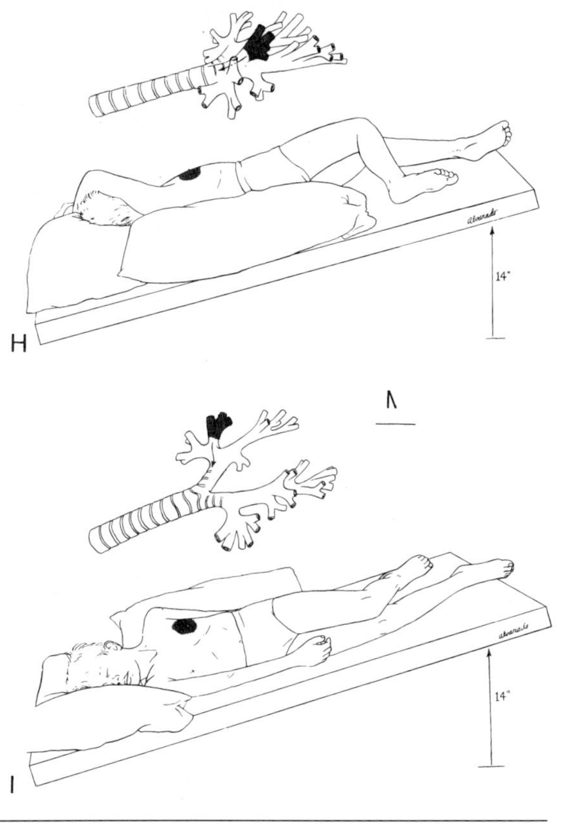

chest illustrates the area to be percussed or vibrated. The area is described in the parentheses. *A,* Apical segment of right upper lobe; apical subsegment of apical-posterior segment of left upper lobe (area between the clavicle and top of the scapula). *B,* Posterior segment of right upper lobe; posterior subsegment of apical-posterior segment of left upper lobe (area over the upper back). *C,* Anterior segments of right and left upper lobes (area between clavicle and nipple). *D,* Superior segments of both lower lobes (area over middle of back at tip of scapula, beside spine). *E,* Posterior basal segments of both lower lobes (area over lower rib cage, beside spine). *F,* Lateral basal segment of right lower lobe. Segment on left is drained in a similar fashion but with the right side down (area over middle portion of rib cage). *G,* Anterior basal segment of left lower lobe. Segment on right is drained in a similar fashion but with the left side down (area over lower ribs, below the armpit). *H,* Right middle lobe (area over right nipple; below breast in developing females). *I,* Left lingular segment of lower lobe (area over left nipple; below breast in developing females). (From Waring WW: Diagnostic and therapeutic procedures. *In* Chernick V [ed]: Kendig's Disorders of the Respiratory Tract in Children, 5th ed. Philadelphia, WB Saunders, 1990, pp 84–85.)

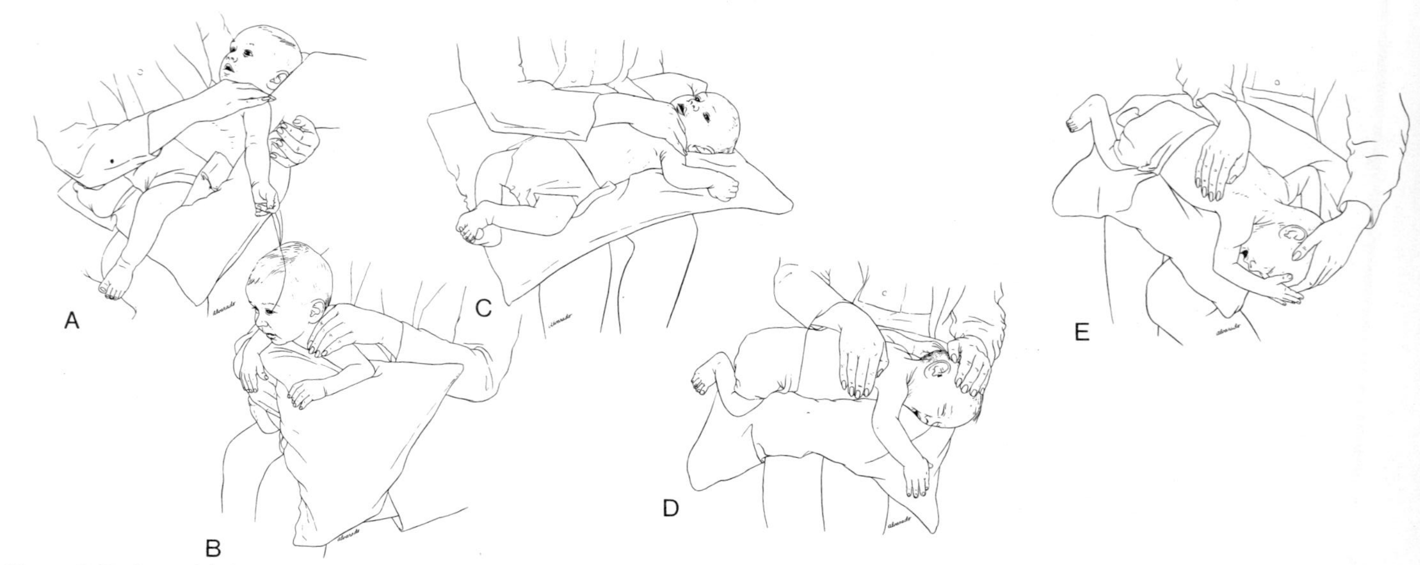

Figure 8–7 Postural drainage positions for infants. *A,* Apical segment of the right upper lobe, and apical subsegment of the apical-posterior segment of the left upper lobe. *B,* Posterior segment of the right upper lobe and posterior subsegment of the apical-posterior segment of the left upper lobe. *C,* Anterior segments of right and left upper lobes. *D,* Superior segments of both lower lobes. *E,* Posterior basal segments of both

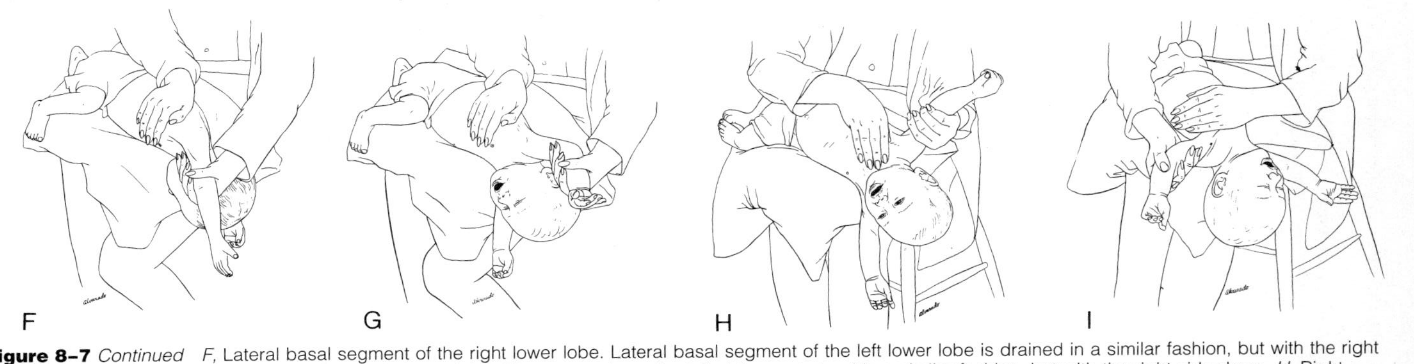

Figure 8–7 *Continued* *F,* Lateral basal segment of the right lower lobe. Lateral basal segment of the left lower lobe is drained in a similar fashion, but with the right side down, *G,* Anterior basal segment of the right lower lobe. The segments on the left side are drained in a similar fashion, but with the right side down. *H,* Right middle lobe. *I,* Left lingular segment of lower lobe. (From Waring WW: Diagnostic and therapeutic procedures. *In* Chernick V [ed]: Kendig's Disorders of the Respiratory Tract in Children, 5th ed. Philadelphia, WB Sanders, 1990, pp 86–87.)

deficiency of alveolar surfactant. In 1961, dipalmitoylphosphatidylcholine (DPPC) was discovered to be the major surface-active phospholipid in natural surfactant. Aerosolized DPPC was used in the treatment of RDS but was found to be ineffective when used alone. In the 1970s it was determined that natural surfactant is a complex substance with several proteins critical to its function. It was not until 1980, when Fujiwara and colleagues reported that a mixture of bovine surfactant and synthetic lipids improved oxygenation and ventilator settings in preterm infants, that the interest in surfactant replacement rose again. Widespread clinical trials of various exogenous surfactants that began in the late 1980s have resulted in the Food and Drug Administration's approval of a commercially available synthetic surfactant (Exosurf) and a modified natural surfactant (Survanta).

Function and Composition of Surfactant

Surfactant lowers alveolar surface tension and stabilizes the alveolar volume, reducing the alveoli's tendency to collapse at low lung volumes. This maintains a residual volume of gas in the lungs and increases the functional residual capacity and alveolar surface area. Surfactant is composed of the following:

- Phospholipids
  - Phosphatidylcholine (DPPC or lecithin)
  - Phosphatidylglycerol (PG)
  - Phosphatidylinositol and phosphatidylserine
  - Phosphatidylethanolamine
  - Sphingomyelin
- Neutral lipids
  - Cholesterol
  - Free fatty acids
- Surfactant-associated proteins
  - SP-A (surfactant protein A)
  - SP-B (surfactant protein B)
  - SP-C (surfactant protein C)
  - SP-D (surfactant protein D)

Types of Exogenous Surfactants

Table 8–14 lists the source and components of the various exogenous surfactants that have been used in the treatment of RDS in infants.

Indications

There are currently two indications for surfactant replacement.

TABLE 8–14 Types of Exogenous Surfactant

SURFACTANT	SOURCE	COMPONENTS
Human surfactant	Human amniotic fluid	SP-A, SP-B, SP-C
Curosurf	Pig lungs	DPPC, SP-B, SP-C
CLSE (calf lung surfactant extract)	Calf lungs	DPPC, SP-B, SP-C
Survanta*	Cow lungs	DPPC, SP-B, SP-C, palmitic acid, tripalmitin
Exosurf*	Artificial (synthetic)	DPPC, tyloxapol, hexadecanol
ALEC (artificial lung expanding compound)	Artificial (synthetic)	DPPC, PG

* Currently approved by the Food and Drug Administration and commercially available.
DPPC, dipalmitoylphosphatidylcholine; SP-A, surfactant-associated protein A; SP-B, surfactant-associated protein B; SP-C, surfactant-associated protein C; PG, phosphatidylglycerol.

Prophylaxis

When given as a preventive agent, surfactant is administered before the onset of RDS (at or shortly after birth) in infants who are at high risk for the development of RDS. This includes those with

- Low birth weight (<1300 g)
- Gestational age of less than 32 weeks
- Laboratory evidence of surfactant deficiency
    - A lecithin : sphingomyelin ratio of less than 2 : 1
    - Absence of PG
    - Bubble stability test indicating lung immaturity

Rescue Therapy

After the diagnosis of RDS has been made, rescue therapy is given to infants who have clinical and radiologic evidence of RDS:

- Increased work of breathing

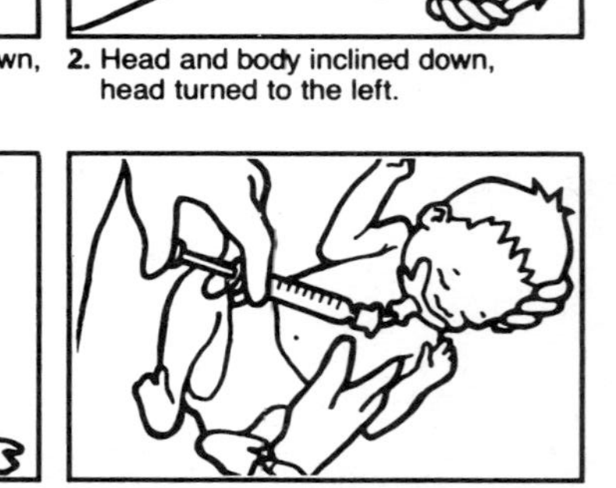

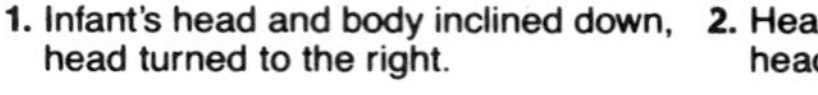

1. Infant's head and body inclined down, head turned to the right.

2. Head and body inclined down, head turned to the left.

3. Head and body inclined up, head turned to the right.

4. Head and body inclined up, head turned to the left.

Figure 8–8 *See legend on opposite page*

- Increased oxygen requirements
- Endotracheal intubation and assisted ventilation
- Chest radiograph characteristic of RDS

Contraindications

Surfactant replacement therapy is generally not given to infants who have

- Evidence of fetal lung maturity
- Major congenital or chromosomal anomalies considered to be incompatible with life

Administration

Administration varies with the type of surfactant used.

Exosurf

1. Exosurf is delivered through a side port adaptor that fits into the ETT.
2. It is given as a 5-ml/kg bolus over 5 minutes.
3. Positive pressure ventilation is maintained during instillation.
4. The infant is placed supine in the midline position for the first half-dose. Midway through dosing, the infant is turned 45 degrees to the right for 30 seconds, after which he or she is returned to the midline position and the second half-dose is given. The infant is then turned 45 degrees to the left for 30 seconds.

Survanta

1. Survanta is thawed before use by being kept at room temperature for 20 minutes or by being held in the hand for at least 8 minutes.
2. It is delivered through a 5 French end-hole catheter (feeding tube) with the tip placed just beyond the end of the ETT (above the carina).
3. It is given as a 4-ml/kg dose.
4. One-quarter doses are given in the positions illustrated in Figure 8–8.
5. Positive pressure ventilation is maintained after each one-quarter dose is administered.

Figure 8–8 Positioning of infant for instillation of Survanta exogenous surfactant. (Used with permission of Ross Products Division, Abbott Laboratories. Columbus, OH 43216. From Clinical Education Aid, ©1970 Ross Products Division, Abbott Laboratories.)

Dosage Frequency

The frequency of surfactant replacement depends on the patient's clinical status. A total of four additional doses can be given within the first 48 hours, no sooner than 6 hours apart, if the infant remains on mechanical ventilation and requires an FIO_2 of 0.3 or greater.

Monitoring During Therapy

Table 8–15 lists the variables that should be monitored during surfactant replacement therapy.

TABLE 8–15 Monitoring During Surfactant Replacement Therapy

VARIABLES MONITORED DURING ADMINISTRATION
Oxygenation (pulse oximetry or transcutaneous monitoring)
Heart rate
Respiratory rate
Blood pressure
Chest expansion
Skin color
Placement and position of delivery device (catheter, tube)
FIO_2
Ventilator settings
Reflux of surfactant into ETT
VARIABLES MONITORED AFTER ADMINISTRATION
Arterial blood gas values
Heart rate
Respiratory rate
Blood pressure
Skin color
Chest expansion
Breath sounds
FIO_2
Ventilator settings
Pulmonary mechanics
Lung volumes
Chest radiograph

ETT, endotracheal tube.

TABLE 8–16 Complications Associated With Surfactant Replacement Therapy

Pulmonary hemorrhage
Apnea
Mucus plugging
Bradycardia
Tachycardia
Decreased oxygen saturation
Barotrauma resulting from increased lung compliance following surfactant replacement and failure to change ventilator settings accordingly
Reflux of surfactant into the oropharynx or nasopharynx
Nosocomial infection

Complications

Complications associated with surfactant replacement therapy are listed in Table 8–16.

Surfactant Replacement Therapy for Other Disorders

Exogenous surfactant therapy is being investigated for use in the following disorders:

- Adult respiratory distress syndrome
- Congenital pneumonias
- Meconium aspiration

EXTRACORPOREAL MEMBRANE OXYGENATION

Extracorporeal circulation is the technique of supporting the function of the heart or lungs, or both, with external artificial organs. This support is known as extracorporeal membrane oxygenation (ECMO) or extracorporeal life support (ECLS).

Neonatal Extracorporeal Membrane Oxygenation

Neonatal disorders treated with ECMO are listed in Table 8–17. The decision to institute ECMO depends largely on the selection criteria that each individual ECMO center has

TABLE 8–17 Neonatal Disorders Treated With Extracorporeal Membrane Oxygenation
Meconium aspiration syndrome
Congenital diaphragmatic hernia
Persistent pulmonary hypertension of the newborn
Sepsis
Pneumonia
Respiratory distress syndrome
Air leak syndrome

established. Table 8–18 lists selection criteria commonly used in ECMO centers. The oxygen index (OI) is currently the most widely accepted predictor of mortality in neonates with respiratory failure on conventional ventilators. An OI greater than 40 is indicative of greater than 80% mortality.

$$OI = \frac{MAP \times F\text{IO}_2}{Pa\text{O}_2} \times 100$$

Pediatric Extracorporeal Membrane Oxygenation

ECMO in pediatric patients has been indicated most often in those whose condition was potentially reversible and in whom death was certain otherwise. Table 8–19 lists the disorders in which ECMO may be employed. Although it is impossible to provide specific recommendations for the institution of ECMO in older patients, the selection criteria

TABLE 8–18 Neonatal Extracorporeal Life Support Selection Criteria
Oxygen index >40
No major cardiac defect
Reversible lung disease
Gestational age >33 weeks
Mechanical ventilation <14 days
No major intraventricular hemorrhage
No significant coagulopathy or bleeding complications (relative contraindication)

TABLE 8–19 Pediatric Disorders Treated With Extracorporeal Membrane Oxygenation
Pneumonia
Viral
Bacterial
Adult respiratory distress syndrome
Aspiration
Intrapulmonary hemorrhage
Pneumocystis
Cardiac failure following heart surgery

provided by the University of Michigan are suggested as guidelines (Table 8–20).

Blood Flow During Extracorporeal Membrane Oxygenation and the Extracorporeal Membrane Oxygenation Circuit

Blood flow through a typical venoarterial (VA) ECMO circuit is illustrated in Figure 8–9. The circuit begins and ends with the cannulas. Blood is drained by gravity from the venous cannula to the bladder box system. This consists of a small reservoir situated between the patient and the pump. Fluids and heparin are infused here. The pump serves to maintain blood flow through the circuit. The blood is pumped through the membrane oxygenator where a sweep gas provides a constant fresh source gas of oxygen and constantly flushes out diffused carbon dioxide. The last component of the circuit is the heat exchanger, which warms the blood and maintains the body temperature immediately before the blood is reinfused into the patient.

Venoarterial Extracorporeal Membrane Oxygenation

In VA ECMO, a venous cannula is inserted into the right internal jugular vein and blood is drained from the right atrium (Fig. 8–10). The cannula has port holes that open at the end, and it removes blood from the right atrium. The blood then flows through the ECMO circuit. An arterial cannula inserted in the right common carotid artery serves to reinfuse the oxygenated blood into the aortic arch.

Venovenous Extracorporeal Membrane Oxygenation

In venovenous (VV) ECMO, a double-lumen cannula is inserted into the right atrium via the right internal jugular

TABLE 8–20 University of Michigan Pediatric and Adult Extracorporeal Membrane Oxygenation Criteria

INDICATIONS	
Poor gas exchange despite "optimal" ventilator and pharmacologic therapy	
Age <60 years	
Ventilator support <6 days	
Neurologic status responsive	
Oxygenation decreased:	shunt >30% $Pa_{O_2}/F_{IO_2} \leq 100$
and/or	
CO_2 clearance decreased:	Pa_{CO_2} >45 mm Hg despite minute ventilation >0.2 L/kg

CONTRAINDICATIONS

Relative	Absolute
Ventilator support 6–10 days	Ventilator >10 days
Immunosuppression	Septic shock
Systemic sepsis	Cardiac arrest
Active bleeding	Brain injury
	Terminal disease
	Metabolic acidosis (base deficit >5 mEq/L for 12 hours)

From Bartlett RH: Extracorporeal Life Support Manual for Adult and Pediatric Patients. Ann Arbor, MI, University of Michigan Medical Center, 1993.

vein. The cannula has two lumens. One is used to drain blood from the right atrium. This blood flows through the ECMO circuit. The other lumen is used to reinfuse the oxygenated blood into the right atrium. A comparison of the VA and VV systems is presented in Table 8–21.

Patient Management During Extracorporeal Membrane Oxygenation

Various factors are monitored during ECMO. The main goal of ECMO is to provide adequate oxygen delivery. This

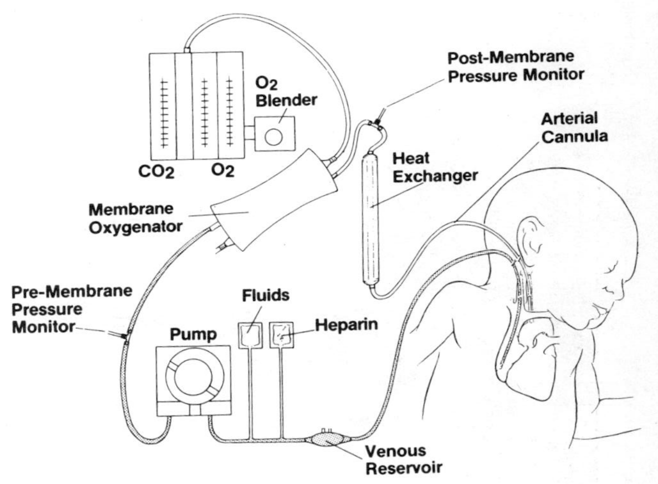

Figure 8–9 Circuit for extracorporeal life support. (From Short BL: Physiology of extracorporeal membrane oxygenation. *In* Polin RA, Fox WW [eds]: Fetal and Neonatal Physiology. Philadelphia, WB Saunders, 1992.)

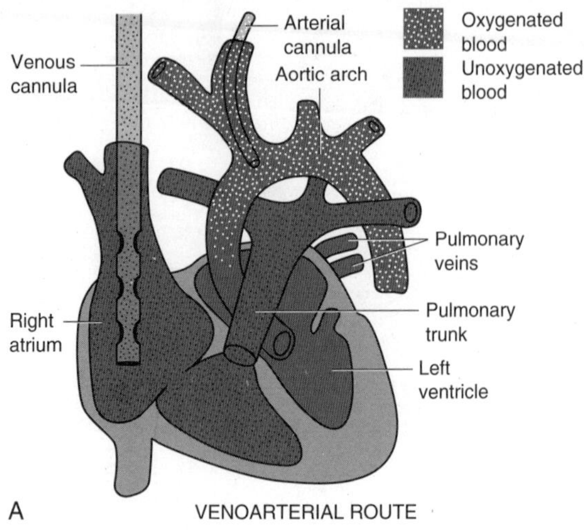

A VENOARTERIAL ROUTE

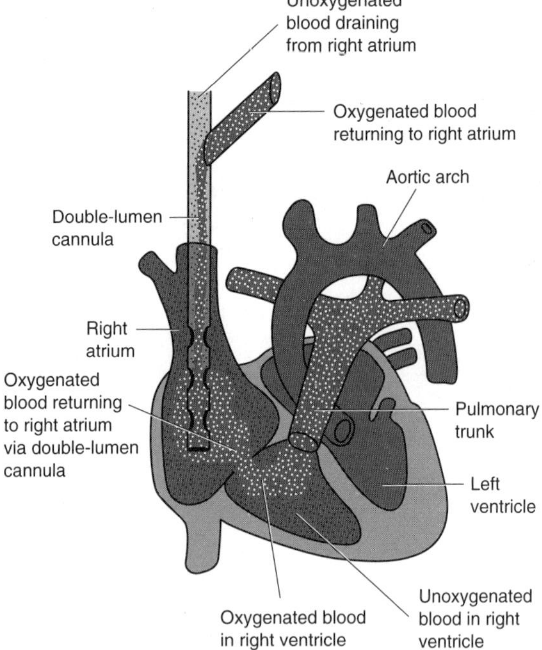

B VENOVENOUS ROUTE

Figure 8–10 Illustration of mechanisms of blood flow during extracorporeal membrane oxygenation (ECMO). In the venoarterial route, blood is removed from the right atrium via a cannula inserted in the right internal jugular vein. Oxygenated blood is returned to the aortic arch via a cannula in the right common carotid artery. In the venovenous route, blood is also removed from the right atrium via a cannula inserted in the right internal jugular vein, but the oxygenated blood is returned to the venous circulation.

TABLE 8–21 Advantages and Disadvantages of Venovenous and Venoarterial Extracorporeal Life Support

VENOVENOUS EXTRACORPOREAL LIFE SUPPORT	VENOARTERIAL EXTRACORPOREAL LIFE SUPPORT
Advantages	**Advantages**
Sparing of carotid artery	Provides cardiac support
Preservation of pulsatile flow	Excellent gas exchange
Normal pulmonary blood flow	Rapid stabilization
Perfusion of lungs with oxygenated blood	**Disadvantages**
Perfusion of coronaries with oxygenated blood	Carotid artery ligation
Avoidance of infusion of possible emboli directly into arterial circulation	Nonpulsatile flow
Central venous pressure accurate	Reduced pulmonary blood flow
Selective limb perfusion does not occur	Lower myocardial oxygen delivery
Disadvantages	Direct infusion of possible emboli into arterial circulation
No cardiac support	Central venous pressure inaccurate
Lower systemic PaO_2	
Recirculation issues	

is assessed by monitoring the SvO_2 via a catheter inserted into the circuit and by monitoring the SaO_2 via pulse oximetry. The FIO_2 and flow rate of the sweep gas are monitored and adjusted.

Heparin is administered to prevent clotting within the circuit, and activated clotting times are monitored to assess heparin administration. Because platelets are continuously consumed during ECMO, they are administered daily directly to the patient or into the circuit. Guidelines concerning the blood components are listed in Table 8–22.

Patients are sedated while on ECMO to prevent accidental decannulation or hypertension secondary to agitation and to provide comfort. Because of the high risk of intraventricular hemorrhage, daily head ultrasounds are performed. The

TABLE 8–22 Hematologic Guidelines for Extracorporeal Life Support

Hematocrit:	>38 ml/dl
Platelets:	>100,000/mm^3
Fibrinogen:	>195 g/dl
Prothrombin time:	<17 seconds
Activated clotting times:	180–200 seconds

Courtesy of Children's Hospital, Boston, MA.

TABLE 8–23 Complications Associated With Extracorporeal Membrane Oxygenation

PATIENT COMPLICATIONS
Seizures
Intraventricular hemorrhage
Pulmonary hemorrhage
Pneumothorax
Infection
Dialysis-hemofiltration
Hemolysis
Hypertension
Abnormal creatinine value
Electrolyte abnormalities
Hyperbilirubinemia
Cardiac dysfunction
Cardiac arrhythmias
Myocardial stun
Cannula site bleeding
Surgical site bleeding
MECHANICAL COMPLICATIONS
Clots in circuit
Air in circuit
Cannula problems
Oxygenator failure
Pump malfunction
Heat exchanger malfunction
Tubing rupture

patient's head is maintained in the midline position to assure adequate cerebral drainage and perfusion.

Ventilator settings during ECMO are maintained to allow the lung to heal. Respiratory care includes chest vibration, manual ventilation with an inspiratory hold, normal saline lavage, and suctioning. Chest radiographs are taken daily.

Complications

Complications seen in patients on ECMO are divided into patient and mechanical issues. The central nervous system and the risk of intraventricular hemorrhage are the major areas of concern in neonates. Table 8–23 lists these complications. The Extracorporeal Life Support Organization (ELSO) registry contains information from ECMO cases and maintains data concerning complications.

Bibliography

American Association for Respiratory Care: Clinical practice guideline: Surfactant replacement therapy. Respir Care 1994; 39:824.

American Association for Respiratory Care: Clinical practic guideline: Delivery of aerosols to the upper airway. Respir Care 1994; 39:803.

American Association for Respiratory Care: Clinical practice guideline: Endotracheal suctioning of mechanically ventilated adults and children with artificial airways. Respir Care 1993; 38:501.

American Association for Respiratory Care: Clinical practice guideline: Intermittent positive pressure breathing. Respir Care 1993; 38:1189.

American Association for Respiratory Care: Clinical practice guideline: Humidification during mechanical ventilation. Respir Care 1992; 37:887.

American Association for Respiratory Care: Clinical practice guideline: Selection of aerosol delivery device. Respir Care 1992; 37:891.

American Association for Respiratory Care: Clinical practice guideline: Oxygen therapy in the acute care hospital. Respir Care 1991; 36:1410.

American Association for Respiratory Care: Clinical practice guideline: Incentive spirometry. Respir Care 1991; 36:1402.

Asher MI, Douglas C, Airy M, et al: Effects of chest physical therapy on lung function in children recovering from acute severe asthma. Pediatr Pulmonol 1990; 9:146.

Bartlett RH: Extracorporeal Membrane Oxygenation Technical Specialist Manual, 9th ed. Ann Arbor, MI, University of Michigan, 1988.

Beckham RW, Mishoe SC: Sound levels inside incubators and oxygen hoods used with nebulizers and humidifiers. Respir Care 1982; 27:33.

Boeckling AC: Exogenous surfactant therapy for premature infants. Neonatal Intensive Care 1992; 5:22.

Coffman JA, McManus KP: Oxygen therapy via nasal catheter for infants with bronchopulmonary dysplasia. Crit Care Nurs 1984; 4:22.

Desmond J, Schwenk WF, Thomas E, et al: Immediate and long-term effects of chest physiotherapy in patients with cystic fibrosis. J Pediatr 1983; 103:538.

Fujiwara T, Maeta H, Chida S, et al: Artificial surfactant therapy in hyaline membrane disease. Lancet 1980; 1:55.

Gomella TL: Neonatology Management, Procedures, On-Call Problems, Diseases, Drugs, 2nd ed. Norwalk, CT, Appleton & Lange, 1992.

Grim PS, Gottlieb LJ, Boddie A, Batson E: Hyperbaric oxygen therapy. JAMA 1990; 263:2216.

Hazinski MF: Nursing Care of the Critically Ill Child, 2nd ed. St. Louis, Mosby-Year Book, 1992.

Kanto WP: A decade of experience with neonatal extracorporeal membrane oxygenation. J Pediatr 1994; 124:335.

Kersten LD: Comprehensive Respiratory Nursing. Philadelphia, WB Saunders, 1989.

Mahlmeister MJ, Fink JB, Horrman GL, et al: Positive expiratory pressure mask therapy: Theoretical and practical considerations and a review of the literature. Respir Care 1991; 36:1218.

Neonatal ECMO Registry of the Extracorporeal Life Support Organization (ELSO). Ann Arbor, MI, Extracorporeal Life Support Organization, April, 1994.

Newhouse MT, Dolovich M: Aerosol Therapy in Children. Basic Mechanisms of Pediatric Respiratory Disease: Cellular and Integrative. New York, BC Decker, 1991.

Pramanik AK, Holtzman RB, Merritt TA: Surfactant replacement therapy for pulmonary diseases. Pediatr Clin North Am 1993; 40:913.

Pryor JA: International Perspectives in Physical Therapy, 7: Respiratory Care. Edinburgh, Churchill Livingstone, 1991.

Rau JL: Delivery of aerosolized drugs to neonatal and pediatric patients. Respir Care 1991; 36:514.

Raval D, Cuevas D, Mora A, et al: Chest physiotherapy in preterm infants with RDS in the first 24 hours of life. J Perinatol 1986; 7:301.

Reines DH, Sade RM, Bradford BF, et al: Chest physiotherapy fails to prevent postoperative atelectasis in children after cardiac surgery. Ann Surg 1982; 195:451.

Reisman J, Rivington-Law B, Corey M, et al: Role of conventional physiotherapy in cystic fibrosis. J Pediatr 1988; 113:632.

Schumacher RE: Extracorporeal membrane oxygenation: Will this therapy continue to be as efficacious in the future? Pediatr Clin North Am 1993; 40:1005.

Skale N: Manual of Pediatric Nursing Procedures. Philadelphia, JB Lippincott, 1992.

Vain NE, Prudent LM, Stevens SP, et al: Regulation of oxygen concentration delivered to infants via nasal cannulas. Am J Dis Child 1989; 143:1458.

Vazquez RL, Spahr RC: Hyperbaric oxygen use in neonates: A report of four patients. Am J Dis Child 1990; 144:1022.

Waring WW: Diagnostic and therapeutic procedures. *In* Chernick V (ed): Kendig's Disorders of the Respiratory Tract in Children, 5th ed. Philadelphia, WB Saunders, 1990, pp 77–95.

Warwick WJ, Hansen LG: The long-term efficacy of high-frequency chest compression on pulmonary complications of cystic fibrosis. Pediatr Pulmonol 1991; 11:265.

SECTION 9

Diagnostic and Monitoring Procedures

I. Pulmonary Function and Mechanics

A. Terminology

B. Interpretation of pulmonary function and mechanics

C. Formulas used to predict normal values

D. Ventilator-patient management using pulmonary mechanics

II. Blood Gas Analysis

A. Normal values

B. Acid-base balance

1. Equations illustrating acid-base relationships
2. Acid-base interpretation

C. Oxygen delivery and ventilation

1. Oxygen deficiency
2. Oxyhemoglobin dissociation curve
3. 30-60-90 rule for estimating oxygen saturation
4. Equations

D. Arterial puncture

1. Puncture sites
2. Procedure
3. Complications

E. Capillary puncture

1. Puncture sites
2. Procedure
3. Contraindications
4. Complications

III. Hemodynamic Monitoring

A. Cardiac output

B. Cardiac output measurement methods

1. Thermal dilution
2. Dye dilution
3. Fick equation

C. Equations

D. Cardiac catheterization waveforms

IV. Indirect Calorimetry and Nutritional Assessment

A. Terminology

B. Equations

V. Noninvasive Monitoring

A. Pulse oximetry

1. Patient application
2. Relationship between functional and fractional saturation

B. Transcutaneous Po_2 and Pco_2 monitoring

1. Patient application

C. Capnometry
   1. Patient application
   2. Capnogram
D. Impedance pneumography
   1. Patient application

VI. Radiographic Assessment
A. Densities
B. Systematic approach to evaluating a chest x-ray film
C. Advanced imaging methods

VII. Bronchoscopy
A. Rigid and flexible bronchoscopy
B. Indications
C. Complications

Abbreviations

BMR–basal metabolic rate
CI–cardiac index
CL–lung compliance
CL_{dyn}–dynamic lung compliance
CO–cardiac output
COHb–carboxyhemoglobin (carbon monoxide)
Crs–respiratory system compliance
CVP–central venous pressure
2,3 DPG–2,3-diphosphoglycerate
EIB–exercise-induced bronchospasm
ERV–expiratory residual volume
FEF_{25-75}–forced expiratory flow between 25% and 75% of vital capacity
FEV_1–forced expiratory volume in 1 second
FRC–functional residual capacity
F-V–flow-volume
FVC–forced vital capacity
Hb–hemoglobin
IC–inspiratory capacity
MAP–mean arterial pressure
MEE–metabolic energy expenditure
MetHb–methemoglobin (unoxygenated iron)
MIP–maximum inspiratory pressure
MPAP–mean pulmonary artery pressure
NIF–negative inspiratory force
O_2Hb–oxygenated hemoglobin
OHDC–oxyhemoglobin dissociation curve
P_{100}–respiratory drive
PCWP–pulmonary capillary wedge pressure
PEFR–peak expiratory flow rate
PM–pulmonary mechanics
P_{TCCO_2}–transcutaneous P_{CO_2}

P_{TCO_2}–transcutaneous P_{O_2}
PTI–pressure time index
PTP–pressure time product
PVR–pulmonary vascular resistance
PVRI–pulmonary vascular resistance index
Raw–airway resistance
REE–resting energy expenditure
RHb–reduced (unoxygenated) hemoglobin
RMR–resting metabolic rate
RV–residual volume
RVP–right ventricular pressure
S_{PO_2}–oxygen saturation by pulse oximetry measurement
SVR–systemic vascular resistance
SVRI–systemic vascular resistance index
TC–time constant
T_e–expiratory time
TEE–total energy expenditure
TGV–thoracic gas volume
T_i–inspiratory time
T_i/T_{total}–respiratory time fraction
TLC–total lung capacity
T_{total}–total cycle time
V_{CO_2}–carbon dioxide production
V_D–dead space
V_E–minute ventilation per unit time
V_{O_2}–oxygen consumption
V-P–volume-pressure
V/Q–ventilation to perfusion ratio
V_T–tidal volume
WOB–work of breathing
WOB_M–mechanical ventilation work of breathing
WOB_P–patient work of breathing during spontaneous breathing
$WOB_{P\&V}$–work of breathing during ventilator-assisted spontaneous breaths

PULMONARY FUNCTION AND MECHANICS

Terminology

Lung Volumes. Lung volume measurements include tidal volume (V_T), inspiratory capacity (IC), expiratory reserve volume (ERV), functional residual capacity (FRC), residual volume (RV), vital capacity (VC), total lung capacity (TLC), and thoracic gas volume (TGV). Figure 9–1 illustrates the subdivisions of lung volumes.

Spirometry. Spirometry consists of flow-volume (F-V) or time volume measurements. Figure 9–2 illustrates time-volume spirometry. Figures 9–3 through 9–5 illustrate F-V loops with various patterns that may occur.

Volume-Pressure Loops. The volume-pressure (V-P) loop is a graphic loop display of a tidal breath with volume on the vertical axis and airway or transpulmonary pressure change on the horizontal axis. The more compliant the lung

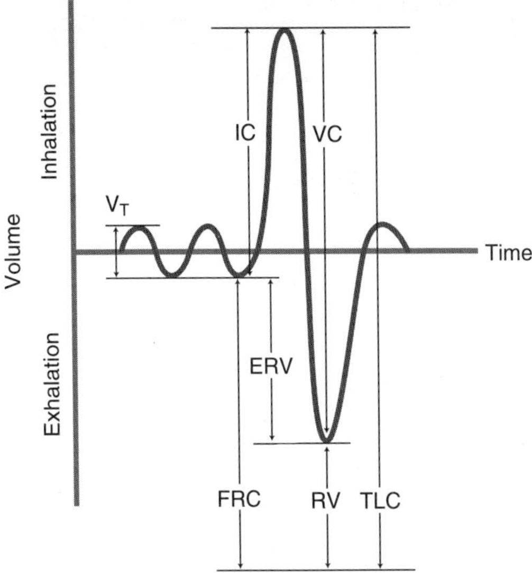

Figure 9–1 A graphic display of the subdivisions of total lung capacity, from quiet tidal breathing on the left to maximal inhalation and exhalation on the right. V_T, tidal volume; TLC, total lung capacity; VC, vital capacity; RV, residual volume; FRC, functional residual capacity; IC, inspiratory capacity; ERV, expiratory reserve volume.

is, the more vertical the V-P loop appears. Figures 9–6 through 9–8 illustrate V-P loops and patterns that may be displayed.

Restrictive Lung Process. A disease or anatomic process that results in reduced lung volumes is a restrictive lung process.

Obstructive Lung Process. A disease or anatomic process that results in reduced flow rates into and out of the lungs is an obstructive lung process.

Diffusing Capacity. A test measuring the diffusion of carbon monoxide (CO) across the alveolar capillary junction is the diffusing capacity. It is increased in interstitial disease processes.

Maximum Voluntary Ventilation. MVV is rapid, full inspiratory and expiratory breaths measured over 10 or 15 seconds and reported in liters per minute.

Maximum Inspiratory Pressure. MIP is the maximum negative pressure measured during inspiration against an

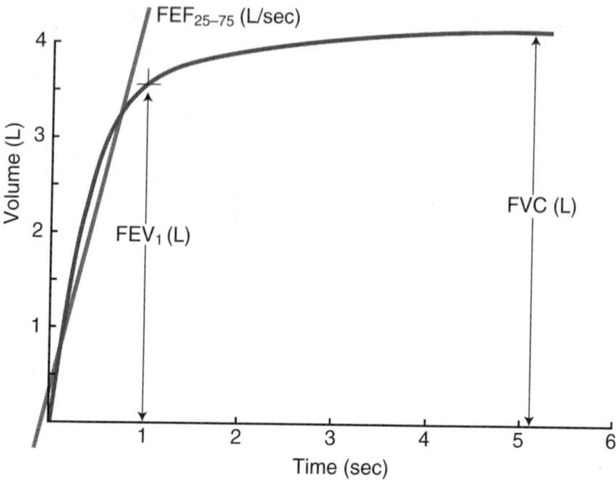

Calculation of FEF_{25-75}: 1. Determine 25% and 75% of FVC

2. Slope of line through 25% and 75% =

$$\frac{(V_{75}) - (V_{25})}{(T_{75}) - (T_{25})} \text{ (L/sec)}$$

Figure 9–2 Demonstration of a normal standard time-volume spirometry graph depicting the forced vital capacity (FVC), the forced expiratory volume in 1 second (FEV_1), and the forced expiratory flow between 25% and 75% of the vital capacity (FEF_{25-75}).

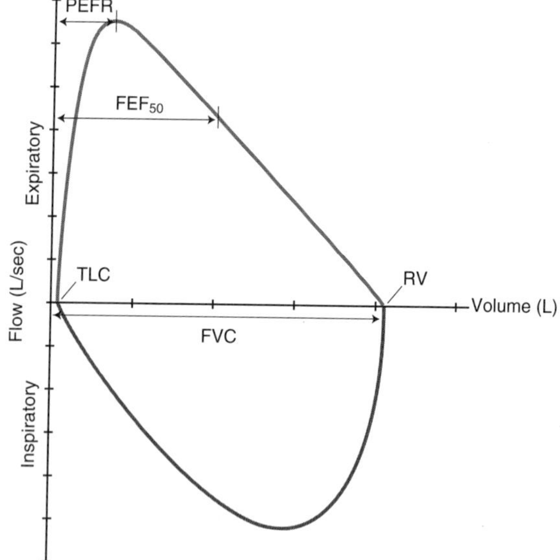

Figure 9–3 Demonstration of a normal flow-volume loop, showing both the expiratory and inspiratory loops. The usual flow rates are identified. Note that no FEV_1 is evident because there is no time axis.

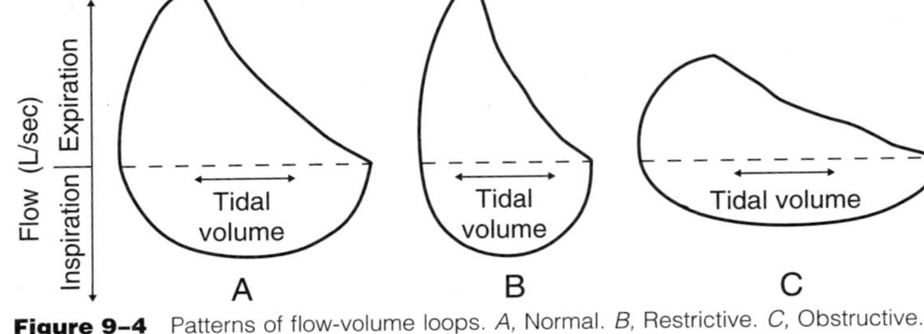

Figure 9–4 Patterns of flow-volume loops. *A*, Normal. *B*, Restrictive. *C*, Obstructive.

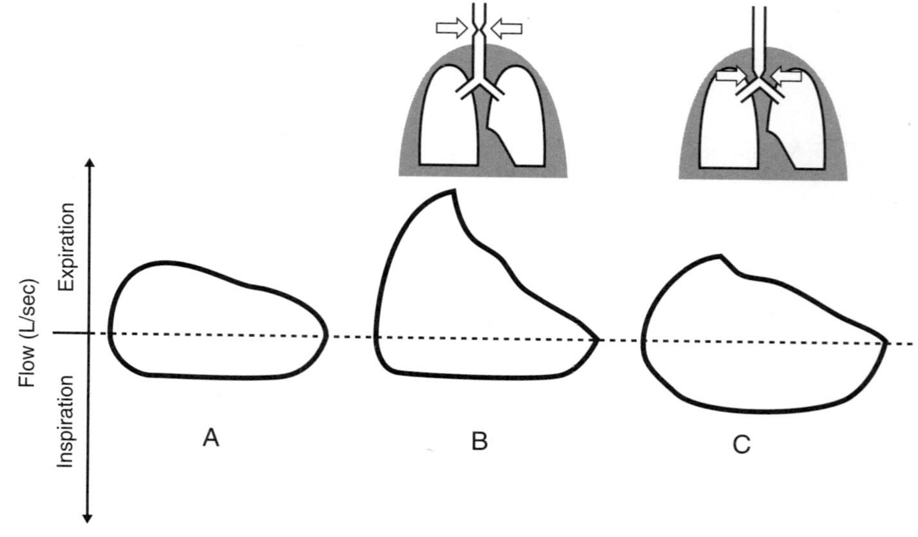

Figure 9–5 *See legend on opposite page*

occluded orifice. It is useful in differentiating respiratory muscle weakness from other causes of restrictive lung disease. It is highly effort-dependent.

Pulmonary Mechanics. PM is the interaction of forces and physical principles that determine the characteristics of gas movement into and out of the lungs.

Transpulmonary Pressure. This is the difference in intrapleural and airway pressures—the pressure exerted on the lungs that is responsible for inspiration.

Inspiratory Time. T_i is the measured time, in seconds, in which gas flows into the lungs.

Expiratory Time. T_e is the measured time, in seconds, in which gas flows out of the lungs.

Total Cycle Time. T_{total} is the sum of T_i and T_e.

Time Constant. TC is the mathematical product of compliance (C) and resistance (R) expressed in seconds. A TC is an interval over which a given change occurs as a percentage of total change. Measured T_i and T_e should be at least three respiratory TCs for complete inspiration or expiration to occur.

Lung Compliance. CL is the change in lung volume for a given amount of applied pressure change and is reported in milliliters per centimeters of water.

Respiratory System Compliance. Crs is an assessment of the elasticity of the total respiratory system by measuring CL under conditions of no gas flow into or out of the lungs.

Dynamic Lung Compliance. CL_{dyn} is an assessment of airway resistance by measuring CL during resting tidal breathing.

Specific Lung Compliance. This is lung compliance measured at known levels of total lung capacity (TLC).

Airway Resistance. Raw is the energy (pressure) needed to move gas through the pulmonary conducting airways and is expressed in centimeters of water per liter per second.

Figure 9–5 Flow-volume loops showing various forms of airway obstruction. *A*, Fixed obstruction. *B*, Variable extrathoracic obstruction. *C*, Variable intrathoracic obstruction.

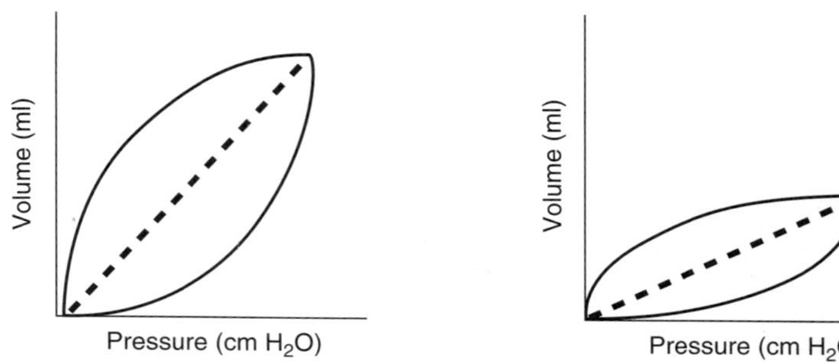

Figure 9–6 Volume-pressure loops demonstrating normal and decreased lung compliance. *A,* Normal lung compliance. *B,* Decreased lung compliance.

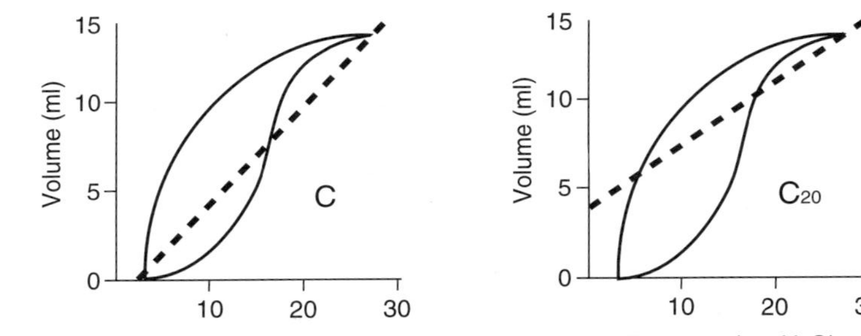

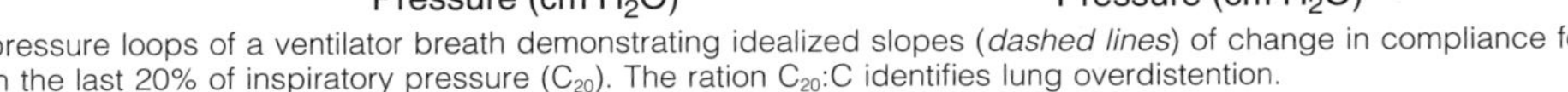

Figure 9–7 Volume-pressure loops of a ventilator breath demonstrating idealized slopes (*dashed lines*) of change in compliance for the entire breath (C) and change in compliance in the last 20% of inspiratory pressure (C_{20}). The ration C_{20}:C identifies lung overdistention.

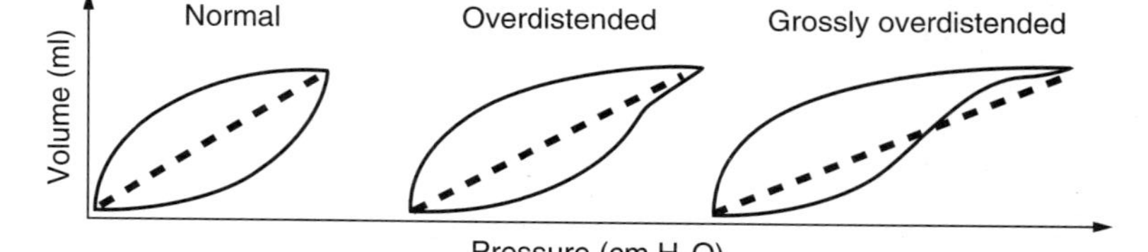

Figure 9–8 Volume-pressure loops demonstrating lung overdistention during positive pressure ventilation.

Peak Expiratory Flow Rate. PEFR is the maximum flow that can be achieved during a rapid, forced expiration and is expressed in liters per minute. Note that the PEFR on an F-V loop is reported in liters per second. It is used commonly in the management of asthmatic patients.

Negative Inspiratory Force. NIF is the maximum negative pressure generated during inspiration against an occlusion and is expressed in centimeters of water. It is also known as the MIP.

Forced Expiratory Flow Between 25% and 75% of Vital Capacity. FEF_{25-75} reflects primarily the function of small airways.

Minute Ventilation. $\dot{V}_E$ is V_T multiplied by the number of breaths per minute and is expressed in liters per minute.

Respiratory Time Fraction. T_i/T_{total} is a dimensionless parameter related to endurance and derived by dividing T_i by T_{total}.

Respiratory Drive. P_{100} is the neural drive to stimulate diaphragmatic contraction which is derived by measuring the negative airway pressure 100 msec after airway occlusion and is expressed in centimeters of water. A low value represents reduced drive.

Pressure Time Product. PTP is the computation related to metabolic work (oxygen consumption) of respiratory muscles and is expressed in centimeters per second per minute. The value decreases during optimal positive pressure support of spontaneous breaths.

Pressure Time Index. PTI is a dimensionless parameter computed by combining strength and endurance and esophageal pressure and MIP with T_i/T_{total}.

Interpretation of Pulmonary Function and Mechanics

Tables 9–1 through 9–7 provide information that may be used for interpretation in pulmonary function testing.

Formulas Used to Predict Normal Values

TGV $= 2.04 \times \text{cm Ht}^{2.7361} \times 10^{-6}$

FRC $= 1.57 \times \text{cm Ht}^{2.238} \times 10^{-2}$ (infants)

$0.75 \times \text{cm Ht}^{2.92} \times 10^{-3}$ (male child, adolescent)

TABLE 9–1 Lung Volume Measurements in Infants and Children

AGE	THORACIC GAS VOLUME (ml)	FUNCTIONAL RESIDUAL CAPACITY (ml)
Birth	20–25 ±3	—
Preterm < 2.5 kg	29–32 ±7	20–25 ±9
Preterm healthy	35–48 ±4	24–29 ±5
Preterm RDS	44–57 ±10	29–34 ±7
Term	29–38 ±7	25–30 ±4
Infants	30–40 ±6	20–30 ±5

RDS, respiratory distress syndrome.

FRC $= 1.78 \times \text{cm Ht}^{2.74} \times 10^{-3}$ (female child, adolescent)

FVC $= 4.4 \times \text{cm Ht}^{2.67} \times 10^{-3}$ (white male)

$3.3 \times \text{cm Ht}^{2.72} \times 10^{-3}$ (white female)

TABLE 9–2 Pulmonary Function Measurements in Children

MEASUREMENT	VARIABILITY (%)	NORMAL RANGE (% PREDICTED)	IMPORTANT CHANGE (%)
FVC	5–7	80–120	>10
FEV_1	8	80–120	>15
FEV_1 : FVC	—	*	—
FEF_{25-75}	15	60–140	>30
FEF_{50}	15	60–140	>30
TLC	7	80–120	>10
RV	7	80–120	>10
RV : TLC	7	†	—

* Absolute value is used; normal range for children is 82% to 95%.
† Absolute value is used; normal range for children is 20% to 30%.
FVC, forced vital capacity; FEV_1, forced expiratory volume in 1 second; FEV_1 : FVC, ratio of forced expiratory volume in 1 second to forced vital capacity; FEF_{25-75}, forced expiratory flow between 25% and 75% of the vital capacity; FEF_{50}, forced expiratory flow at 50% of the vital capacity; TLC, total lung capacity; RV, residual volume; RV : TLC, ratio of residual volume to total lung capacity.

TABLE 9–3 Characterization of Obstructive and Restrictive Patterns in Pulmonary Function Testing

MEASUREMENT	OBSTRUCTIVE	RESTRICTIVE
FVC	Normal or decreased	Decreased
FEV_1	Decreased	Decreased
FEV_1 : FVC	Decreased	Normal or increased
TLC	Normal or increased	Decreased
RV	Increased	Normal or decreased
RV : TLC	Increased	Normal or increased

FVC, forced vital capacity; FEV_1, forced expiratory volume in 1 second; FEV_1 : FVC, ratio of forced expiratory volume in 1 second to forced vital capacity; TLC, total lung capacity; RV, residual volume; RV : TLC, ratio of residual volume to total lung capacity.

FVC	$= 1.07 \times \text{cm Ht}^{2.93} \times 10^{-3}$	(black male)
	$8.34 \times \text{cm Ht}^{2.97} \times 10^{-4}$	(black female)
	$1.06 \times \text{cm Ht}^{2.97} \times 10^{-3}$	(Hispanic male)
	$1.25 \times \text{cm Ht}^{2.92} \times 10^{-3}$	(Hispanic female)
FEV_1	$= 2.1 \times \text{cm Ht}^{2.8} \times 10^{-3}$	(white, male and female)
	$1.03 \times \text{cm Ht}^{2.92} \times 10^{-3}$	(black male)
	$1.14 \times \text{cm Ht}^{2.89} \times 10^{-3}$	(black female)
	$1.73 \times \text{cm Ht}^{2.85} \times 10^{-3}$	(Hispanic male)
	$1.61 \times \text{cm Ht}^{2.85} \times 10^{-3}$	(Hispanic female)

TABLE 9–4 Static Lung Compliance As It Varies With Age

Birth:	1–2 cm H_2O
Newborn:	3–6 cm H_2O
Infant:	9–12 cm H_2O
Child:	55–65 cm H_2O
Preadolescent:	90–110 cm H_2O

TABLE 9–5 Predicted Average Normal Peak Expiratory Flow Rate (L/min) Using a Wright Peak Flowmeter, Ages 4 to 18 Years

HEIGHT (cm)	FLOW RATE	HEIGHT (cm)	FLOW RATE
104	120	142	320
107	134	145	333
109	147	147	347
112	160	150	360
114	174	152	373
117	187	155	387
119	200	157	400
122	214	160	413
124	227	163	427
127	240	165	440
130	254	168	453
132	267	170	467
135	280	173	480
137	294	175	493
140	307	178	507

$FEF_{27-75} = 7.89 \times \text{cm Ht}^{2.46} \times 10^{-4}$ (white male)

$3.79 \times \text{cm Ht}^{2.16} \times 10^{-3}$ (white female)

$3.61 \times \text{cm Ht}^{2.6} \times 10^{-4}$ (black male)

$1.45 \times \text{cm Ht}^{2.34} \times 10^{-3}$ (black female)

$9.13 \times \text{cm Ht}^{2.45} \times 10^{-4}$ (Hispanic male)

$1.20 \times \text{cm Ht}^{2.4} \times 10^{-3}$ (Hispanic female)

PEFR (Wright's) $= 2.26 \times \text{cm Ht}^{2.39} \times 10^{-3}$ (male)

$4.59 \times \text{cm Ht}^{2.35} \times 10^{-3}$ (female)

Ventilator-Patient Management Using Pulmonary Mechanics

Pulmonary mechanics may be used in the determination of optimal ventilatory settings, identification of lung overdistention, and ability to wean the patient from mechanical ventilation. Figures 9–7 and 9–8 illustrate the effect overdis-

TABLE 9–6 Positive Methacholine Challenge in a Seven-Year-Old Girl With a Chronic Cough

METHACHOLINE		PULMONARY FUNCTION		
Concentration	Cumulative Dose	FVC (L) (% Predicted)	FEV_1 (L) (% Predicted)	% Change FEV_1
Saline	0	1.51 (83)	1.4 (82)	
0.025	0.125	1.51	1.38	−1
0.25	1.375	1.64	1.53	+9
2.5	13.875	1.54	1.39	−1
10	63.875	1.33	1.07	−24
Albuterol		1.41	1.26	−10

FVC, forced vital capacity; FEV_1, forced expiratory volume in 1 second.

TABLE 9–7 Exercise Testing Protocol for the Diagnosis of Exercise-Induced Bronchospasm

PRETEST PREPARATION

1. Patient must avoid exertion for at least $2\frac{1}{2}$ to 3 hours before testing.
2. Climatic conditions (temperature and humidity) should be standardized.
3. For a given patient, tests and retests should be at the same time of day.
4. Retesting, if necessary, should be performed between 1 day and 1 week of the original test.
5. A medical history should be obtained and a physical examination performed.
6. The child should be familiarized with the objectives of the test and the laboratory.
7. Baseline pulmonary function should be obtained.

WITHDRAWAL OF MEDICATION

1. All $beta_2$-sympathomimetics, methylxanthines, and anticholinergics should be discontinued at least 8 hours before testing.
2. Long-acting methylxanthines should be withdrawn 24 hours before testing.
3. Disodium cromoglycate should be withdrawn 24 hours before testing.

EXERCISE PROTOCOL

1. Running up and down stairs in the office, hospital, or clinic is not sufficient.
2. Cycle ergometer or treadmill exercise is recommended.
3. Continuous monitoring of heart rate is necessary; monitoring of gas exchange is recommended.
4. Bar-Or recommends that a successful test consist of *at least* 5 minutes of constant work rate exercise at 80% to 90% of the heart rate maximum. Thus the appropriate work rate must be estimated before testing by using normal values. The investigator may then have to adjust the work rate within the first several minutes.

PULMONARY FUNCTION TESTS

1. Baseline (preexercise) testing (e.g., FVC and FEV_1) is done immediately before the exercise challenge.
2. Testing is repeated at 2, 5, and 10 minutes after the initial exercise and then repeated every 5 minutes until EIB subsides.
3. The most common calculation is the percent value of the ratio:

$$\frac{\text{Preexercise pulmonary function value} - \text{Lowest postexercise value}}{\text{Preexercise value}}$$

4. A positive test is usually defined as a drop in pulmonary function of more than 15 percent.

Adapted from Chernick V (ed): Kendig's Disorders of the Respiratory Tract in Children. Philadelphia, WB Saunders, p 171; based on Bar-Or O: Pediatric Sports Medicine. New York, Springer Verlag, 1983, pp 102–104.
FVC, forced vital capacity; FEV_1, forced expiratory volume in 1 second.

tention has on V-P loops. Through pulmonary mechanics, Figure 9–9 compares the work of breathing that occurs during mechanical ventilation (WOB_M) with that occurring during spontaneous breathing (WOB_P). Table 9–8 lists normal values of various pulmonary mechanics and the values that indicate that weaning from mechanical ventilation may be considered.

BLOOD GAS ANALYSIS

Normal Values

Table 9–9 lists the normal values of parameters commonly measured from arterial and capillary blood samples.

Acid-Base Balance

Equations Illustrating Acid-Base Relationships

Law of Mass Action

$$CO_2 + H_2O \leftrightharpoons H_2CO_3 \leftrightharpoons H^+ + HCO_3^-$$

Henderson-Hasselbalch

$$pH = 6.1 + \log [HCO_3^-/(Paco_2 \times 0.03)]$$

Acid-Base Interpretation. Table 9–10 demonstrates the trends in arterial blood gas values for metabolic and respiratory acid-base disorders. Tables 9–11 and 9–12 list common causes of acidosis and alkalosis.

Oxygen Delivery and Ventilation

Oxygen Deficiency. Hypoxemia refers to a decrease in the amount of oxygen in the arterial blood. Table 9–13 lists the reasons for hypoxemia.

Oxyhemoglobin Dissociation Curve. The shape and shift of the oxyhemoglobin dissociation curve (OHCD) affect the oxygen binding to hemoglobin in the lungs and the unloading of oxygen to the tissue sites (Fig. 9–10; Table 9–14). The P_{50} is defined as the Po_2 at which hemoglobin is 50% saturated with oxygen.

30-60-90 Rule for Estimating Oxygen Saturation

Pao_2 of 30 mm Hg = Sao_2 of 60% and
Pao_2 of 60 mm Hg = Sao_2 of 90%

Equations

Arterial Oxygen Content

$$Cao_2 = [Hb \times 1.39 \times (\%Sao_2/100)] + (0.0031 \times Pao_2)$$

Mixed Venous Oxygen Content

$$C\bar{v}o_2 = [Hb \times 1.39 \times (\%S\bar{v}o_2/100)] + (0.0031 \times P\bar{v}o_2)$$

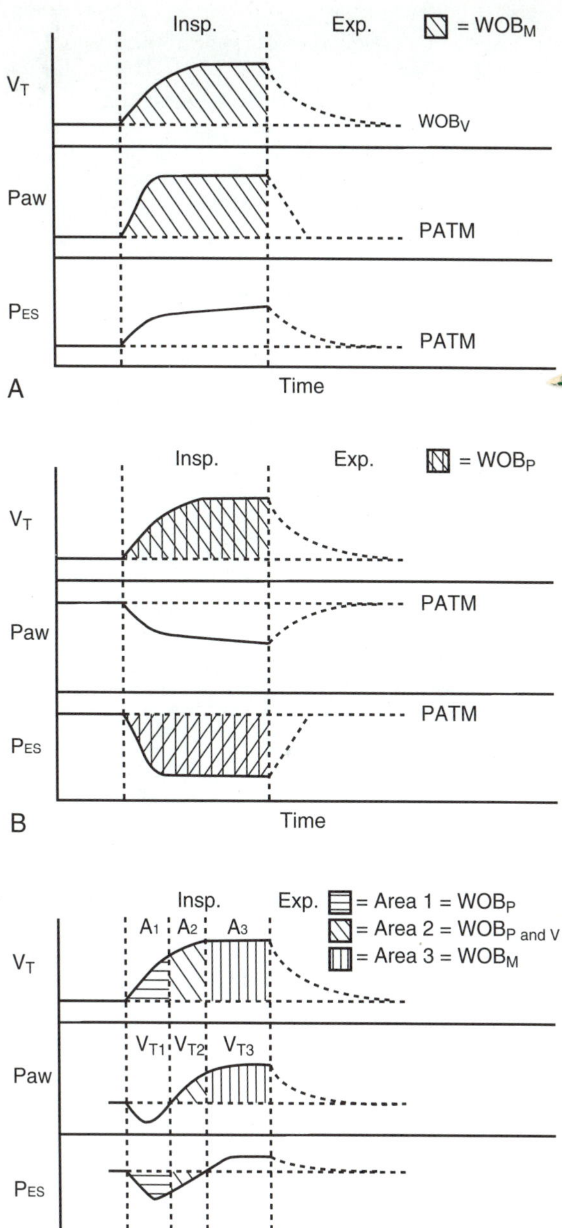

Figure 9–9 *A,* Mechanical ventilator work of breathing (WOB$_M$). *B,* Patient WOB during spontaneous breaths (WOB$_P$). *C,* WOB during ventilator-assisted spontaneous breaths (WOB$_{P\ and\ V}$). Paw, airway pressure; P_{ES}, esophageal pressure; PATM, atmospheric pressure; V_T, tidal volume. (Adapted from Pulmonary Monitoring. Bicore Monitoring Systems, Irvine, CA.)

TABLE 9–8 Normal Values and Indications for Weaning*

PARAMETER	NORMAL RANGE	INDICATIONS FOR WEANING
f	10–20 bpm	<30 bpm
Esophageal pressure change	5–10 cm H_2O	<15 cm H_2O
V_T	7–10 ml/kg	>4–5ml/kg
Minute ventilation	5–10 L/min	<10 L/min
T_i/T_{total}	0.3–0.4	Increase >0.1†
WOB_P	0.3–0.6 J/L	<0.75 J.L†
PTI	0.05–0.12	<0.15†
Raw	2–5 cm H_2O/L/second	<15 cm H_2O/L/second
CL	50–125 ml/cm H_2O	>25 ml/cm H_2O
PTP	200–300 cm H_2O sec/min†	—
MIP	−30 cm H_2O	−20 cm H_2O
Auto-PEEP	0	<3 cm H_2O
P_{100}	2–4 cm H_2O	<6 cm H_2O†
f/V_T	60–90	<105

Adapted from Pulmonary Monitoring. Bicore Monitoring Systems, Irvine, CA.

f, frequency; V_T, tidal volume; T_i/T_{total}, respiratory time fraction; WOB_P, patient work of breathing during spontaneous breathing; PTI, pressure time index; Raw, airway resistance; CL, lung compliance; PTP, pressure time product; MIP, maximum inspiratory pressure; PEEP, positive end-expiratory pressure; P_{100}, respiratory drive; f/V_T, frequency per tidal volume

* Reported adult values.

† Research indicates these parameters may aid in evaluating weaning potential. If values exceed acceptable ranges, successful weaning may be less likely. Ranges are not intended as a substitute for proper clinical assessment.

Alveolar Air Equation

$$P_{AO_2} = [(Pb - P_{H_2O}) \times F_{IO_2}] - Pa_{CO_2}[F_{IO_2} + (1 - F_{IO_2})/R]$$

Alveolar Air Equation (Clinical Form)

$$P_{AO_2} = [(Pb - P_{H_2O}) \times F_{IO_2}] - (Pa_{CO_2}/R)$$

where Pb = barometric pressure, P_{H_2O} = water vapor pressure (47 at 37° C), and R = respiratory quotient (0.8 average).

TABLE 9–9 Normal Value Ranges for Age-Related Arterial Blood Gas Measurements

MEASUREMENT	BIRTH	HOUR 1	>8 HOURS	INFANT >1 DAY	CHILD-ADULT
pH	7.2–7.3	7.3–7.35	7.3–7.4	7.3–7.4	7.35–7.45
P_{CO_2} (mm Hg)	45–55	40–55	30–40	30–40	35–45
P_{O_2} (mm Hg)	<60	60–70	60–90	80–100	80–100
HCO_3^- (mEq/L)	20–24	18–22	19–23	20–22	22–24
BE	−5–−2	−5–−2	−6–−2	−6–−1	−2–+2

BE, base excess.

TABLE 9–10 Laboratory Values for Acid-Base Disturbances

DISORDER	pH	$Paco_2$	HCO_3^-
Metabolic acidosis			
Uncompensated	↓	N	↓
Partially compensated	↓	↓	↓
Compensated	N	↓	↓
Metabolic alkalosis			
Uncompensated	↑	N	↑
Partially compensated	↑	↑	↑
Compensated	N	↑	↑
Respiratory acidosis			
Uncompensated	↓	↑	N
Partially compensated	↓	↑	↑
Compensated	N	↑	↑
Respiratory alkalosis			
Uncompensated	↑	↓	N
Partially compensated	↑	↓	↓
Compensated	N	↓	↓
Mixed acidosis	↓	↑	↓
Mixed alkalosis	↑	↓	↑

Adapted from Boyda EK, Kee JL, Monaghan FD: Knowledge basic to the nursing care of adults with fluid, electrolyte, and acid-base imbalance. *In* Monaghan FD, Drake T, Neighbors M (eds): Nursing Care of Adults. Philadelphia, WB Saunders, 1994.
N = normal, ↓ = below normal range, ↑ = above normal range.

Alveolar-Arterial Oxygen Gradient

$$P(A\text{-}a)O_2 = [((Pb - P_{H_2O}) \times F_{IO_2}) - (Pa_{CO_2}/R)] - Pa_{O_2}$$

Arterial-Alveolar Oxygen Fraction

$$P(a/A)O_2 = Pa_{O_2}/P_{AO_2}$$

Oxygen Index

$$OI = Pa_{O_2}/F_{IO_2}$$

Shunt Equation

$$\dot{Q}_s/\dot{Q}_t = (Cc_{O_2} - Ca_{O_2})/(Cc_{O_2} - C\bar{v}_{O_2}),\ \text{normal} < 5\%$$

Cc_{O_2} (pulmonary capillary oxygen content) is assumed to equal C_{AO_2} derived from the alveolar oxygen equation.

Minute Ventilation

$$\dot{V}_E = V_T \times f$$

Physiologic Dead Space

$$V_D/V_T = (Paco_2 - P\bar{e}co_2)/(Paco_2 - P\bar{v}o_2)$$

TABLE 9–11 Causes of Acidosis

RESPIRATORY ACIDOSIS	METABOLIC ACIDOSIS
Lung disease	Diarrhea
Upper airway obstruction (laryngotracheobronchitis, epiglottitis, foreign body)	Small bowel, biliary, or pancreatic tube or fistula drainage
Small airway obstruction (asthma, bronchiolitis)	Hyperalimentation
Chronic obstructive disease (cystic fibrosis, bronchopulmonary dysplasia, bronchiectasis)	Ingestion of chloride-containing compounds
Pneumonia	Calcium chloride
Pulmonary edema	Magnesium chloride
Respiratory distress syndrome, adult respiratory distress syndrome	Ammonium chloride
Aspiration (meconium, foreign body)	Hydrochloric acid
Pulmonary hypoplasia	Renal tubular acidosis
Impaired lung motion	Renal failure
Pleural effusion	Deficiency of carbonic anhydrase
Pneumothorax	Lactic acidosis
Thoracic cage abnormalities (flail chest, scoliosis, osteogenesis imperfecta congenita, thoracic dystrophy)	Tissue hypoxia
	Sepsis
	Neonatal cold stress
	Ketoacidosis
	Diabetes mellitus
	Starvation
	Toxic ingestions
	Salicylate poisoning
	Methanol poisoning
	Ethylene glycol poisoning
	Prolonged use of paraldehyde
	Inborn errors of metabolism

Table continued on following page

TABLE 9–11 Causes of Acidosis *Continued*

RESPIRATORY ACIDOSIS	METABOLIC ACIDOSIS
Apnea	
Neurologic-neuromuscular disorders	
Brainstem or spinal cord injury-tumor	
Paralysis of diaphragm	
Drug overdose-oversedation	
Muscular dystrophy	
Guillain-Barré syndrome	
Myasthenia gravis	
Poliomyelitis	
Botulism	
Extreme obesity	
Complications of mechanical ventilation	

Adapted from Brewer ED: Disorders of acid-base balance. Pediatr Clin N Am 1990; 37:429–447.

Oxygen Delivery

$$Do_2 = Cao_2 \times (Cco_2 - C\bar{v}o_2)$$

$$Do_2 = \text{cardiac output} \times Cao_2$$

Arterial Puncture

Puncture Sites. Puncture sites are illustrated in Figure 9–11. Punctures are not performed in the following areas:

- Sites at which there has been a previous incident of blanching of the extremity (result of arterial obstruction or spasm)
- On limbs that are infected or have evidence of peripheral vascular disease
- Through or distal to shunts in a dialysis patient

Procedure. Steps in performing an arterial puncture are as follows:

1. Hands are washed on entering the patient's room.
2. The pulse is palpated to determine the optimal site. An Allen's test is performed if the radial artery, posterior tibial artery, or dorsal artery of the foot is to be used.

TABLE 9–12 Causes of Alkalosis

RESPIRATORY ALKALOSIS	METABOLIC ALKALOSIS
Anxiety	Vomiting
Fever	Nasogastric suctioning
Sepsis	Congenital Cl^- wasting diarrhea
Hypoxemia Pneumonia Atelectasis Pulmonary emboli Congestive heart failure Asthma	Dehydration
Central nervous system disorders Head injury Brain tumor Infection Cerebrovascular accident High altitude	Diuretic administration
Liver failure	Steroid administration
Reye's syndrome	Cushing's syndrome
Hyperthyroidism	Bartter's syndrome
Salicylate poisoning	HCO_3^- administration
Mechanical ventilation	Hypokalemia
	Hypochloremia
	Chewing tobacco
	Massive blood transfusion
	Cystic fibrosis infants fed regular formula or breast milk (low in sodium)

Adapted from Brewer ED: Disorders of acid-base balance. Pediatr Clin N Am 1990; 37:429–447.

TABLE 9–13 Classifications of Hypoxemia

- Hypoventilation
- V/Q mismatch
- Shunt
  - Cardiac
  - Intrapulmonary
- Diffusion defect
- Altitude

V/Q, ventilation to perfusion ratio.

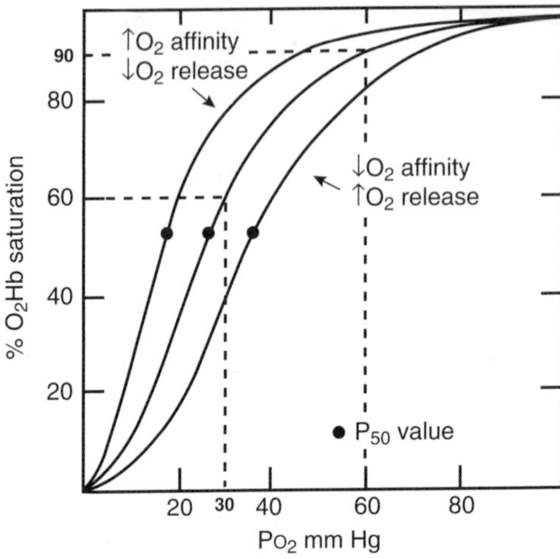

Figure 9–10 An oxyhemoglobin dissociation curve with the normal P_{50} illustrated and the effect of right and left shifts of the curve. As the curve shifts to the right, the oxygen affinity of hemoglobin decreases, more oxygen is released at a given oxygen tension, and the P_{50} value increases. When the curve shifts to the left, there is increased oxygen affinity, less oxygen is released at a given oxygen tension, and the P_{50} value decreases. The dashed lines correlate the landmarks of the 30-60-90 rule for estimating oxygen saturation. (Adapted from Oski FA: Fetal hemoglobin, the neonatal red cell, and 2,3-diphosphoglycerate. Pediatr Clin N Am 1972; 19:907–917.)

TABLE 9–14 Factors That Shift the Oxyhemoglobin Dissociation Curve

INCREASED AFFINITY (Left Shift)	DECREASED AFFINITY (Right shift)
Increased pH	Decreased pH
Decreased $Paco_2$	Increased $Paco_2$
Decreased temperature	Increased temperature
Decreased 2,3 DPG	Increased 2,3 DPG
Fetal hemoglobin	
Carboxyhemoglobin	
Methemoglobin	

2,3 DPG, 2,3-diphosphoglycerate.

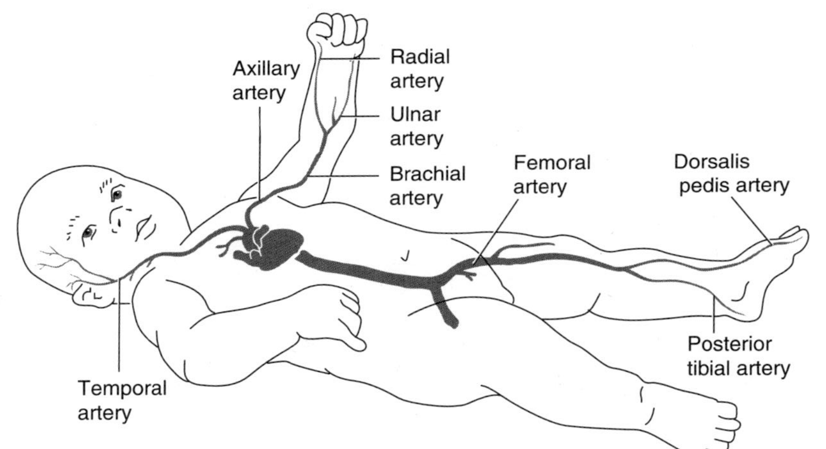

Figure 9–11 Arterial sites that may be used for peripheral artery puncture in infants and children.

3. Well-fitting gloves are donned.
4. The puncture area is scrubbed with antiseptic and allowed to air dry.
5. The limb to be used is immobilized and the small child or uncooperative patient is restrained.
6. The artery is again palpated and positioned with the index and middle finger of the clinician's least dominant hand.
7. The needle or butterfly catheter is inserted into the artery, bevel up, at a 30- to 45-degree angle and is advanced slowly.
8. The amount of blood needed is obtained and the needle or catheter is withdrawn. Using a sterile gauze pad, firm pressure is applied immediately to the site for at least 5 minutes until the bleeding stops. Pressure may need to be applied longer in patients receiving anticoagulation therapy. Pressure dressings are not used.
9. The sample is analyzed immediately or is placed on ice and analyzed within 1 hour.

Complications

- Hematoma formation
- Thrombosis and necrosis of head of femoral bone
- Infection
- Scarring
- Laceration of an artery
- Nerve damage
- Bleeding
- Obstruction of an artery by clots or spasm
- Pain

Capillary Puncture

Puncture Sites. Preferred sites include

- Posterolateral portion of the foot, just anterior to the heel (Fig. 9–12)
- Palmar or fleshy surface of the distal aspects of the fingers and toes (Fig. 9–13)

Puncture is avoided in the following areas:

- Posterior heel curvature (back of heel)
- Fingers of neonates
- Through previous puncture sites
- Through inflamed sites with apparent or possible infection present
- Extremities with localized swelling or edema
- Cyanotic areas

Procedure. Steps in performing a capillary puncture are as follows:

1. The puncture site is selected and the area is warmed for 5 to 10 minutes. A chemical heating pad is preferred, but

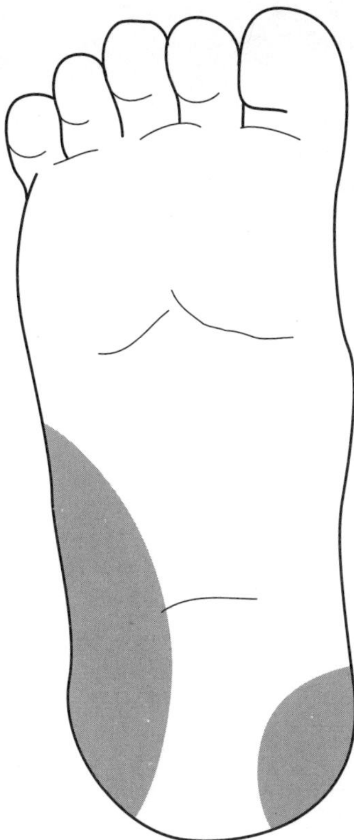

Figure 9–12 Shaded areas represent the recommended puncture sites in the infant's heel to obtain capillary blood for analysis.

a towel soaked in warm water (approximately 40° C, not hot to touch) can be used.

2. Hands are washed and well-fitting gloves are donned.
3. The warming device is removed and the puncture site is cleansed with an antiseptic. The area is dried with a sterile gauze pad.
4. The area to be punctured is immobilized (Figs. 9–13 and 9–14).
5. Holding the lancet (maximum tip length of 2.4 mm) between the thumb and index finger, it is positioned perpendicular to and above the puncture site. The lancet is inserted into the skin with one continuous, deliberate motion.
6. The first drop of blood is wiped away with a dry, sterile gauze pad.
7. Moderate, firm pressure is applied to the site and the blood is collected with a capillary tube (colored ring held away from patient). The tube is held in a slightly

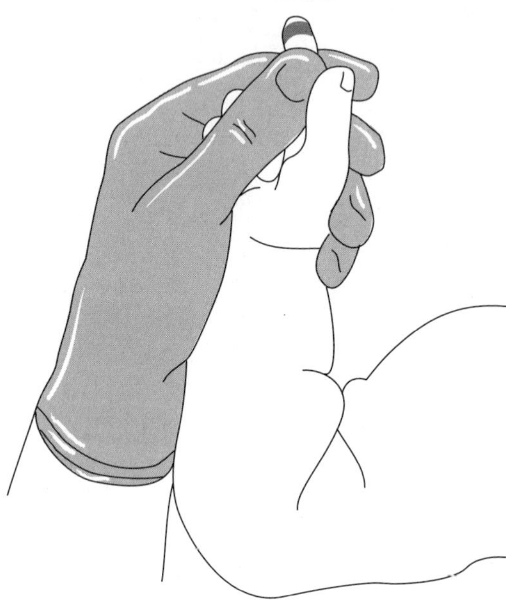

Figure 9–13 Technique for grasping the finger for a capillary puncture. The shaded area represents the recommended site for the puncture.

downward, horizontal position with the tip placed as near to the puncture site as possible without actually touching the site. The required amount of blood is collected.

8. Pressure is applied to the puncture site with a sterile gauze pad until the bleeding stops.
9. The sample is analyzed immediately or a metal flea is inserted and the tube sealed. The flea is removed prior to analyzing the blood.

Contraindications

- Decreased peripheral blood flow (e.g., hypotension, hypothermia)
- Polycythemia (hematocrit value >70%)
- Patients younger than 24 hours of age

Complications

- Infection
- Scarring
- Calcaneous osteomyelitis
- Calcifications
- Nerve damage
- Arterial laceration
- Bruising
- Cellulitis

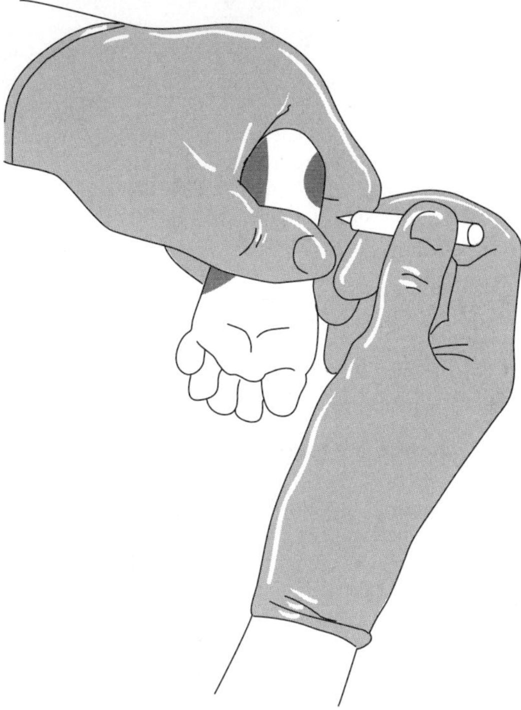

Figure 9–14 Technique of stabilizing the heel for a capillary puncture.

- Bleeding
- Burns

HEMODYNAMIC MONITORING

Cardiac Output

Cardiac output (CO) is the amount of blood ejected by the left ventricle (systole) over time. Resting, repolarization, or the refilling period is referred to as diastole. CO is expressed in liters per minute and is obtained using the following equation:

$$CO = \text{stroke volume} \times \text{heart rate}$$

Stroke volume is affected by the following:

1. Myocardial contraction, which is the shortening of heart muscle fibers causing ejection and filling of the heart.
2. Distensibility, which is the expandibility or stretchability of the myocardial fibers. As filling volume increases, CO

improves until overdistention occurs, after which CO decreases (Fig. 9–15).

3. Preload, which is diastolic filling; if there is insufficient volume, there is reduced contraction force. It is usually the result of high pulmonary vascular resistance (PVR) or right ventricular or valvular dysfunction. Excessive filling volume results in loss of distensibility.
4. Afterload, which is the forces opposing the ejection of blood from the left ventricle; it is mainly affected by systemic vascular resistance (SVR) or valvular dysfunction. High SVR results in reduced stroke volume. If chronic, the problem results in myocardial hypertrophy and loss of distensibility.

Factors that affect cardiac output are listed in Table 9–15.

Cardiac Output Measurement Methods

Thermal Dilution. A known volume of cold fluid is rapidly injected into the right atrium from a multilumen catheter that measures the temperature decay (warming or thermal dilution) at the distal end of the catheter. A computer converts the rate of decay to CO.

Dye Dilution. A known concentration of dye (indium green or methylene blue) is rapidly injected into the right atrium from a multilumen catheter. Blood samples are frequently drawn from the distal end of the catheter. Each sample is analyzed by photospectrometry to determine the

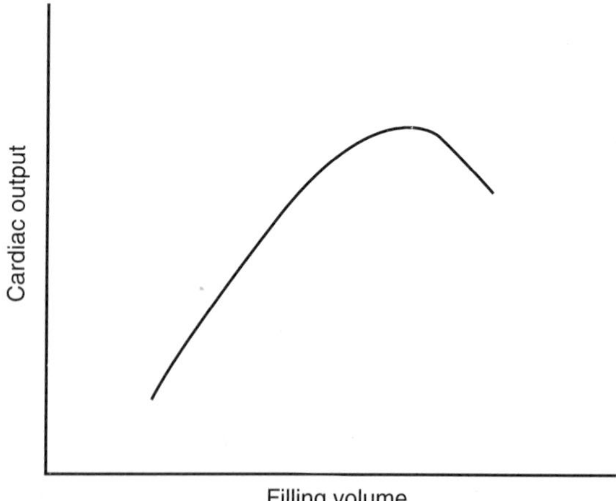

Figure 9–15 The Frank-Starling curve, demonstrating that the greater the muscle is stretched (filling volume), the greater the force of the contraction, until a critical point is reached and the contraction and cardiac output diminish.

TABLE 9–15 Factors That Affect Cardiac Output

DECREASE	INCREASE
Bradycardia	Tachycardia*
Hypovolemia	Intravascular fluids
PEEP-CPAP	Sepsis
Valvular dysfuction	Aortic assist devices
Pulmonary vascular resistance	Inotropic drugs
Congenital anomalies	Nitrates-vasodilators
Myocardial dysfunction	Intracardiac shunts
Pericardial dysfunction	
Hypertension	

* Infants have a limited ability to alter myocardial contractility, so cardiac output is mainly regulated by heart rate and intravascular fluid volume.
PEEP, positive end-expiratory pressure; CPAP, continuous positive airway pressure.

decay rate of the dye concentration (dilution). The rate of decay is plotted on a graph to calculate CO.

Fick Equation

$$CO = \dot{V}O_2/(CaO_2 - CvO_2)$$

$$\text{Oxygen consumption: } \dot{V}O_2 = \dot{V}E \times \left[FIO_2 \times \left(\frac{1 - FECO_2 - FEO_2}{1 - FIO_2} \right) - FEO_2 \right]$$

FEO_2 and $FECO_2$ are measured by collecting mixed exhaled gases.

Equations

Cardiac Index (CI)

$$CI = CO/\text{body surface area}$$

Mean Arterial Pressure (MAP)

$$MAP = [(2 \times \text{diastolic pressure}) + (\text{systolic pressure})]/3$$

MAP is an indicator of afterload. The same formula is applied to the pulmonary artery to derive mean pulmonary artery pressure (MPAP), which is an indicator of preload.

TABLE 9–16 Hemodynamic Variables and Normal Measurements

MEASUREMENT	SYSTOLIC (mm Hg)	DIASTOLIC (mm Hg)	MEAN (mm Hg)
Systemic	90–140	60–90	70–105
CVP	—	—	2–7
RVP	15–30	0–8	—
PAP	15–30	5–15	10–20
PCWP	—	—	5–15
MEASUREMENT	**UNIT**	**INFANT**	**ADULT-CHILD**
CO	L/min	—	4–8
CI	L/min/m^2	—	2.5–5
SVR	mm Hg/L/min	—	10–20
SVRI	mm Hg/L/min/m^2	10–15	20–35
PVR	mm Hg/L/min	—	1–3
SVRI	mm Hg/L/min/m^2	3–10	0.5–3

CVP, central venous pressure; RVP, right ventricular pressure; PAP, pulmonary artery pressure; PCWP, pulmonary capillary wedge pressure; CO, cardiac output; CI, cardiac index; SVR, systemic vascular resistance; SVRI, systemic vascular resistance index; PVR, pulmonary vascular resistance.

Systemic Vascular Resistance (SVR)

$$SVR = (MAP - CVP)/CO$$

Systemic Vascular Resistance Index (SVRI)

$$SVRI = (MAP - CVP)/CI$$

Pulmonary Vascular Resistance (PVR)

$$PVR = (MPAP - PCWP)/CO$$

Pulmonary Vascular Resistance Index (PVRI)

$$PVRI = (MPAP - PCWP)/CI$$

Normal values for hemodynamic variables are listed in Table 9–16.

Cardiac Catheterization Waveforms

Figure 9–16 illustrates examples of pressure waveforms produced as a right-sided heart catheter (Swan-Ganz) moves through the heart and wedges in the pulmonary capillaries.

INDIRECT CALORIMETRY AND NUTRITIONAL ASSESSMENT

Terminology

Basal Metabolic Rate. BMR is the lowest state of energy expenditure. Measurements are taken during fasting, resting, and neutral thermal environment conditions.

Resting Metabolic Rate (RMR) or Resting Energy Expenditure (REE). This is the BMR plus energy expenditure during a resting state.

Total Energy Expenditure (TEE). TEE is the energy expenditure measurement when corrections are made for activity and other metabolic expenditure.

Metabolic Energy Expenditure (MEE). MEE is the indirect calorimetry measurement of TEE.

Table 9–17 lists the cardiorespiratory and metabolic information that is available from exercise testing.

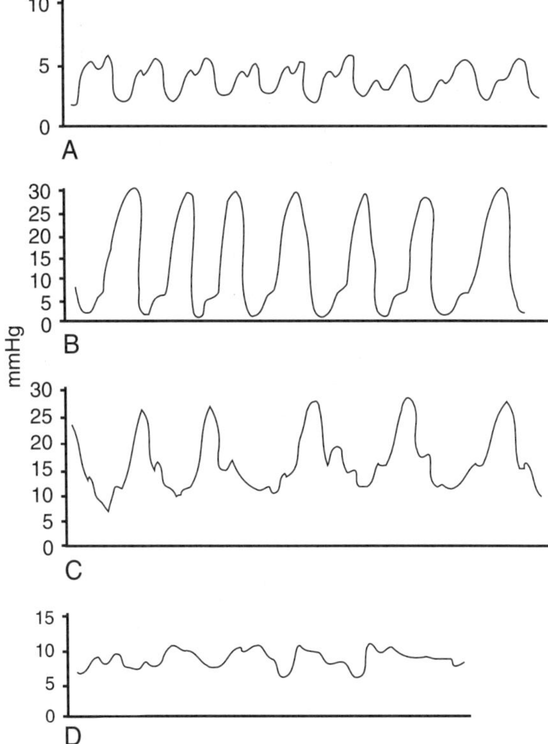

Figure 9–16 Examples of pressure waveform patterns at various locations surrounding the right heart. *A*, Central venous pressure. *B*, Right ventricular pressure. *C*, Pulmonary artery pressure. *D*, Pulmonary capillary wedge pressure.

TABLE 9–17 Cardiorespiratory and Metabolic Information Available From Exercise Testing

TERM	SYMBOL	DEFINITION
Maximal oxygen uptake	$\dot{V}O_{2max}$	A plateau or decrease in $\dot{V}O_2$ despite a continuing increase in work rate. Care must be taken to distinguish the peak $\dot{V}O_2$ (the largest $\dot{V}O_2$ achieved by the subject) from the true $\dot{V}O_{max}$.
Anaerobic, lactate, or ventilatory threshold	AT, LT, VAT	The point during progressive exercise when lactate concentration begins to increase in the blood. The usual gas exchange manifestations of the AT are hyperventilation with respect to $\dot{V}O_2$ (increase in $\dot{V}_E/\dot{V}O_2$ and end-tidal PO_2), which occurs when $\dot{V}_E/\dot{V}CO_2$ and end-tidal PCO_2 are constant.
Work efficiency, oxygen cost of exercise	—	These variables are determined from the relationship of $\dot{V}O_2$ to the work rate.
Response time of gas exchange adaptations to exercise (mean response time, time constant)	RT. MRT, τ	The mathematically derived descriptor of the time required for $\dot{V}O_2$, $\dot{V}_E$, and $\dot{V}CO_2$ to achieve a steady state in response to a work rate input.

Ventilatory response to exercise	$\Delta\dot{V}_E/\Delta\dot{V}CO_2$	Slope of the linear portion of the relationship between $\dot{V}_E$ and $\dot{V}CO_2$ during progressive exercise. (n.b., the ventilatory equivalent of CO_2 is the ratio $\dot{V}_E/\dot{V}CO_2$ and is not the same as the slope.)
Respiratory compensation point	RCP	The point during AT exercise when hyperventilation for $\dot{V}CO_2$ occurs. Presumably, the RCP occurs when the bicarbonate is no longer able to adequately buffer the lactic acid produced during high-intensity exercise and pH changes. This stimulates the peripheral chemoreceptors.
Oxygen pulse	O_2 pulse	The ratio $\dot{V}O_2$/HR. This ratio represents the amount of oxygen extracted per heart beat, which is not the same as the slope of the $\dot{V}O_2$-heart rate relationship during progressive exercise.
$\dot{V}O_2$ to heart rate relationship	$\Delta\dot{V}O_2/\Delta HR$	This ratio represents the slope of the linear portion of the relationship between $\dot{V}O_2$ and HR during progressive exercise.
Exercise-induced bronchospasm	EIB	A fall of at least 15% in the ratio FEV_1/FVC following a bout of exercise.

Adapted from Chernick V (ed): Kendig's Disorders of the Respiratory Tract in Children. Philadelphia, WB Saunders, 1990, p 158.

Equations

Metabolic Energy Expenditure

$$MEE = (3.94 \times \dot{V}O_2) + (1.106 \times \dot{V}CO_2)$$

Oxygen Consumption

$$\dot{V}O_2 = CO \times (CaO_2 - C\bar{v}O_2) \text{ (See Fick equation)}$$

$$\text{Adult} = 3.5 \text{ ml/kg}$$

$$\text{Child} = 6 \text{ to } 8 \text{ ml/kg}$$

Caloric Need

An approximate increase in caloric need is directly proportional to oxygen uptake.

$$MEE \times \text{weight} = \text{kcal/day}$$

NONINVASIVE MONITORING

Pulse Oximetry

Pulse oximetry provides continuous monitoring of oxygenation by noninvasively measuring the saturation of oxygen, pulse rate, and pulse amplitude.

Patient Application. The pulse oximeter sensor should be applied to vascular areas (Fig. 9–17). Sites must be large enough to accommodate the sensor. Possible sites in neonates are

- Wrist
- Ball of foot
- Palm of hand
- Ankle

Possible sites in larger infants and children include

- Fingers
- Toes
- Forehead
- Bridge of nose

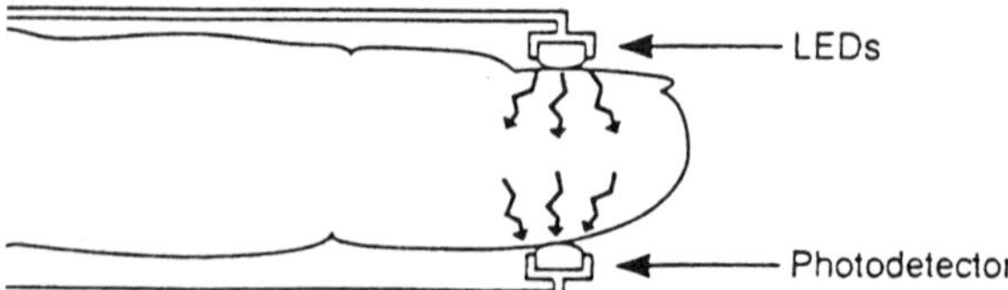

Figure 9–17 Proper alignment of light-emitting diodes (LEDs) opposite the photodetector in a sensor applied to a finger. (From Pulse Oximetry: Technical, Note Number 7. Hayward, CA, Nellcor, Inc., 1991.)

Monitoring sites are changed routinely to avoid pressure sores or tissue injury (risk is highest in neonates).

Relationship Between Functional and Fractional Saturation

Functional saturation is measured by pulse oximetry as

$$\% \text{ functional } O_2Hb = O_2Hb/(O_2Hb + RHb)$$

Fractional saturation is measured by co-oximetry as

$$\% \text{ fractional } O_2Hb = O_2Hb/(O_2Hb + RHb + COHb + MetHb)$$

The difference in the two saturations is important to note when comparing pulse oximetry and co-oximeter calculations, especially when monitoring patients with elevated COHb or MetHb saturations.

Transcutaneous Po_2 and Pco_2 Monitoring

Transcutaneous monitoring provides the measurement of partial pressure of oxygen and carbon dioxide on the skin surface (Figs. 9–18 and 9–19).

Patient Application. Calibration of the monitor is performed prior to applying the electrode on the skin. Monitor-

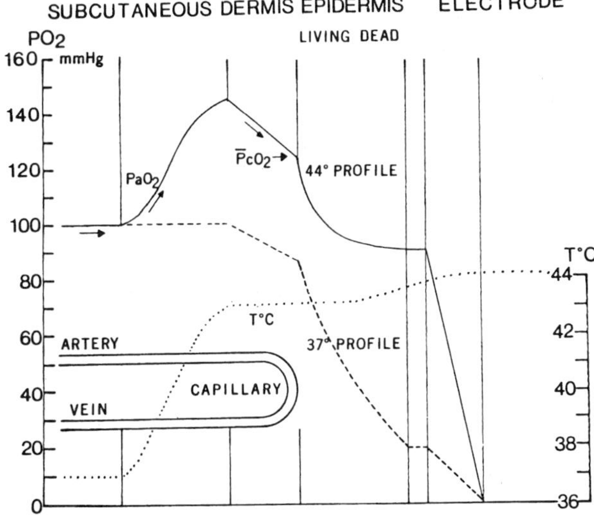

Figure 9–18 Skin surface Po_2. Dashed line represents unheated Po_2, whereas the solid line represents the cumulative effects of a heated electrode on Po_2. (Adapted from Thunstrom AM, Stafford NJ, Severinghaus JW: A two temperature, two Po_2 method of estimating the determinants of $Tcpo_2$. *In* Huch A, Huch R, Lucey JF [eds]: Continuous Transcutaneous Blood Gas Monitoring: Birth Defects, Volume XV. New York, Alan R Liss, 1979, p 168.)

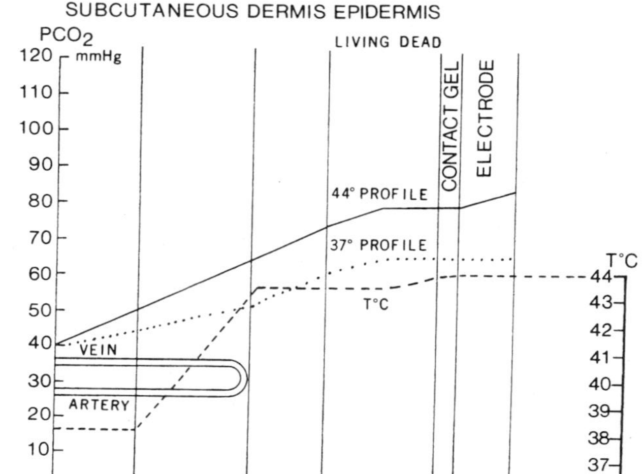

Figure 9–19 Skin surface P_{CO_2}. Dotted line represents unheated P_{CO_2}, whereas the solid line represents the cumulative effects of a heated electrode on P_{CO_2}. (Adapted from Thunstrom AM, Stafford MJ, Severinghaus JW: A two temperature, two P_{O_2} method of estimating the determinants of T_{CPO_2}. *In* Huch A, Huch R, Lucey JF [eds]: Continuous Transcutaneous Blood Gas Monitoring: Birth Defects, Volume XV. New York, Alan R. Liss, 1979, p 168.)

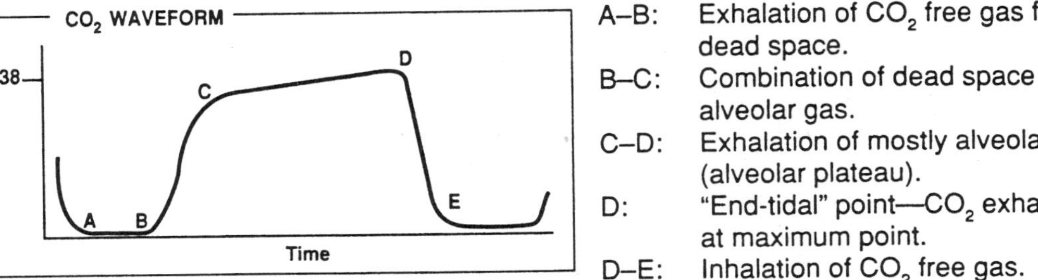

A–B: Exhalation of CO_2 free gas from dead space.

B–C: Combination of dead space and alveolar gas.

C–D: Exhalation of mostly alveolar gas (alveolar plateau).

D: "End-tidal" point—CO_2 exhalation at maximum point.

D–E: Inhalation of CO_2 free gas.

Figure 9–20 Normal capnogram. (From Advanced Concepts in Capnography. Hayward, CA, Nellcor, Inc., 1988.)

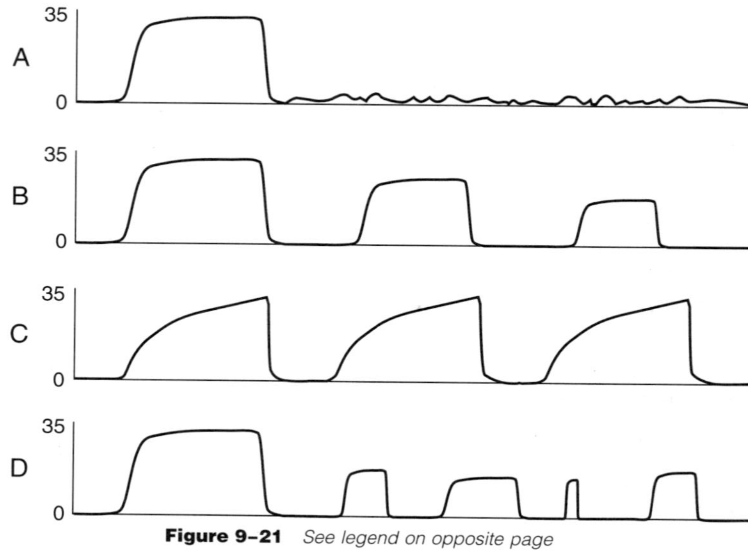

Figure 9–21 *See legend on opposite page*

See legend on opposite page

ing sites should be flat, nonbony areas. To prevent thermal injuries, the sensor is repositioned every 2 to 4 hours (more often if a blister or burn develops).

Capnometry

Capnometry, or end-tidal carbon dioxide monitoring, is a noninvasive method of measuring the partial pressure of carbon dioxide in the expired air.

Patient Application. Gas samples are obtained from the patient through the following:

- An adapter attached to an endotracheal tube
- A catheter placed in the posterior nasopharynx
- A mask
- A mouthpiece

Capnogram. The capnogram (waveform display of exhaled carbon dioxide) provides a graphic representation of exhaled carbon dioxide (Fig. 9–20). The shape of the waveform characterizes various clinical conditions (Fig. 9–21).

The advantages and disadvantages of using pulse oximetry, capnometry, and transcutaneous monitoring are listed in Table 9–18.

Impedance Pneumography

Impedance pneumography uses a set of electrodes for noninvasive monitoring of breathing rate and pattern of chest movement. It is used most often in home care apnea and event monitors. Measurement is based on the difference in resistance (impedance) to electric current when the thorax expands with gas volume (Fig. 9–22). The main disadvantage of impedance pneumography is that if airway obstruction occurs and airflow stops, chest and abdominal movements may still occur and the apnea alarm will not be triggered.

Patient Application

1. All soap, oil, powder, and lotion is cleansed from the patient's chest.

Figure 9–21 End-tidal CO_2 recordings. *A,* Abrupt disconnection from the ventilator. *B,* Falling P_{ETCO_2}, possibly an increase in tidal volume, or if Pa_{CO_2} is unchanged, a reduction in pulmonary blood flow from overdistention or low cardiac output. *C,* Dampened waveform from severe airflow obstruction or side stream sampling tube obstruction. *D,* System leak or secretions in the sampling chamber. (Adapted from Advanced Concepts in Capnography. Hayward, CA, Nellcor, Inc., 1988.)

TABLE 9–18 Advantages and Disadvantages of Noninvasive Monitoring Systems*

MONITOR	ADVANTAGE	DISADVANTAGE
Pulse oximetry	Continuous and noninvasive Prevents frequent blood gas punctures Measurements in real time No calibration required Effective for all age ranges Cost-effective	Imprecise for determining Pa_{O_2} because of shape of oxyhemoglobin dissociation curve Loses accuracy at low saturation levels Motion and light artifact Affected by perfusion and skin pigmentation Measures functional HbO_2 Allergy to adhesive

Transcutaneous oxygen–carbon dioxide monitoring	Prevents frequent blood gas punctures Monitors multiple gases Continuous and noninvasive Precise measurements Stable measurements Perfusion may be quantified	Frequent calibration and site changes Blistering of measuring site Affected by skin site conditions Relatively expensive supplies Affected by perfusion Allergy to adhesive
Capnometry	Prevents frequent blood gas punctures Waveform analysis Monitors ventilation to perfusion changes as $PaCO_2$-$PETCO_2$ changes Independent of tissue perfusion Rapid results from ventilator adjustments available May be used to measure airflow	Side stream sampling reduces V_T Main stream sampling increases V_D/V_T Underestimates $PaCO_2$ Correlation reduced when patient unintubated Errors with leaks Lag time with side stream Older sensors may cause burns

* All noninvasive monitors may lead to clinical judgments that are based on inaccurate values being reported. Most monitors are used to report trends and should reliably correlate with arterial gas measurements. It is crucial to understand the limitations and specifications of each individual monitor being used.

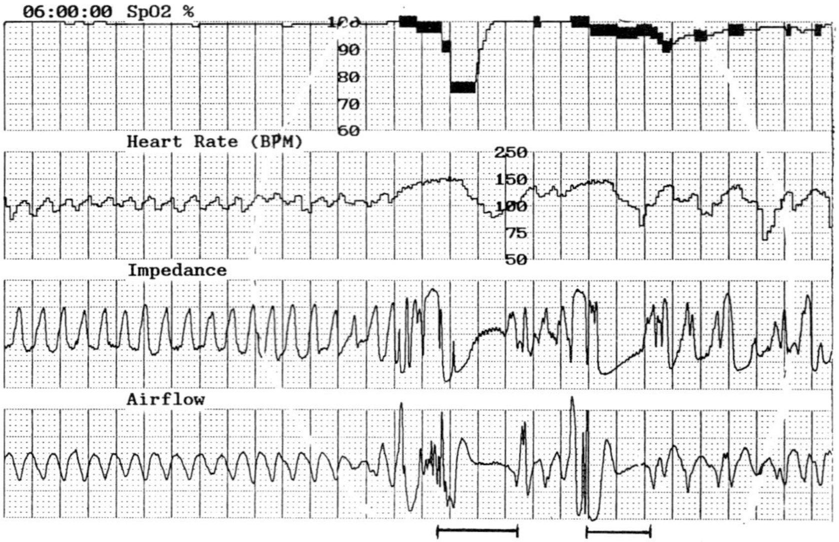

06:00:00 SpO2 %

100
90
80
70
60

Heart Rate (BPM)

250
150
100
75
50

Impedance

Airflow

Figure 9–22 *See legend on opposite page*

2. The soft foam belt is placed under the patient's back (Fig. 9–23).
3. Electrode pads are applied on both sides of the thorax along the intersection of the nipple line with the axillary line. Adhesive pads may be used in the hospital setting.
4. The belt is wrapped snugly around the patient's chest to hold the electrodes in place. The belt is fastened with velcro so that one finger can slide under it. Excessive overlap that blocks electrode contact with the chest under the belt is not allowed.

RADIOGRAPHIC ASSESSMENT

Basic concepts concerning the nature of x-rays include

- Matter that absorbs all x-ray energy is white.
- Matter that absorbs some of the x-ray energy is gray.
- Matter that does not absorb x-ray energy is black.

Densities

Images on a chest film consist of one or more of the four basic densities listed further on. As tissue becomes denser, the color on the film becomes lighter (i.e., the black color of an aerated lung to the white color of ribs).

Air. Air is black and radiolucent. Examples are gas in the trachea, bronchi, stomach, and intestines.

Fat. Fat is gray. Examples are skin and soft tissue around muscle.

Fluid. Fluid is whitish (lighter than gray). Examples are heart, blood vessels, and diaphragm.

Bone-Metal. These are white and radiopaque. Examples are ribs, vertebrae, prostheses, and surgical clips.

Systematic Approach to Evaluating a Chest X-ray Film

1. The type of position the patient was placed in is identified.
2. The radiographic view (anteroposterior, posteroanterior, oblique) is identified.
3. One begins at the center of the x-ray film.

Figure 9–22 Example of an impedance pneumogram showing periodic breathing.

4. The anatomy is identified (e.g., heart, diaphragm, ribs, trachea).
5. The size of the heart and mediastinum is evaluated.
6. One works out to the periphery
   a. The posterior aspects of the ribs are counted to determine if the film is a normal inspiratory, poor inspiratory, or expiratory film.
   b. The size, shape, and symmetry of the chest cage are noted.
   c. The trachea is examined for deviation and endotracheal tube placement.
   d. The position of the diaphragm is noted (elevated, flat).
   e. Pathologic conditions are identified (Table 9–19).
   f. Progression is compared with previous films.

Advanced Imaging Methods

Advanced methods used in evaluation include

- Fluoroscopy
- Magnetic resonance imaging (MRI)
- Computerized tomography (CT) scanning
- Ultrasound imaging
- Vascular cinetography
- Nuclear radiotide imaging

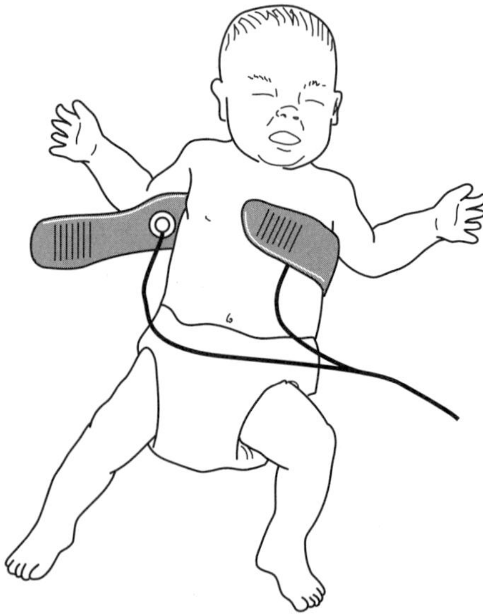

Figure 9–23 With the infant on a flat surface, the belt is positioned in line with the infant's nipples. After the electrodes are placed, the belt is wrapped snugly around the infant's chest.

BRONCHOSCOPY

Rigid and Flexible Bronchoscopy

Rigid and flexible bronchoscopy are compared in Table 9–20.

Indications

Indications for bronchoscopy may be classified as diagnostic or therapeutic and are listed in Table 9–21.

Complications

Complications that may be encountered with bronchoscopy include

1. Oxygen desaturation
2. Hypoventilation
3. Adverse reactions to sedatives
   a. Oversedation resulting in hypoventilation or apnea
   b. Hypotension in response to narcotic analgesics
   c. Allergic reactions and seizures
4. Infection
5. Bleeding, particularly from nasal mucosa
6. Hemoptysis
7. Fever
8. Airway edema
9. Sore throat
10. Stridor

TABLE 9–19 Radiographic Features of Pathologic Conditions

CONDITION	VIEW	RADIOGRAPHIC FEATURES
Croup	Lateral neck	Narrowed subglottic airway, steeple sign, ballooning hypopharyngeal space, normal oval epiglottis
Epiglottitis	Lateral neck	Enlarged, rounded epiglottis—steeple sign, normal subglottic airway, ballooning hypopharyngeal space
Foreign body	AP chest	Inspiratory film likely normal, possible atelectasis from complete bronchi obstruction; expiratory film shows hyperinflation and possible mediastinal shift to unaffected lung
RDS	AP chest	Hazy infiltrates, reticular pattern (ground glass), low lung volume, atelectasis possible

Pneumothorax	AP chest	Air collection, shift of mediastinum to opposite side; dissection of air into mediastinum, peritoneum, or pericardial spaces
PIE	AP chest	Small circular cyst formations along dissected airways
Pleural effusion	PA chest	Air fluid level, possible mediastinal shift
Asthma	PA chest	Hyperinflated lung volume, depressed diaphragm; atelectasis possible from mucus plugging
Pneumonia	AP chest	Segmental or patchy infiltrates
ARDS	AP chest	Consolidation, air bronchograms
Congenital heart disease	AP chest	Enlarged cardiac silhouette, vascular markings
Diaphragmatic hernia	AP chest	Bowel and gas in thorax, shifted mediastinum
Paralyzed diaphragm	Fluoroscopy	Unilateral diaphragm movement during inspiration, usually sniffing if patient can perform maneuver

AP, anteroposterior; RDS, respiratory distress syndrome; PA, posteroanterior; PIE, pulmonary interstitial emphysema; ARDS, adult respiratory distress syndrome.

TABLE 9-20 Comparison of Rigid and Flexible Bronchoscopy

RIGID BRONCHOSCOPY

- Rigid steel tube construction
- Fitted with an anesthesia circuit, a telescope, and grasping instruments
- Requires general anesthesia
- Performed in the operating room
- Patient is ventilated by anesthesiologist
- Comparatively expensive
- Slightly better optics
- Larger suction channels for thick secretions
- Special instruments for removal of foreign bodies, manipulation of the airway, laser attachments
- Distends and distorts the shape of the airways during visualization

FLEXIBLE BRONCHOSCOPY

- Flexible fiberoptic construction
- Requires sedation
- Performed in treatment room or intensive care unit with monitors
- Comparatively less expensive
- Patient is breathing spontaneously
- Specimens and cultures from the lower airways and peripheral sites
- Views upper airways
- Allows a dynamic view and gives a better idea of the true shape of the airways
- Larynx and vocal cord structures without distortion
- May be used to intubate
- Suction channels of limited diameter on smaller scopes

TABLE 9-21 Indications for Bronchoscopy

THERAPEUTIC
Foreign body aspiration
Surgical removal of granulomas or polyps
Clearing thick secretions
Persistent atelectasis, right middle lobe syndrome
Evaluating tracheostomy or endotracheal tube
Guiding intubation
Guiding surgery on airway, aortopexy
DIAGNOSTIC
Congenital stridor
Laryngomalacia
Laryngeal polyposis
Vocal cord paralysis
Congenital laryngeal webs
Visualizing airway anatomy
Tracheomalacia
Tracheitis
Persistent pneumonitis
Obtaining biopsy specimen
Obtaining bronchoalveolar lavage specimen
Measuring transbronchial drug levels

Bibliography

Advanced Concepts in Capnography. Hayward, CA, Nellcor, Inc., 1988.

Alexander CM, Teller LE, Gross JB: Principles of pulse oximetry: Theoretical and practical considerations. Anesth Analg 1989; 68:368.

Aloan CA: Laboratory and radiologic assessment. *In* Aloan CA (ed): Respiratory Care of the Newborn. Philadelphia, JB Lippincott, 1987, pp 61–81.

Al-Saidy W, Hill DW: The importance of an elevated skin temperature in transcutaneous oxygen tension measurements. *In* Huch A, Huch R, Lucey JF (eds): Continuous Transcutaneous Blood Gas Monitoring: Birth Defects Volume XV. New York, Alan R. Liss, 1979, p 149.

Amar D, Neidzwski J, Wald A, Finck AD: Fluorescent light interferes with pulse oximetry. J Clin Monit 1989; 5:135–136.

American Association for Respiratory Care: Clinical Practice Guideline for Bronchial Provocation. Respir Care 1992; 37:902–906.

American Association for Respiratory Care: Clinical Practice Guideline: Sampling for arterial blood gas analysis. Respir Care 1992; 37:913–917.

American Association for Respiratory Care: Clinical Practice Guideline for Pulse Oximetry. Respir Care 1991; 36:1406–1409.

Boyda EK, Kee JL, Monaghan FD: Knowledge basic to the nursing care of adults with fluid, electrolyte, and acid-base imbalance. *In* Monaghan FD, Drake T, Neighbors M (eds): Nursing Care of Adults. Philadelphia, WB Saunders, 1994.

Brouillette RT, Morrow AS, Mayre DE: Comparison of respiratory inductive plethysmography and thoracic impedance for apnea monitoring. J Pediatr 1987; 111:377.

Brown M, Vender JS: Noninvasive oxygen monitoring. Crit Care Clin 1988; 4:493–509.

Brutocao DP, O'Rourke PP: Monitoring in pediatric care. *In* Kacmarek RM, Hess D, Stoller JK (eds): Monitoring in Respiratory Care. St. Louis, Mosby-Year Book, 1994, pp 621–647.

Chatburn RL: Evaluation of pediatric pulmonary function: Theory and application. Respir Care 1989; 34:597–610.

Connors AF: Hemodynamic monitoring. *In* Kacmarek RM, Hess D, Stoller JK (eds): Monitoring in respiratory care. St. Louis, Mosby-Year Book, 1994, pp 227–265.

Courtney SE, Weber KR, Breakie LA, et al: Capillary blood gases in the neonate. A reassessment and review of the literature. Am J Dis Child 1990; 144:168–172.

Czervinske MP: Arterial blood gas analysis and other cardiopulmonary monitoring. *In* Koff PB, Eitzman DV, Neu J (eds): Neonatal and Pediatric Respiratory Care, St. Louis, CV Mosby, 1988, pp 260–281.

Dascalova L, Gueorguieva E: Respiratory pauses in normal prematurely born infants. Biol Neonat 1983; 44:325.

DuBois AB, Botelho SY, Comroe JH Jr: A new method for measuring airway resistance in man using a body plethysmograph: Values in normal subjects and in patients with respiratory disease. J Clin Invest 1956; 35:327–335.

Hilman BC, Allen JL: Clinical application of pulmonary function testing in children and adolescents. *In* Hilman BC (ed): Pediatric Respiratory Disease: Diagnosis and Treatment. Philadelphia, WB Saunders, 1993, pp 98–107.

Kirplani H, Kechagias S, Lerman J: Technical and clinical aspects of capnography in neonates. J Med Eng Technol 1991; 15:154.

Knudson RJ, Slatin RC, Lebowitz MD, et al: The maximal expiratory flow volume curve. Am Rev Respir Dis 1976; 113:587–600.

Lemen RJ: Pulmonary function testing in the office, clinic, and home. *In* Chernick V (ed): Kendig's Disorders of the Respiratory Tract in Children. Philadelphia, WB Saunders, 1990, pp 147–154.

Mogue LR, Rantala B: Capnometers. J Clin Monit 1988; 4:115.

Monaco F, McQuitty JC: Transcutaneous measurements of carbon dioxide partial pressure in sick neonates. Crit Care Med 1981; 9:756.

Monaco F, Nickerson BG, McQuitty JC: Continuous transcutaneous oxygen and carbon dioxide monitoring in the pediatric ICU. Crit Care Med 1982; 10:765.

Nellcor: Pulse Oximetry: Technical Note Number 7. Hayward, CA, Nellcor, Inc., 1991.

Nellcor: Technical Note Number 2. Hayward, CA, Nellcor, Inc., 1987.

Romes ES, Stork EK, Carlo WA, Martin RJ: Limitations of transcutaneous Po_2 and Pco_2 monitoring in infants with bronchopulmonary dysplasia. Pediatrics 1984; 74:217.

Russell RI, Helms PJ: Comparative accuracy of pulse oximetry and transcutaneous oxygen in assessing arterial saturation in pediatric intensive care. Crit Care Med 1990; 18:725.

Severinghaus JW: Transcutaneous monitoring of arterial Pco_2. *In* Spence AA (ed): Respiratory Monitoring in Intensive Care. New York, Churchill Livingstone, 1982, p 85.

Severinghaus JW, Spellman MJ: Pulse oximeter failure threshold in hypotension and ischemia. Anesthesiology 1990; 73:532.

Smallhout B, Kalenda Z: An Atlas of Capnography. Zeist, Netherlands, Kerkebosch, 1975.

Stock MD: Noninvasive carbon dioxide monitoring. Crit Care Clin 1988; 4:511.

Taussig LM, Chernick V, Wood R, et al: Standardization of lung function testing in children. J Pediatr 1980; 97:668–676.

Tobin MJ: Monitoring pressure, flow and volume during mechanical ventilation. Respir Care 1992; 37:1081–1096.

Welch JP, DeCesare R, Hess D: Pulse oximetry: Instrumentation and clinical applications. Respir Care 1990; 35:584.

Weng T, Levison H: Standards of pulmonary function testing in children. Am Rev Respir Dis 1969; 99:879–894.

Wood RE: Diagnostic and therapeutic procedures in pediatric pulmonary disease. *In* Lough MD, Doershuk CF, Stern RC (eds): Pediatric Respiratory Therapy, 3rd ed. Chicago, Year Book Medical, 1985, pp 209–225.

SECTION 10

Pharmacology

Abbreviations

BID–twice daily
CNS–central nervous system
DPI–dry powder inhaler
ET–endotracheal
g–gram
IC–intracardiac
IM–intramuscular
IO–intraosseus
IV–intravenous
L–liter
LVN–large-volume nebulizer
MDI–metered dose inhaler
mg–milligram
ml–milliliter
PRN–as needed
q–every
QID–four times daily
SPAG–small-particle aerosol generator
SVN–small-volume nebulizer
Tab–tablet
TID–three times daily
μg–microgram

EQUIVALENTS

Volume: 1 L = 1000 ml
0.001 L = 1 ml

Weight:

$1\ g = 1000\ mg$ or $10^3\ mg$
$1\ g = 1{,}000{,}000\ \mu g$ or $10^6\ \mu g$
$1\ mg = 1000\ \mu g$ or $10^3\ \mu g$
$= 0.001\ g$ or $10^{-3}\ g$
$1\ \mu g = 0.001\ mg$ or $10^{-3}\ mg$
$= 0.000001\ g$ or $10^{-6}\ g$

$1\ g = 1000\ mg = 1{,}000{,}000\ \mu g$
$1\ mg = 1000\ \mu g = 0.001\ g$
$1\ \mu g = 0.001\ mg = 0.000001\ g$
$1\ g = 10^3\ mg = 10^6\ \mu g$
$1\ mg = 10^{-3}\ g = 10^3\ \mu g$
$1\ \mu g = 10^{-6}\ g = 10^{-3} mg$

DRUG DOSAGE CALCULATIONS

To calculate milligrams per milliliter from a percent (%) solution:

1. Determine the amount of milligrams in 1 ml in a % solution:
   - Since $x\% = x$ g/100 ml solution and
   - Since 1000 mg = 1 g, then
   - Moving the decimal point of the % solution value over one space to the right gives the amount of milligrams in 1 ml
2. Example using 0.5% solution:
   - 0.5% = 5 g/100 ml solution and
   - Moving the decimal point of 0.5% over one space to the right results in 5%
   - Therefore, a 0.5% solution is equivalent to 5 mg/ml
3. Another method of determining milligrams per milliliter in a % solution:
   - Change the % solution to a dilution factor
   - Example: 0.5% = 0.5 : 100 = 5 : 1000

$$\frac{\begin{array}{c}0.5:100\\ \times 10:\times 10\end{array}}{5:1000} = 5:1000$$

↳always reveals milligrams per milliliter

To calculate a % solution from a dilution:

1. Remember that 1 : 100 = 1%
   Use this as a tool and compare all calculations to 100.
2. Example:

$$\frac{\begin{array}{c}1:200\\ \times .5:\times .5\end{array}}{0.5:100}$$

↳always reveals the % solution

OR

1. Remember that 1 : 1000 = 0.1%
   Use this as a tool; compare all calculations to 1000.

2. Example:

$$\begin{array}{r} 1:200 \\ \times 5:\times 5 \\ \hline 5:1000 \end{array} \qquad \begin{array}{r} 1:100 \\ \times 10:\times 10 \\ \hline 10:1000 \end{array}$$

Move the decimal over one space to the left to find the %.

$5:1000 = 0.5\%$ $\qquad$ $10:1000 = 1\%$

To calculate a volume dose from a known concentration of drug:

1. Remember that

Desired milliliters = (desired dose/known dose) × known volume

2. Example: How many milliliters are needed to deliver 0.5 mg from a known 5 mg/ml supply? (Remember that 5 mg/ml = 5 mg in 1 ml)

   The desired dose is 0.5 mg, the known dose is 5 mg, and the known volume is 1 ml. Therefore, the desired milliliters are

$$\text{ml} = (0.5\ \text{mg}/5\ \text{mg}) \times 1\ \text{ml}$$

$$= 0.1\ \text{ml}$$

To calculate a weight dose from a known volume dose of drug:

1. Remember that

Amount in milligrams = (known dose/known volume) × desired volume

2. Example: What is the weight in milligrams when delivering 0.1 ml from a 5 mg/ml supply?

   The known dose is 5 mg, the known volume is 1 ml, and the desired volume is 0.1 ml. Therefore, the weight in milligrams is

$$\text{mg} = (5\ \text{mg}/1\ \text{ml}) \times 0.1\ \text{ml}$$

$$= 0.5\ \text{mg}$$

Text continued on page 356

TABLE 10–1 Pulmonary Medications

MEDICATION	ROUTE	DOSE-FREQUENCY	ACTION-REMARKS
Albuterol	MDI	2 puffs q 4–6 hours	Bronchodilator sympathomimetic
	Rotacaps	200 μg q 4–6 hours	
	SVN	0.1–0.15 mg/kg; 0.03 ml/kg q 4–6 hours 0.25–0.5 ml q 15 minutes × 3 for acute distress	0.5% aerosol solution; intermittent nebulization, diluted in 2–3 ml normal saline
	LVN	5–15 mg/hour	Status asthmaticus; 0.5% aerosol solution, continuous administration,* requires continuous cardiac monitoring
	Elixir	0.1–0.15 mg/kg q 4–6 hours	
	Tab	2–4 mg q 4–6 hours	
Beclomethasone	MDI	1–2 puffs q 6–8 hours	Inhaled steroid
Beractant phospholipids (Survanta)	ET	100 mg/kg	Surfactant (bovine); single dose, subsequent dose after 6 hours
	ET	4 ml/kg	

Table continued on following page

TABLE 10–1 Pulmonary Medications *Continued*

MEDICATION	ROUTE	DOSE-FREQUENCY	ACTION-REMARKS
Caffeine	PO	20 mg/kg (loading) 5 mg/kg (subsequent)	Respiratory stimulant for apnea of prematurity; oral administration daily to maintain serum level of 10–15 μg/ml
Colfosceril palmitate (Exosurf)	ET	5 ml/kg	Synthetic surfactant; single dose, subsequent dose after 12 hours
Cromolyn sodium	MDI SVN or DPI	2 puffs q 6 hours 20 mg q 6 hours	Prophylactic mast cell stabilizer
Recombinant human DNase	SVN	2.5 mg daily	Mucolytic, nebulized daily in a separate clean nebulizer
Flunisolide	MDI	1–2 puffs q 12 hours	Inhaled steroid
Ipratropium bromide	MDI SVN	1–2 puffs q 6–8 hours 25 μg/kg q 6–8 hours	Bronchodilator, parasympatholytic
Isoetharine	SVN	0.1–0.2 mg/kg q 4–6 hours 2.5–5 mg	Bronchodilator, sympathomimetic; 1% aerosol solution for intermittent nebulization diluted in normal saline
Metaproterenol	SVN	0.1–0.3 ml q 4–6 hours	Bronchodilator, sympathomimetic; 5% aerosol solution, intermittent nebulization, diluted in normal saline

	MDI	1–3 puffs q 3–4 hours	Maximum 12 puffs/day
	Elixir	0.3–0.5 mg/kg q 4–6 hours	
	Tab	10–20 mg q 4–6 hours	
N-acetylcysteine	SVN	3–5 ml TID or QID	Mucolytic; 10% solution, usually mixed with a bronchodilator
Nedocromil	MDI	2 puffs q 6 hours	Mast cell stabilizer, weak bronchodilator
Prednisolone	Elixir or Tab	5–15 mg/day	Oral steroid; taper decreasing doses
Prednisone	Elixir or Tab	1–50 mg/day	Oral steroid; taper decreasing doses
Racemic epinephrine	SVN	0.05 ml/kg; 0.25–0.5 ml	Sympathomimetic, vasoconstrictor; 2.25% aerosol solution, diluted in saline; caution for rebound effect
Salmeterol	MDI	2 puffs q 10–12 hours	Bronchodilator
Terbutaline	MDI	2 puffs q 4–6 hours	Bronchodilator, sympathomimetic; 5% aerosol solution, intermittent nebulization
	SVN	0.5–1.5 mg q 4–6 hours	
	SVN	0.25–0.5 ml q 15 min × 3 for acute distress	Intermittent nebulization, diluted in 2–3 ml normal saline
	LVN	1–3 mg/hour	Status asthmaticus, 1 mg/ml solution, continuous administration,† requires continuous cardiac monitoring

Table continued on following page

TABLE 10–1 Pulmonary Medications *Continued*

MEDICATION	ROUTE	DOSE-FREQUENCY	ACTION-REMARKS
Terbutaline	Tab	2.5–5 mg q 4–6 hours	
Theophylline	IV or PO	*Loading dose:* Infant, 1–3 mg/kg Child-adult, 5–7 mg/kg *Maintenance dose:* Infant, 1–1.2 mg/kg Child-adult, 0.5 mg/kg	Bronchodilator; maintain serum level of 10–20 μg/ml, q 12 hours
	IV or PO	*Loading dose:* 1 mg/kg per 2 μg/ml *Maintenance dose:* 2 mg/kg	CNS stimulant, increase diaphragm contractility; IV or oral doses; maintain serum level of 5–10 μg/ml q 12 hours

* Use total of 210 ml solution plus diluent in large-volume nebulizer with output of 30 ml/hour. Calculate amount of albuterol; 1.4 × (desired mg/hour). Calculate amount of diluent; 210 ml (amount albuterol) = amount diluent.

† Use total of 210 ml solution plus diluent in large-volume nebulizer with output of 30 ml/hour. Calculate amount of terbutaline; 7 × (desired mg/hour). Calculate amount of diluent; 210 ml (amount terbutaline) = amount diluent.

MDI, metered dose inhaler; q, every; SVN, small-volume nebulizer; LVN, large-volume nebulizer; Tab, tablet; ET, endotracheal; PO, by mouth; DPI, dry powder inhaler; CNS, central nervous system.

TABLE 10–2 Cardiovascular Medications

MEDICATION	DOSE	ACTION-REMARKS
Amrinone	*Loading dose:* 0.75–0.3 mg *Maintenance dose:* 1–10 μg/kg/minute	Sympathomimetic vasodilator; loading dose IV slow push; monitor platelets
Captopril	0.1–0.4 mg/kg	Antihypertensive, angiotension-converting enzyme inhibitor
Diazoxide	4–5 mg/kg	Antihypertensive; IV
Digoxin	Age- and weight-dependent	Cardiac inotrope; serum potassium must be >3.5 mmol/L
Esmolol	25–300 μg/kg/minute	Beta-blocker, decrease blood pressure
Furosemide	1–2 mg/kg	Diuretic; IV, IM, oral preparations; q 4 hours to daily, or PRN
Glucose	0.5–1 g/kg 1 ml/kg D10W	Monitor blood glucose levels >60 mg/dl Hypoglycemia crisis
Hydralazine	1.5–3.6 mg/kg/minute/day 0.1–0.5 mg/kg maximum, 10–20 mg	Vasodilator; given in 4 to 6 doses IM or IV Given in one dose
Indomethacin	0.2–0.3 mg/kg/dose; max 3 doses/24 hours	Ductal closure; 24- to 48-hour closure time

Table continued on following page

TABLE 10–2 Cardiovascular Medications *Continued*

MEDICATION	DOSE	ACTION-REMARKS
Nitroglycerine	1–3 μg/kg/minute 3–25 μg/kg/minute	Vasodilator, preload reduction Afterload reduction
Nitroprusside	0.1–8 μg/kg/minute	Vasodilator, preload and afterload reduction
Norepinephrine	0.02–1 μg/kg/minute	Alpha- and beta-agonist
Phentolamine	1 μg/kg/minute	Alpha-blocker; usually given in conjunction with norepinephrine to improve beta activity
Phenylephrine	0.1–0.5 mg/kg 0.05–0.2 mg/minute	Alpha-adrenergic; titrate to blood pressure
Phentolamine	0.15–2 mg/minute	Alpha-blocker, antihypertensive; IV

Potassium chloride	0.1 mEq/kg/hour	Maintain serum potassium >4 mmol/L
Procainamide	1.5–10 mg/kg 20–50 μg/kg/minute	Anti-arrhythmic; very slow IV push IV infusion
Propranolol	0.5–6 mg/kg/day	Antihypertensive, anti-arrhythmic beta-blocker; may induce bronchospasm
Prostaglandin	0.05–0.2 μg/kg/minute	Pulmonary vasodilator
Tromethamine (THAM)	1 ml/kg/0.1 pH correction desired	Alkalinizing agent
Tolazoline	1 mg/kg test dose 1 mg/kg/hour	Vasodilator for PPHN
Verapamil	0.1–0.3 mg/kg	Calcium channel blocker, antihypotensive; slow infusion

IV, intravenous; IM, intramuscular; PRN, as needed; PPHN, persistent pulmonary hypertension of the newborn.

TABLE 10–3 Sedatives and Anesthesia-Related Medications

MEDICATION	DOSE	ACTION-REMARKS
Chloral hydrate	20–50 mg/kg	Sedative; less respiratory depression than with other narcotics/sedatives
Diazepam	0.1 mg/kg	Benzodiazepine, sedative; IV, q 3–4 hours or PRN
Fentanyl	1–10 μg/kg/hour	Synthetic narcotic
Midazolam	0.1–0.3 mg/kg/hour	Benzodiazepine, sedative; short-acting, q 2–3 hours or PRN
Morphine	0.1 mg/kg	Narcotic; IV, q 2–3 hours or PRN
Pancuronium	0.1–0.15 mg/kg	Nondepolarizing neuromuscular blockade; longer acting, less bradycardia
Phenobarbitol	10–20 mg/kg up to 60 mg/kg	Status epilepticus; IV push
Succinylcholine	1–2 mg/kg	Depolarizing neuromuscular blockade; short-acting, may cause bradycardia
Thiopental	2–7 mg/kg	Sedative for use with increased ICP
Vecuronium	0.1 mg/kg	Nondepolarizing neuromuscular blockade

IV, intravenous; PRN, as needed; q, every; ICP, intracranial pressure.

TABLE 10–4 Antituberculous and Antiviral Medications

MEDICATION	REMARKS
Antituberculosis*	
Isoniazid	May cause hepatic dysfunction
Rifampin	Orange discoloration of secretions; may cause hepatic dysfunction
Streptomycin	Oto- and nephrotoxic
Pyrazinamide	May cause hepatic dysfunction
Ethambutol	May have gastrointestinal and visual side effects
Aerosolized Antiviral Agents†	
Pentamidine	Administered via small-particle hand-held nebulizer, usually monthly
Ribavarin	Nebulized via SPAG-2 for 8–16 hours at a time for 3–5 days

* Medications in the treatment of tuberculosis are frequently used in combination.
† Antiviral agents may cause side effects in the caregiver. Universal precautions and special air filtering equipment are used during aerosol delivery of these medications.
SPAG, small-particle aerosol generator.

TABLE 10–5 Antimicrobial Medications for the Treatment of Specific Infectious Agents in Critically Ill Children

ORGANISM	ANTIMICROBIAL AGENT OF CHOICE*	ALTERNATIVE AGENTS
Bacteria		
Gram-positive cocci (aerobic)		
Staphylococcus aureus		
Non–penicillinase-producing	Penicillin	Cephalothin, vancomycin
Penicillinase-producing	Nafcillin or vancomycin + aminoglycoside or rifampin	Cephalothin, oxacillin + rifampin, or oxacillin + aminoglycoside
Staphylococcus epidermidis	Vancomycin	Imipenem, trimethoprim-sulfamethoxazole
Alpha-streptococci (*Streptococcus viridans*)	Penicillin	Clindamycin, cephalothin, vancomycin
Beta-streptococci (A,B,C,G)	Penicillin	Cephalothin, vancomycin
Enterococcus fecalis		
Serious infection	Ampicillin + aminoglycoside	Vancomycin + aminoglycoside
Uncomplicated urinary infection	Ampicillin, ciprofloxacin, norfloxacin	Vancomycin
Enterococcus bovis	Penicillin	Cephalothin, vancomycin
Streptococcus pneumoniae	Penicillin	Erythromycin, vancomycin, cephalothin

Gram-negative cocci (aerobic)		
Neisseria meningitidis	Penicillin	Ceftriaxone, chloramphenicol
Neisseria gonorrhoeae	Ceftriaxone	Ciprofloxacin
Branhamella catarrhalis	Ceftriaxone	Ceftazidime, ciprofloxacin, imipenem, aztreonam
Gram-positive bacilli (aerobic)		
Corynebacterium JK	Vancomycin	Ciprofloxacin
Gram-negative bacilli (aerobic)		
Acinetobacter sp.	Aminoglycoside + piperacillin	Imipenem, ciprofloxacin
Campylobacter jejuni	Erythromycin	Tetracycline
Campylobacter fetus	Aminoglycoside	Chloramphenicol, imipenem
Enterobacter spp.	Aminoglycoside	Ceftazidime, timentin, imipenem, aztreonam
Escherichia coli	Aminoglycoside	Cefuroxime, ceftriaxone
Haemophilus influenzae	Cefuroxime, ceftriaxone	Chloramphenicol
Klebsiella pneumoniae	Aminoglycoside	Aztreonam, ceftazidime, imipenem
Legionella spp.	Erythromycin + rifampin	Ciprofloxacin + rifampin
Listeria monocytogenes	Ampicillin + aminoglycoside	Chloramphenicol
Proteus mirabilis	Ampicillin	Aminoglycoside, cephalosporin
Other *Proteus* spp.	Aminoglycoside	Aztreonam, imipenem

Table continued on following page

TABLE 10–5 Antimicrobial Medications for the Treatment of Specific Infectious Agents in Critically Ill Children *Continued*

ORGANISM	ANTIMICROBIAL AGENT OF CHOICE*	ALTERNATIVE AGENTS
Providencia spp.	Aminoglycoside	Aztreonam, imipenem
Pseudomonas aeruginosa	Aminoglycoside + piperacillin	Aztreonam, ceftazidime, timentin, imipenem
Other *Pseudomonas* spp.	Aminoglycoside + piperacillin	Aztreonam, ceftazidime, timentin, imipenem
Salmonella spp.	Ceftriaxone	Chloramphenicol, imipenem, ciprofloxacin
Serratia marcescens	Aminoglycoside	Ceftazidime, ciprofloxacin, imipenem, aztreonam
Shigella spp.	Ceftriaxone	Chloramphenicol, ciprofloxacin
Anaerobes		
Anaerobic streptococci	Penicillin	Metronidazole, imipenem
Bacteroides spp.		
Oropharyngeal strains	Penicillin	Imipenem, timentin
Gastrointestinal strains	Metronidazole	Imipenem, timentin
Clostridium spp. (except *C. difficile*)	Penicillin	Imipenem, metronidazole
Clostridium difficile	Vancomycin (oral)	Metronidazole (IV or oral)

Other bacteria		
Actinomyces and *Arachnia*	Penicillin G	Tetracycline, clindamycin
Nocardia spp.	Trimethoprim-sulfamethoxazole	Minocycline, amikacin
Mycobacterium tuberculosis	Isoniazid (INH) + rifampin + pyrazinamide	Ethambutol, streptomycin
Fungi (Invasive)		
Aspergillus spp.	Amphotericin B	—
Blastomyces dermatitidis	Amphotericin B	—
Candida spp.	Amphotericin B	—
Coccidioides immitis	Amphotericin B	—
Cryptococcus neoformans	Amphotericin B + flucytosine	Fluconazole
Histoplasma capsulatum	Amphotericin B	Itraconazole†
Mucor-Absidia-Rhizopus	Amphotericin B	—
Protozoa		
Pneumocystis carinii	Trimethoprim-sulfamethoxazole	Pentamidine
Toxoplasma gondii	Sulfadiazine + pyrimethamine	Clindamycin + pyrimethamine

Table continued on following page

TABLE 10–5 Antimicrobial Medications for the Treatment of Specific Infectious Agents in Critically Ill Children *Continued*

ORGANISM	ANTIMICROBIAL AGENT OF CHOICE*	ALTERNATIVE AGENTS
Viruses		
Herpes simplex	Acyclovir	Ganciclovir, foscarnet†
Influenza A	Amantadine	—
Herpes zoster	Acyclovir	Ganciclovir, foscarnet†
Cytomegalovirus	Ganciclovir	Foscarnet
Respiratory syncytial virus	Ribavirin	—
Human immunodeficiency virus	Azidothymidine (AZT)	2′,3′-Dideoxyinosine (ddI)†
Other Organisms		
Borrelia burgdorferi	Tetracycline (early disease) Ceftriaxone (late disease)	Penicillin G
Mycoplasma pneumoniae	Erythromycin	Tetracycline

Chlamydia (psittaci, trachomatis, pneumoniae)	Tetracycline	Chloramphenicol
Leptospira spp.	Penicillin G	Tetracycline
Rickettsia spp.	Tetracycline	Chloramphenicol

From Masur H: Principles of antimicrobial therapy. *In* Holbrook PR (ed): Textbook of Pediatric Critical Care. Philadelphia, WB Saunders, 1993, pp 887–888.
* Susceptibility testing of specific isolates must be considered in addition to these recommendations.
†Investigational drug.
IV, intravenous.

Bibliography

American Heart Association and American Academy of Pediatrics: Chaimeides L (ed): Textbook of Neonatal Advanced Life Support. Dallas American Heart Association, 1990.

Bosso JA: Cystic fibrosis. *In* DiPiro JT, Talbert RL, Hayes PE, et al (eds): Pharmacotherapy: A Pathophysiologic Approach. New York, Elsevier, 1992, pp 1183–1194.

Committee on Infectious Diseases: Use of ribavirin in the treatment of respiratory syncytial virus infection. Pediatrics 1993; 92:501–504.

Kelly HW, Hill MR: Asthma. *In* DiPiro JT, Talbert RL, Hayes PE, et al (eds): Pharmacotherapy: A Pathophysiologic Approach. New York, Elsevier, 1992, pp 408–448.

Kemp JP: Nedocromil sodium, a new bronchial anti-inflammatory agent. Today's Therapeutic Trends 1992; 10:39–48.

Malinowski C: Surfactant replacement therapy. RT 1993; 6(6):19–25.

Nahata MC: Pediatrics. *In* DiPiro JT, Talbert RL, Hayes PE, et al (eds): Pharmacotherapy: A Pathophysiologic Approach. New York, Elsevier, 1992, 56–63.

SECTION 11

Cardio-pulmonary Resuscitation and Airway Management

I. Basic Life Support

A. Causes of cardiac arrest

B. Delivery room resuscitation

C. Establishing an airway

D. Ventilation

1. Rescue breathing
2. Resuscitation bag inflation procedure

E. Circulation

1. Pulse assessment
2. Chest compressions

II. Obstructed Airway Management

A. Infants

B. Children

III. Drugs Used During Resuscitation

IV. Advanced Airway Management Techniques

A. Oral airway insertion

1. Indications
2. Procedure
3. Complications

B. Nasal airway insertion

1. Indications
2. Contraindications
3. Procedure
4. Complications

C. Endotracheal intubation

1. Indications
2. Contraindications to nasotracheal intubation
3. Procedure for orotracheal intubation
4. Procedure for nasotracheal intubation
5. Complications
6. Patient and family considerations

D. Extubation

1. Procedure
2. Complications

V. Suctioning

A. Indications

B. Relative contraindications

C. Bulb suctioning

D. Endotracheal suctioning

E. Nasotracheal suctioning

F. Closed suction systems

G. Complications

Abbreviations

AAP–American Academy of Pediatrics
AHA–American Heart Association
CPR–cardiopulmonary resuscitation
ECG–electrocardiogram
ETT–endotracheal tube
ICP–intracranial pressure
mm–millimeters
PEEP–positive end-expiratory pressure
PIP–positive inspiratory pressure

BASIC LIFE SUPPORT

Causes of Cardiac Arrest

Cardiac arrest in the pediatric patient is rarely cardiac in origin. It is more commonly the result of low oxygen levels secondary to respiratory difficulty or arrest. Tables 11–1 and 11–2 list risk factors and epidemiologic events associated with cardiopulmonary arrest in neonatal and pediatric age groups.

The sequence of cardiopulmonary resuscitation (CPR) procedures is the same for infants, children, and adults; however, there are variations in some techniques because of the differences in development and in the size of the victims. These variations are summarized in Table 11–3.

Delivery Room Resuscitation

Anticipating and preparing for a high-risk delivery is often vital to a successful outcome. The equipment and personnel necessary for neonatal resuscitation should be assembled prior to delivery (Table 11–4). The American Academy of Pediatrics (AAP) and the American Heart Association (AHA) have developed a flow diagram used to direct clinical assessment and resuscitation methods in neonates (Fig. 11–1).

Establishing an Airway

After laying an unconscious patient on his or her back on a flat surface, the airway should be opened using the head tilt–chin lift or jaw thrust maneuver and breathlessness determined (Figs. 11–2 through 11–4). *Caution: The thumb or fingers must not be placed over the soft tissue below the chin. This causes the tongue to obstruct the airway.*

Ventilation

Rescue Breathing

Rescue breathing in an infant and child is illustrated in Figures 11–5 and 11–6. Two initial breaths should be given

TABLE 11–1 Perinatal Factors Associated With Increased Risk of Neonatal Depression

ANTEPARTUM (FETOMATERNAL)
Diabetes
Postterm
Hemorrhage
Substance abuse
No prenatal care
Age >35 years
Multifetal gestation
Diminished fetal activity
Anemia or isoimmunization
Oligohydramnios or hydramnios
Small fetus for maternal dates
Previous fetal or neonatal death
Immature pulmonary maturity studies
Chronic or pregnancy-induced hypertension
Fetal malformation identified by ultrasound
Preterm labor or premature rupture of membranes
Other maternal illness (e.g., cardiovascular, thyroid, neurologic problems)
Drug therapy (e.g., magnesium, adrenergic-blocking drugs, lithium carbonate)
INTRAPARTUM
Infection
Prolapsed cord
Prolonged labor
Maternal sedation
Operative delivery
Meconium-stained fluid
Prolonged rupture of membranes
Breech or other abnormal presentations
Indexes of fetal distress (e.g., abnormal fetal heart rate)

in 1 to 1.5 seconds. If the chest fails to rise, airway obstruction should be suspected and the head should be repositioned. If the chest fails to rise, foreign body obstruction may have occurred (see Obstructed Airway Management).

Ventilation rates during CPR are as follows:

TABLE 11–2 Pediatric Epidemiologic Events Associated With Cardiopulmonary Arrest

Laryngotracheobronchitis
Epiglottitis
Foreign body aspiration
Suffocation
Aspiration
Severe asthma
Pneumonia
Pneumothorax
Pulmonary edema
Smoke inhalation
Cardiac dysrhythmias
Accidental injury
Motor vehicle accident
Electrocution
Congenital heart defects
Anaphylaxis
Hemorrhage
Neurologic infection
Sudden infant death syndrome
Drug-medication overdose

Newborn:	40–60 breaths per minute
Child:	18–20 breaths per minute
Adult (>8 years):	12–16 breaths per minute

Resuscitation Bag Inflation Procedure

Most infants and children can be ventilated using a resuscitation bag and mask. To adequately ventilate a patient with a non–self-inflating resuscitation bag (anesthesia bag), a proper seal must be established around the mouth and nose. Oxygen flow to the bag must be at an appropriate rate, otherwise the bag may be underinflated, which may result in hypoventilation, or it may be hyperinflated, which may result in barotrauma or gastric distention (Fig. 11–7). The steps in ventilating with an anesthesia bag follow:

1. The oxygen tubing is attached to the gas inlet on the bag; the tubing is attached to an oxygen flowmeter or blender. A pressure manometer is attached to the pressure port (Fig. 11–8).
2. Flow to the bag is adjusted so that it fills approximately halfway. If the patient is not intubated, an appropriate-

TABLE 11–3 Summary of Basic Life Support Maneuvers in Infants and Children

MANEUVER	INFANT (<1 y)	CHILD (1 to 8 y)
Airway	Head tilt–chin lift (if trauma is present, use jaw thrust)	Head tilt–chin lift (if trauma is present, use jaw thrust)
Breathing		
Initial	Two breaths at 1 to $1\frac{1}{2}$ s/breath	Two breaths at 1 to $1\frac{1}{2}$ s/breath
Subsequent	20 breaths/min (approximate)	20 breaths/min (approximate)
Circulation		
Pulse check	Brachial/femoral	Carotid
Compression area	Lower half of sternum	Lower half of sternum
Compression width	2 or 3 fingers	Heel of 1 hand
Depth	Approximately one third to one half the depth of the chest	Approximately one third to one half the depth of the chest
Rate	At least 100/min	100/min
Compression-ventilation ratio	5 : 1 (pause for ventilation)	5 : 1 (pause for ventilation)
Foreign-body airway obstruction	Back blows/chest thrusts	Heimlich maneuver

TABLE 11-4 Equipment Used in Neonatal Resuscitation

- Radiant warmer
- Suction equipment
  - Bulb syringe
  - Vacuum
  - Suction catheter
  - DeLee trap
- Ventilation equipment
  - Resuscitation bag
  - Masks
  - Pressure manometer
  - Oxygen tubing
- Oxygen source
- Laryngoscope
  - Handles
  - Batteries
  - Blades
- Endotracheal tubes (sizes 2.5–4 mm)
- Nasogastric tubes
- Umbilical vessel catheter equipment
- Syringes
- Blood gas analysis equipment

sized mask is attached to the bag. The bag is tested by placing it against one's hand and squeezing it, observing for proper inflation.

3. In mask ventilation, the mask is held firmly in place and the bag is squeezed with the operator's free hand (Fig. 11–9). If two individuals are available, one can hold the mask in place while the other controls the bag (Fig. 11–10).
4. The chest should be observed for equal expansion and auscultated for adequate tidal volume.

Circulation

Pulse Assessment

The pulse rate must be assessed to determine if cardiac arrest has occurred. The brachial artery is palpated in infants and the carotid artery is palpated in children. The airway must be maintained while the artery is palpated.

Chest Compressions

If no pulse is palpated, external chest compressions are begun. Locations for chest compressions in infants are illus-

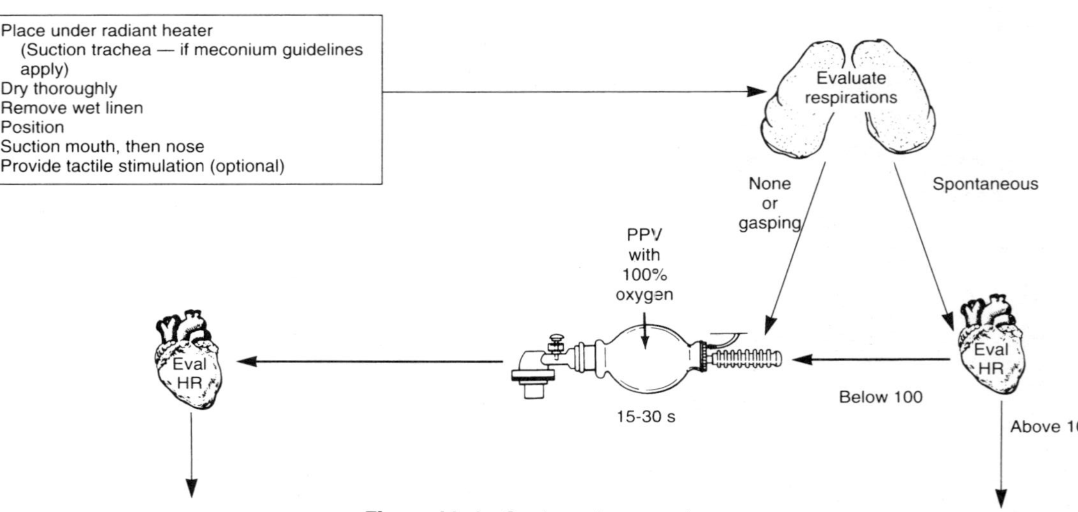

Figure 11–1 *See legend on opposite page*

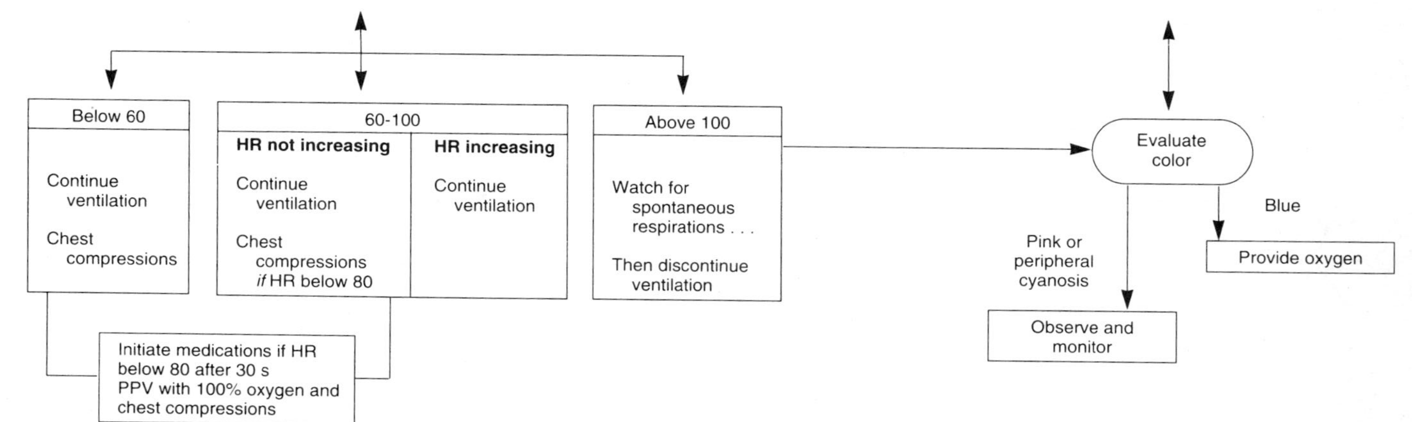

Figure 11–1 Overview of resuscitation in the delivery room. (Reproduced with permission © Textbook of Neonatal Resuscitation, 1987, 1990, 1994. Copyright American Heart Association.)

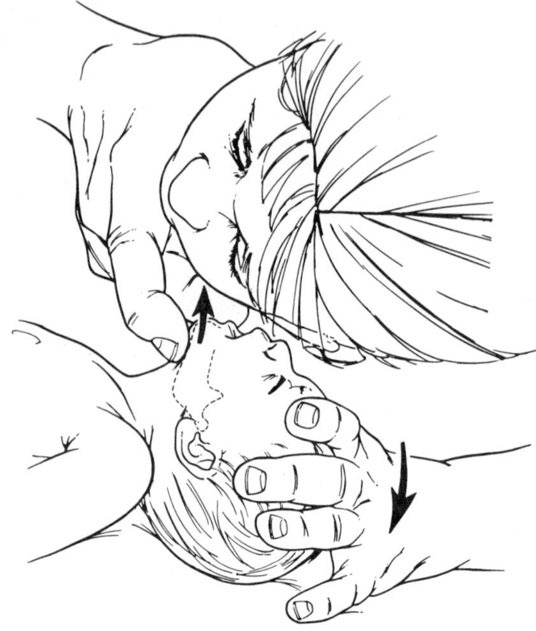

Figure 11–2 Opening the airway with the head tilt–chin lift maneuver. One hand is used to tilt the head, extending the neck. The index finger of the rescuer's other hand lifts the mandible outward by lifting on the chin. Head tilt should not be performed if cervical spine injury is suspected. (Reproduced with permission. © *Guidelines for Cardiopulmonary Resuscitation and Emergency Cardiac Care,* 1992. Copyright American Heart Association.)

trated in Figures 11–11 and 11–12. Chest compressions in children are illustrated in Figure 11–13.

Infant: Compression depth of 0.5 to 1 inch
Compression rate of 100 to 120 per minute
Child: Compression depth of 1 to 1.5 inches
Compression rate of 80 to 100 per minute

A ratio of five compressions to one breath is given in both infants and children.

OBSTRUCTED AIRWAY MANAGEMENT

If the patient is suspected of having airway obstruction caused by a foreign body, maneuvers should be instituted to relieve the obstruction.

Infants

The infant is held head downward on his or her stomach with the legs straddling the rescuer's arm. Four back blows

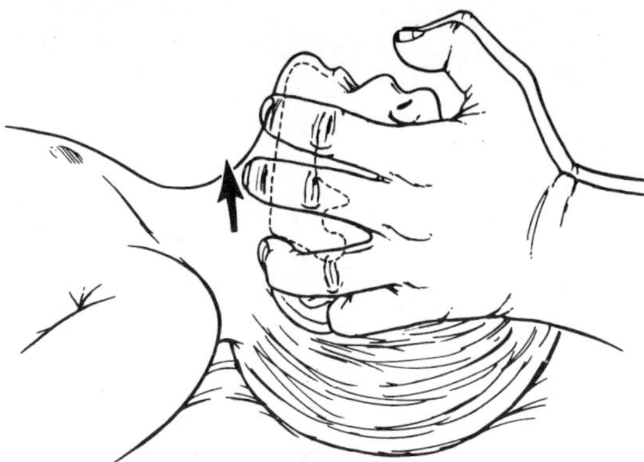

Figure 11–3 Opening the airway with the jaw thrust maneuver. The airway is opened by lifting the angle of the mandible. The rescuer uses two or three fingers of each hand to lift the jaw while other fingers guide the jaw upward and outward. (Reproduced with permission. © *Guidelines for Cardiopulmonary Resuscitation and Emergency Cardiac Care,* 1992. Copyright American Heart Association.)

are applied between the shoulder blades (Fig. 11–14*A*). With the head held downward, the infant is turned onto his or her back, and four chest thrusts are applied in the same location as CPR compressions (Fig. 11–14*B*). The Heimlich maneuver is not used in infants younger than 1 year of age because of the increased risk of intraabdominal injuries.

Children

The Heimlich maneuver is used to relieve airway obstruction in children older than 1 year of age. If the child is conscious and is sitting or standing, the rescuer's arms are wrapped around the child's waist and a fist is made with one hand (Fig. 11–15*A*). The thumb side of the fist is placed midline on the abdomen slightly above the umbilicus and below the xiphoid process. An unconscious child (or one who loses consciousness during the maneuver) is placed supine. With the rescuer straddling the child or standing at the feet, the heel of one hand is placed midline on the abdomen, slightly above the umbilicus and below the xiphoid process, and the other hand is placed on the first hand (Fig. 11–15*B*). Thrusts are made by quickly pressing the thumb side of the fist or the heel of the bottom hand inward and upward.

DRUGS USED DURING RESUSCITATION

Medications used during the resuscitation of infants and children are listed in Tables 11–5 and 11–6. Figure 11–16

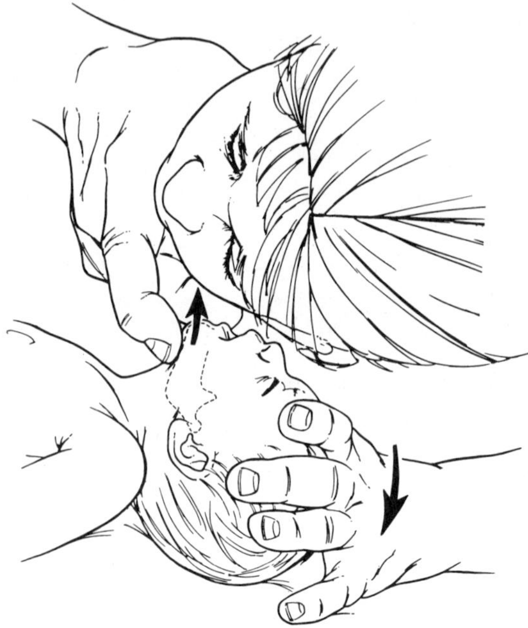

Figure 11–4 Determining breathlessness while opening the airway with the head tilt–chin lift maneuver. The rescuer looks for chest movement, listens for exhaled air, and feels for exhaled air against the cheek. (Reproduced with permission. © *Guidelines for Cardiopulmonary Resuscitation and Emergency Cardiac Care,* 1992. Copyright American Heart Association.)

is a flow diagram illustrating the use of emergency drugs during neonatal resuscitation.

ADVANCED AIRWAY MANAGEMENT TECHNIQUES

Oral Airway Insertion

An oral airway is a tube shaped to follow the curvature of the tongue and soft palate. When inserted correctly in the mouth, it maintains airway patency to the hypopharynx by holding the tongue away from the posterior pharyngeal wall. The tube has a flat outer flange and either a central hollow passageway or two channels along the sides in which a suction catheter can be inserted.

Indications

An oral airway is used to maintain airway patency in the following situations:

- During manual ventilation with a bag-valve-mask device (e.g., CPR, anesthesia)

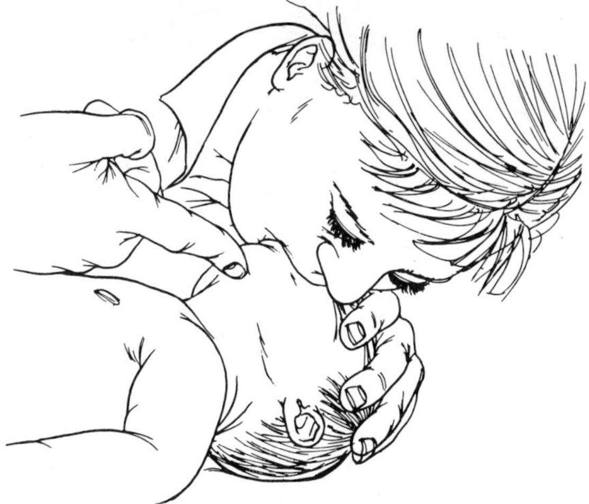

Figure 11–5 Rescue breathing in an infant. The rescuer's mouth covers the infant's nose and mouth, creating a seal. One hand performs head tilt while the other hand lifts the infant's jaw. Avoid head tilt if the infant has sustained head or neck trauma. (Reproduced with permission. © *Guidelines for Cardiopulmonary Resuscitation and Emergency Cardiac Care,* 1992. Copyright American Heart Association.)

- In the unconscious patient with upper airway obstruction
- In the unconscious patient who has lost submandibular muscle tone

Procedure

1. The proper sized airway is selected (Table 11–7). The airway should not be so small that it may be aspirated.
2. The oropharynx is suctioned.
3. With the patient supine, the airway is inserted into the mouth. A tongue blade is used to depress and anteriorly displace the tongue and then the airway is inserted right-side-up into the oropharynx *or* the airway is held sideways or upside down, is inserted into the oropharynx, and is then rotated into the proper position.
4. Breath sounds are auscultated to verify airway patency.
5. Mouth care is provided every 4 to 8 hours, including suctioning of the airway and mouth, repositioning of the airway (to prevent pressure sores), and cleaning of the airway with hydrogen peroxide solution.

Complications

The following complications may occur from an oral airway:

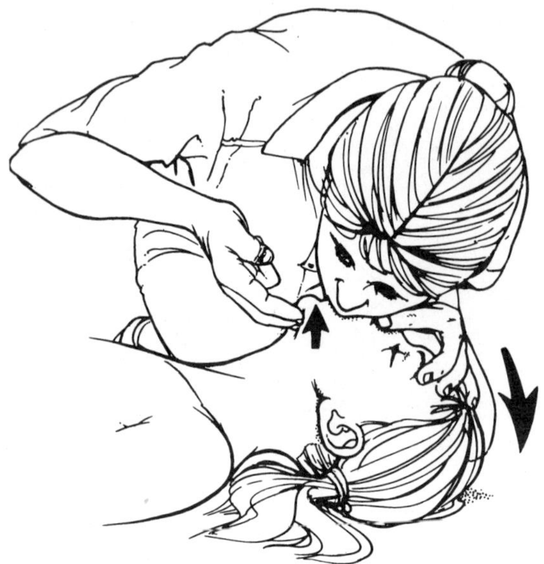

Figure 11–6 Rescue breathing in a child. The rescuer's mouth covers the mouth of the child, creating a mouth-to-mouth seal. One hand maintains the head tilt; the thumb and forefinger of the same hand are used to pinch the child's nose. (Reproduced with permission. © *Guidelines for Cardiopulmonary Resuscitation and Emergency Cardiac Care,* 1992. Copyright American Heart Association.)

- Airway obstruction from improper placement of the airway within the pharynx, aspiration of the oral airway, occlusion of the oral airway passage with secretions, or the tongue's being pushed into the oropharynx
- Gagging, vomiting, and aspiration after stimulation of the gag reflex
- Trauma to the lips, tongue, gums, roof of mouth, or teeth
- Ulcerations and necrosis caused by pressure of the airway
- Infection, usually from poor oral hygiene

Nasal Airway Insertion

A nasal airway is a soft tube that is inserted into the nose and positioned at the base of the tongue. It is used to maintain airway patency to the hypopharynx and can be tolerated by conscious patients.

Indications

A nasal airway is used to maintain airway patency in patients who cannot use an oral airway:

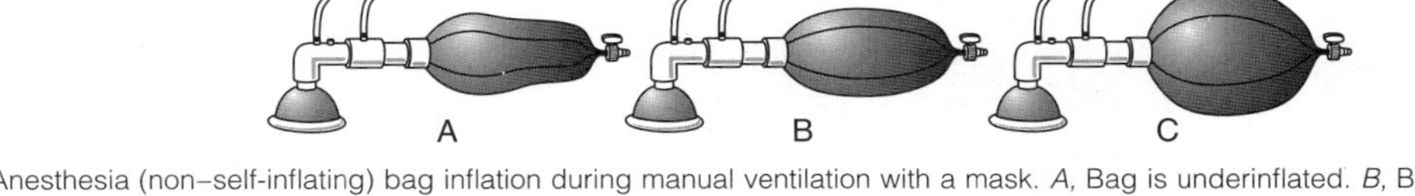

Figure 11–7 Anesthesia (non–self-inflating) bag inflation during manual ventilation with a mask. *A*, Bag is underinflated. *B*, Bag is properly inflated. *C*, Bag is overinflated.

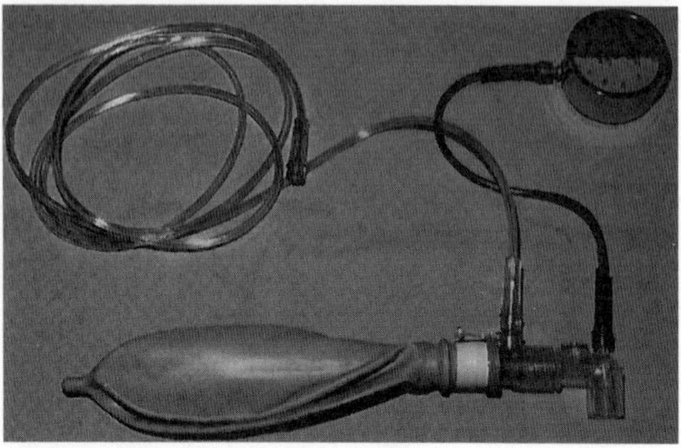

Figure 11–8 Infant non–self-inflating manual resuscitation bag with a pressure manometer in-line.

- Conscious or semiconscious patients
- Patients with a clenched jaw or jaw injury
- Patients with severe facial trauma

Contraindications

The following situations contraindicate a nasal airway:

- Patients receiving anticoagulant therapy (risk of epistaxis)

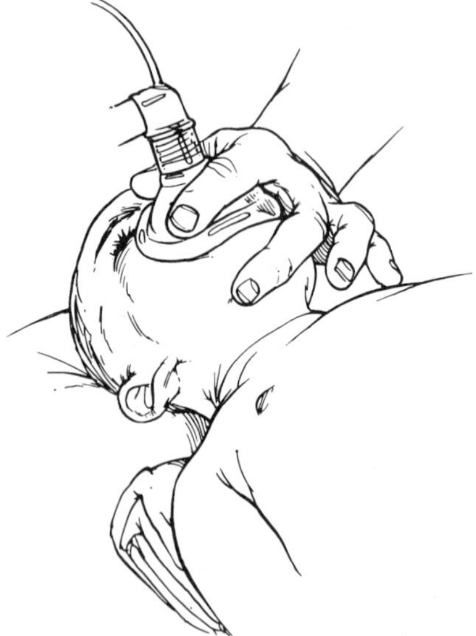

Figure 11–9 One-handed face mask application technique. (Reproduced with permission. © *Textbook of Pediatric Advanced Life Support,* 1988. Copyright American Heart Association.)

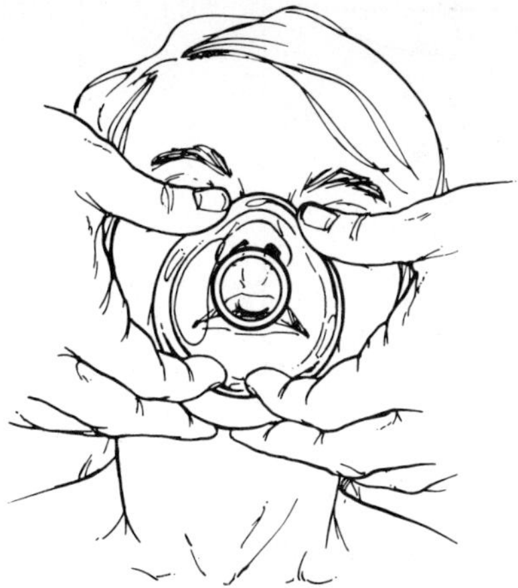

Figure 11–10 Two-handed face mask application technique. A second person is needed to ventilate. (Reproduced with permission. © *Textbook of Pediatric Advanced Life Support,* 1988. Copyright American Heart Association.)

- Patients with hemorrhage disorders (risk of epistaxis)
- Patients with facial fractures causing nasal obstruction or with basal skull fractures (risk of intracranial tube placement)

Procedure

1. The purpose of and the procedure for a nasal airway should be explained to the patient and family.

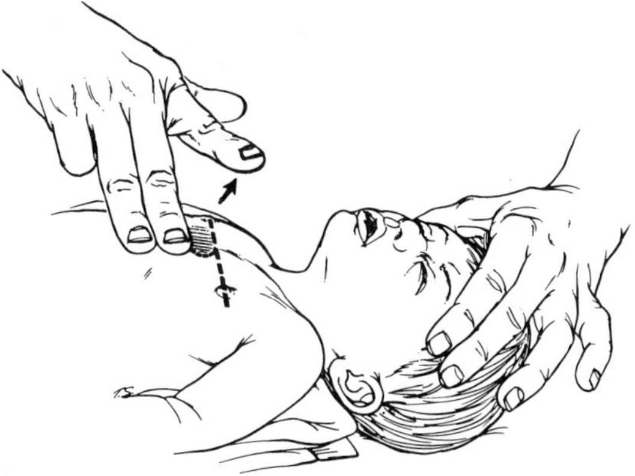

Figure 11–11 Locating proper finger position for chest compression in an infant. Note that the rescuer's other hand is used to maintain head position to facilitate ventilation. (Reproduced with permission. © *Guidelines for Cardiopulmonary Resuscitation and Emergency Cardiac Care,* 1992. Copyright American Heart Association.)

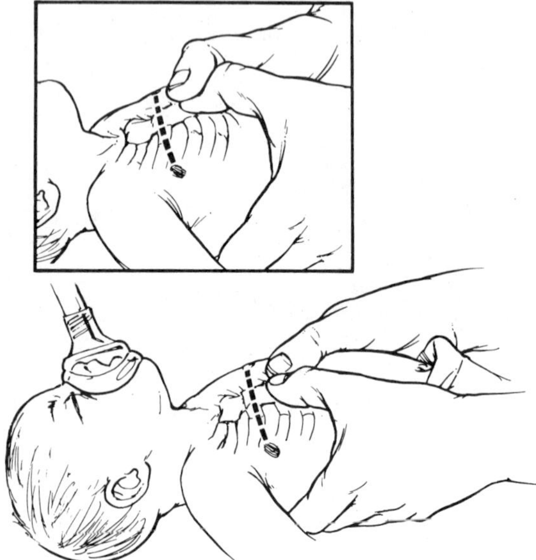

Figure 11–12 Hand position for chest encirclement technique for external chest compressions in neonates. Thumbs are side by side over the midsternum. In the small newborn, thumbs may need to be superimposed. (Reproduced with permission. © *Textbook of Pediatric Advanced Life Support,* 1988. Copyright American Heart Association.)

2. The proper sized tube is selected. The external diameter of the tube should be slightly smaller than the opening of the nares. One should use the largest tube that will easily pass through the nostril.
3. A topical anesthetic (e.g., lidocaine) is applied to the nostril that the tube will be inserted into.
4. The tip and sides of the tube are lubricated with water-soluble jelly.
5. The tube is inset into the nostril posteriorly with the bevel facing the nasal septum. Using an arcing motion, it is gently passed medially and downward along the floor of the nostril. If resistance is met, the tube is slightly rotated.
6. Breath sounds are auscultated to verify airway patency.
7. A safety pin is inserted through a corner of the flange of the tube and taped in place.
8. The tube is changed daily after suctioning, switching from one nostril to the other.
9. The tube is removed during expiration using one smooth pull. If the tube is stuck, lubrication is applied around the nostril and the tube is gently rotated out.

Complications

The following complications may occur:

- Gagging, vomiting, and aspiration after stimulation of the gag reflex

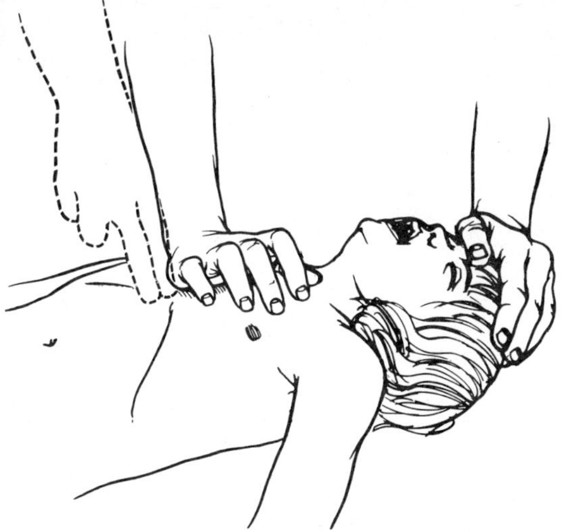

Figure 11–13 Locating hand position for chest compression in the child. Note that the rescuer's other hand is used to maintain head position to facilitate ventilation. (Reproduced with permission. © *Guidelines for Cardiopulmonary Resuscitation and Emergency Cardiac Care,* 1992. Copyright American Heart Association.)

- Gastric insufflation and hypoventilation caused by a tube that is too long entering the esophagus
- Epistaxis
- Infection
- Ulcerations and necrosis from pressure of the airway
- Laryngospasm
- Airway obstruction from occlusion of the tip of the tube with secretions

Endotracheal Intubation

Endotracheal intubation consists of placing an endotracheal tube (ETT) into the trachea. Nasal ETTs are inserted through the nose, and oral tubes are inserted through the mouth.

Indications

Endotracheal intubation is indicated

- To provide an airway for
  Manual or mechanical ventilation (e.g., CPR, apnea)
  Relief of upper airway obstruction (e.g., epiglottitis)
  Direct access to the lungs for suctioning (e.g., persistent atelectasis)

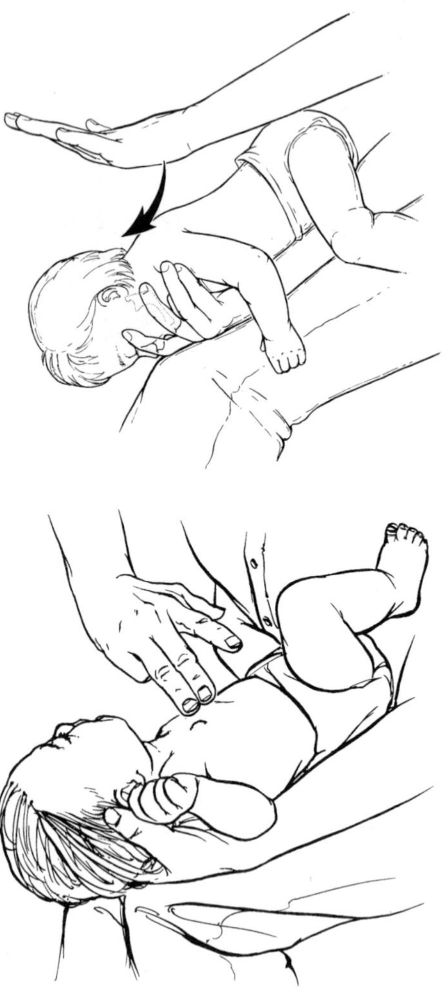

Figure 11–14 In infants with suspected foreign body airway obstruction, four back blows are given (*A*), followed by four chest thrusts (*B*). (Reproduced with permission. © *Instructor's Manual for Pediatric Basic Life Support,* 1994. Copyright American Heart Association.)

- To protect the airway from aspiration (e.g., drug overdose)

Contraindications to Nasotracheal Intubation

Nasotracheal intubation is contraindicated with

- Bleeding diathesis
- Abnormal clotting times or anticoagulant therapy
- Facial or nasal trauma or fractures
- Basilar skull fracture

Text continued on page 383

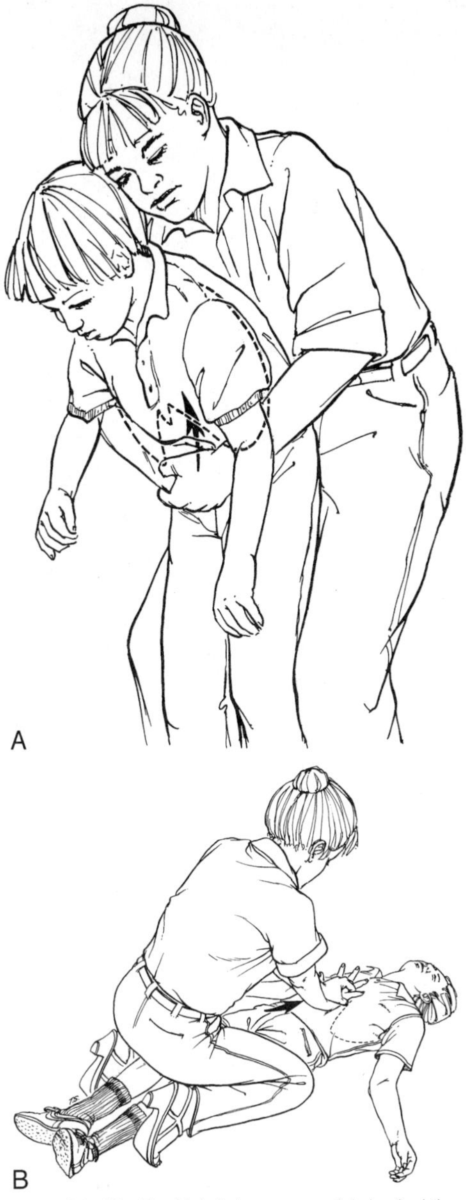

Figure 11–15 The Heimlich maneuver (abdominal thrusts) is performed in children suspected of having foreign body obstruction. *A,* Heimlich maneuver in conscious child, standing. *B,* Heimlich maneuver in unconscious child, lying. (Reproduced with permission. © *Instructor's Manual for Pediatric Basic Life Support,* 1994. Copyright American Heart Association.)

TABLE 11–5 Medications for Neonatal Resuscitation

MEDICATION	CONCENTRATION TO ADMINISTER	PREPARATION	DOSAGE/ ROUTE*	TOTAL DOSE/INFANT		RATE/ PRECAUTIONS
Epinephrine	1 : 10,000	1 ml	0.1–0.3 ml/ kg IV or ET	**Weight**	**Total Ml**	Give rapidly
				1 kg	0.1–0.3 ml	
				2 kg	0.2–0.6 ml	
				3 kg	0.3–0.9 ml	
				4 kg	0.4–1.2 ml	
Volume expanders	Whole blood 5% albumin Normal saline Ringer's lactate	40 ml	10 ml/kg IV	**Weight**	**Total Ml**	Give over 5–10 min
				1 kg	10 ml	
				2 kg	20 ml	
				3 kg	30 ml	
				4 kg	40 ml	

Sodium bicarbonate	0.5 mEq/ml (4.2% solution)	20 ml or two 10-ml prefilled syringes	2 mEq/kg IV	**Weight**	**Total Dose**	**Total Ml**	Give *slowly*, over at least 2 min Give only if infant being effectively ventilated
				1 kg	2 mEq	4 ml	
				2 kg	4 mEq	8 ml	
				3 kg	6 mEq	12 ml	
				4 kg	8 mEq	16 ml	
Naloxone	0.4 mg/ml	1 ml	0.1 mg/kg (0.25 ml/kg) IV, ET, IM, SQ	**Weight**	**Total Dose**	**Total Ml**	Give rapidly; IV, ET preferred; IM, SQ acceptable
				1 kg	0.1 mg	0.25 ml	
				2 kg	0.2 mg	0.50 ml	
				3 kg	0.3 mg	0.75 ml	
				4 kg	0.4 mg	1 ml	
	1 mg/ml	1 ml	0.1 mg/kg (0.1 ml/kg) IV, ET, IM, SQ	1 kg	0.1 mg	0.1 ml	
				2 kg	0.2 mg	0.2 ml	
				3 kg	0.3 mg	0.3 ml	
				4 kg	0.4 mg	0.4 ml	

Table continued on following page

TABLE 11–5 Medications for Neonatal Resuscitation *Continued*

MEDICATION	CONCENTRATION TO ADMINISTER	PREPARATION	DOSAGE/ ROUTE*	TOTAL DOSE/INFANT		RATE/ PRECAUTIONS
				Weight	**Total μg/Min**	
Dopamine	$\frac{6 \times \text{weight (kg)} \times \text{desired dose } (\mu g/kg/min)}{\text{desired fluid (ml/hr)}} =$	mg of dopamine per 100 ml of solution	Begin at 5 μg/kg/min (may increase to 20 μg/kg/min if necessary) IV	1 kg 2 kg 3 kg 4 kg	5–20 μg/min 10–40 μg/min 15–60 μg/min 20–80 μg/min	Give as a continuous infusion using an infusion pump Monitor HR and BP closely Seek consultation

IM, intramuscular; ET, endotracheal; IV, intravenous; SQ, subcutaneous; HR, heart rate; BP, blood pressure.

TABLE 11–6 Medications for Pediatric Resuscitation

MEDICATION	DOSE	INDICATIONS/ADMINISTRATION
Adenosine	0.1–0.2 mg/kg	Precardioversion IV rapid infusion
Atropine	0.02 mg/kg	Bradycardia (do not use if bradycardia is due to hypoxemia; should correct hypoxemia instead) IV, IM, SC, PO, ET
Bretylium	Initial: 5 mg/kg Subsequent: 10 mg/kg	Ventricular arrhythmias IV rapid infusion
Calcium chloride (10%)	20 mg/kg	Hypocalcemia, electromechanical dissociation (questionable) IV slow infusion
Dopamine	Renal: 0.5–2 μg/kg/minute Beta-adrenergic: 5–15 μg/kg/minute Alpha-adrenergic: 15–20 μg/kg/minute	Renal perfusion, hypotension, shock IV continuous infusion

Table continued on following page

TABLE 11–6 Medications for Pediatric Resuscitation *Continued*

MEDICATION	DOSE	INDICATIONS/ADMINISTRATION
Dobutamine	5–20 μg/kg/minute	Increased myocardial contraction Titrate IV infusion
Epinephrine (1:10,000)	0.1 mg/kg	Hypotension, bradycardia, asystole IV, IO, IC, ET
Isoproterenol	0.1–1 μg/kg/minute	Increase myocardial contractility, bradycardia IV continuous infusion
Lidocaine	Bolus: 1 mg/kg Infusion: 20–50 μg/kg/minute	Ventricular arrhythmias IV bolus, then infusion
Sodium bicarbonate	Initial: 1 mEq/kg (0.3 × kg × base excess)	Metabolic acidosis IV slow infusion, repeat after 10 minutes; requires adequate ventilation

ET, endotracheal; IC, intracardiac; IO, intraosseus; IV, intravenous; PO, by mouth; SC, subcutaneous; IM, intramuscular.

Procedure for Orotracheal Intubation

1. The necessary equipment is gathered (Table 11–8). The light source on the laryngoscope and the cuff on the ETT are checked.
2. The appropriate type and size of laryngoscope blade and ETT are selected (Table 11–9). The appropriate size of ETT for any child older than 1 year can be calculated using the following formula:

   Internal diameter in millimeters = (16 + age in years) − 4

   A cuffed ETT usually is not needed in children younger than 8 years of age. An inflated cuff increases the outer diameter of the ETT by approximately 0.5 mm.
3. The purpose of and procedure for orotracheal intubation are explained to the conscious patient (in terms appropriate for age).
4. The patient is placed in the "sniffing" position.
5. The nose and oropharynx are suctioned as needed. One hundred percent oxygen is administered for 2 to 5 minutes, with or without positive pressure.
6. The laryngoscope is held in the left hand and the blade is inserted into the right side of the mouth, sweeping the tongue to the left (Fig. 11–17). The blade is advanced midline with a forward and upward motion. *One must not flex or rotate the wrist.* Gentle external pressure applied to the thyroid cartilage may help to visualize the glottis. After the glottis is visualized, the ETT is held in the right hand and inserted into the right side of the mouth, past the vocal cords, and into the trachea. The tube is positioned midtrachea. If intubation cannot be accomplished within 30 seconds, the equipment is removed and adequate oxygenation is ensured via bag-mask ventilation before reattempting to intubate.
7. Once the ETT has been placed, the patient is ventilated and assessed for proper tube placement by auscultating the chest for bilateral breath sounds. If the chest expands or breath sounds are heard on one side only, main stem intubation has likely occurred; the ETT is slowly withdrawn until bilateral expansion and breath sounds are present.
8. The tube is stabilized against the mouth and then taped in place. *The tube is not released until it is completely taped in place* (Fig. 11–18).
9. The patient's heart rate, respirations, blood pressure, color, and oxygen saturation are monitored throughout the procedure.
10. A chest radiograph is obtained to confirm tube placement.

Medications
Epinephrine
Volume Expander
Sodium Bicarbonate

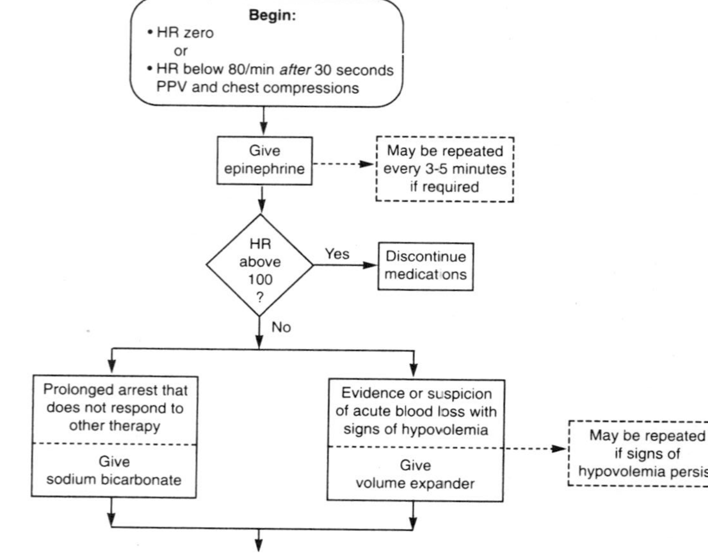

Figure 11–16 *Continued*

Dopamine

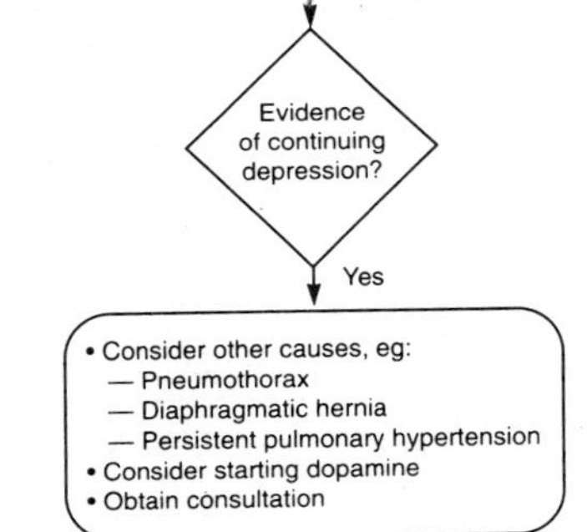

Naloxone Hydrochloride

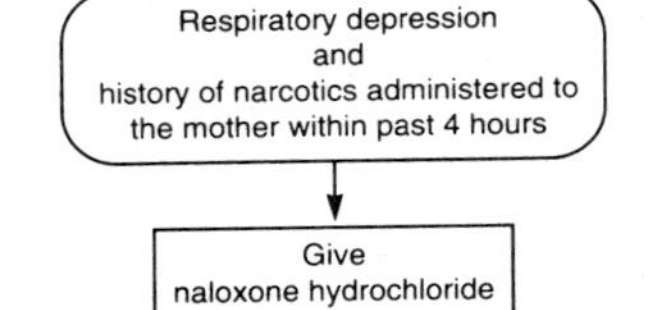

Figure 11–16 *See legend on following page*

TABLE 11–7 Pediatric Oral Airway Sizes

PATIENT SIZE	AIRWAY SIZE
Newborn	00
Infant	0
1 to 3 years	1
3 to 8 years	2
9 years to small adult	3

Procedure for Nasotracheal Intubation

Once a stable airway is established via orotracheal intubation, a nasotracheal tube may be placed. A nasotracheal tube is usually one size smaller than the oral tube.

1. The tube is lubricated with petroleum or 2% lidocaine jelly.
2. The tube is inserted into the nostril until one half of its length has been passed through the nose. With an assistant holding the oral ETT, the glottis is exposed (in the same manner as in orotracheal intubation). Once the tip of the nasal ETT is visualized in the hypopharynx, the tip is grasped with a forceps (held in the right hand). The nasal ETT is lifted up and in front of the glottic opening. The oral ETT is removed and the nasal ETT is immediately advanced into the trachea. Passage of the tube may be made easier by gently rotating the tube to the right or left.
3. Proper tube placement is assessed using the method described in the section on orotracheal intubation.

Complications

The following complications may occur:

- Trauma to lips, teeth, upper airway, trachea, or esophagus

Figure 11–16 A summary of the key points related to the use of medications during neonatal resuscitation. (Reproduced with permission. © *Textbook of Neonatal Resuscitation,* 1987, 1990, 1994. Copyright American Heart Association.)

TABLE 11–8 Essential Airway Equipment for Intubation

Laryngoscope handles (2)
Curved and straight laryngoscope blades
Endotracheal tubes (3 sizes)
Stylet
Bag and mask
Suction set-ups (2)
Suction catheter to fit endotracheal tube
Tonsil suction (Yankauer tube)
Foam donut head rest
Oropharyngeal airway
Magill forceps or Kolodny hemostats
1-inch tape
Benzoin

- Esophageal intubation
- Hypoxia, hypoventilation
- Laryngospasm, bronchospasm
- Cardiac arrhythmias
- Aspiration
- Hypotension

TABLE 11–9 Guidelines for Pediatric Tracheal Tube Size

CHILD'S AGE	INTERNAL DIAMETER (mm)
Premature	
1000 g	2.5
1000–1500 g	3.0
1500–2500 g	3.5
Normal newborns	3.5–4.0
6–12 months	4.0–4.5
1–2 years	4.5
4 years	5.0
6 years	5.5
8 years	6.0
10 years	6.5
Greater than 12 years	
Female	7.0–8.5
Male	8.0–10.0

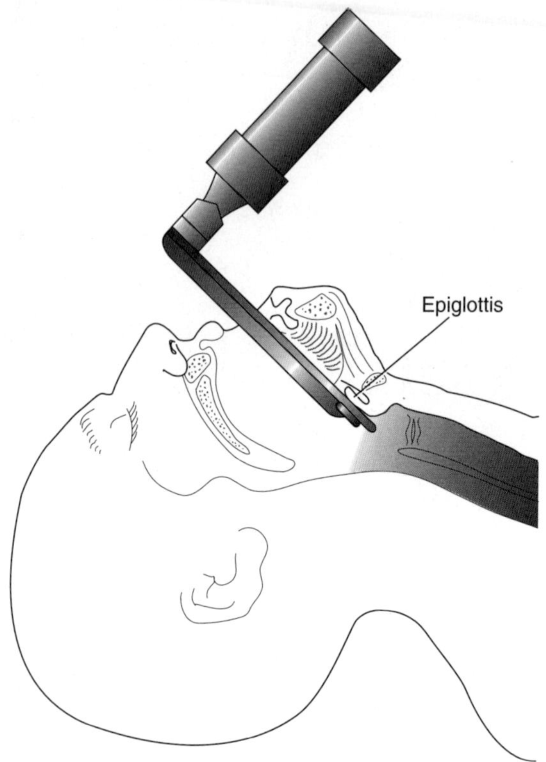

Figure 11-17 Direct laryngoscopy using a straight (Miller) blade.

- Main stem intubation
- Pneumothorax
- ETT obstruction from secretions, blood, kinking, or biting
- Cuff rupture on cuffed ETT
- Accidental extubation
- Laryngeal edema
- Maxillary sinusitis
- Nosocomial pneumonia
- Granuloma of vocal cords
- Necrosis of nasal septum

Patient and Family Considerations

1. It should be explained that the child will not be able to vocalize while the ETT is in place but will be able to do so after extubation.
2. Alternative ways to communicate (e.g., writing, drawing, hand signals, pointing to chart symbols) should be provided.

3. The purpose of and procedure for suctioning should be explained and the discomfort acknowledged.
4. If restraints are used, their purpose is explained (i.e., to prevent accidental extubation).
5. It is explained that swallowing may help decrease gagging.

Extubation

Extubation is indicated when there has been improvement or reversal of the disease process that initially mandated the intubation. Prior to extubation, the patient must be

- Hemodynamically stable
- Able to breathe spontaneously with an adequate tidal volume and minute ventilation
- Have adequate muscle strength to protect the airway

Procedure

1. The procedure is explained to the patient and family.
2. The necessary equipment is assembled:
   - Resuscitation bag and mask
   - Suction equipment
   - Adhesive remover
   - Equipment needed for reintubation
   - Small-volume nebulizer therapy equipment and racemic epinephrine and saline (for postextubation airway edema)
   - Oxygen therapy equipment
3. The oropharynx and trachea are suctioned.
4. The patient is oxygenated with 100% oxygen by bag.
5. The cuff is deflated (if cuffed tube is in place).
6. The ETT is held and the tape is removed from the face and tube with adhesive remover.
7. One large breath is delivered via the bag, and the ETT is withdrawn at peak inflation. *The tube is not removed during a cough or at end-expiration.*
8. Oxygen is administered via an appropriate device (e.g., mask, hood).

Complications

The following complications are possible:

- Sore throat
- Hoarseness
- Laryngeal edema
- Stridor
- Laryngospasm
- Inability to maintain adequate oxygenation (hypoxia)
- Inability to maintain adequate ventilation (hypercarbia)

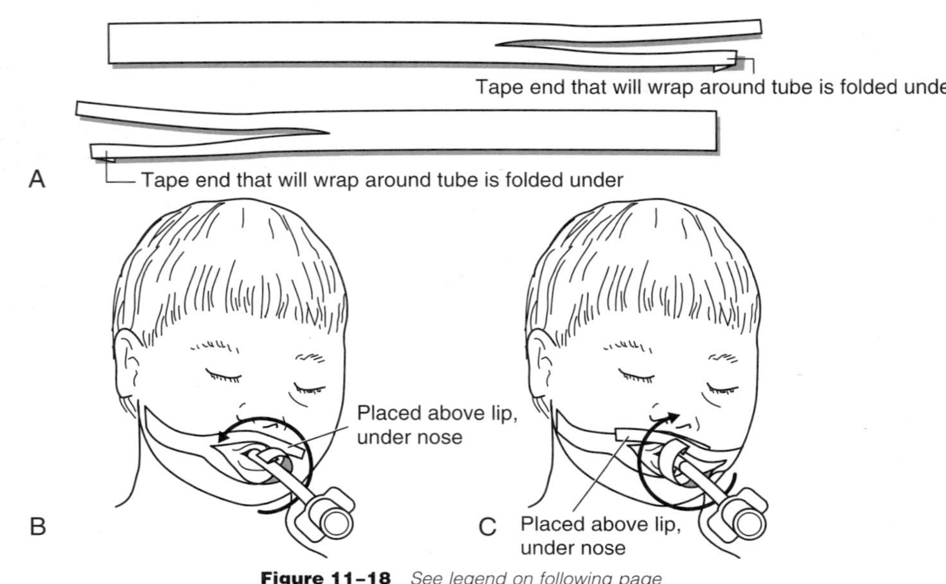

Figure 11–18 *See legend on following page*

SUCTIONING

Suctioning may stimulate a patient to cough, which aids in removing secretions from the airways. Suctioning can also directly remove secretions by exerting a vacuum through a syringe or catheter.

Indications

The following represent indications for suctioning:

- Accumulation of secretions in the airways or ETT
  Visible presence of secretions in the ETT or mouth
  Coarse, gurgling respiratory sounds
  Rales or crackles heard on auscultation
- Obstruction of airways or ETT with mucus plugs
- Inability to cough effectively
  Intubated-tracheostomized patient
  Unconscious patient
  Patient with neuromuscular disorder (e.g., myasthenia gravis, Guillain-Barré syndrome, muscular dystrophy)
- Need to obtain specimens for diagnostic purposes

Relative Contraindications

- Thrombocytopenia
- Epiglottitis and an unsecured airway
- Hemodynamic instability due to inadequate oxygenation and ventilation
- Increased intracranial pressure (ICP)

Bulb Suctioning

The rubber syringe is used to remove mucus from the mouth or nares of an infant. This is not a sterile procedure.

1. The bulb is gently squeezed (depressed) and the syringe is inserted into the mouth or nostril in the area of mucus.

Figure 11–18 Steps used to secure the ET tube with tape. *A* and *B*, Slit two pieces of tape, making a Y on one end of each piece (as shown). Turn under the end of the tape that will be wrapped around the ET tube. This will make tape removal easier. *C*, Apply benzoin to the area below the nose and across the cheeks (where tape will be placed). Attach one piece of tape to the cheek and below the nose, wrapping the bottom of the Y around the ET tube. The tape should be placed under the tube (chin side) first, then wrapped around the top of the tube. *D*, Repeat step B on the other side of the face.

2. The pressure on the bulb is gently released (this suctions the mucus).
3. The syringe is removed from the nostril or mouth and the mucus is cleared by squeezing the bulb.
4. The bulb syringe is cleaned with sterile water and wiped with gauze pads. It is allowed to air dry between uses.

Endotracheal Suctioning

1. The necessary equipment is assembled and the vacuum pressure is set appropriately:

   Neonate: 60 to 80 mm Hg

   Child: 80 to 100 mm Hg

   The vacuum pressure is tested by occluding the suction tubing. The suction catheter should be less than one half the size of the internal diameter of the ETT.
2. Prior to beginning endotracheal suctioning, the purpose and procedure are explained to the patient and family, and the patient's breath sounds, heart rate, respiratory rate, pulse oximetry, and electrocardiogram (ECG) tracing are monitored.
3. The patient is ventilated at the same positive inspiratory pressure (PIP) and positive end-expiratory pressure (PEEP) as that set on the ventilator and with an F_{IO_2} of at least 0.1 to 0.2 greater than that currently being delivered.
4. Normal saline is instilled in small incremental amounts for lavage, and the patient is bagged. Maximum volumes for lavage are

   Neonate: 0.5 ml

   Infant: 1.0 ml
   Child: 2 to 5 ml

   Other solutions used in lavage include sodium bicarbonate and *N*-acetylcysteine (Mucomyst).
5. A sterile suction catheter is held in the dominant hand (gloved and sterile), and the catheter vent and tubing are held in the other gloved, sterile hand. The catheter is lubricated with sterile water and is inserted into the endotracheal or tracheostomy tube until resistance is met. *Vacuum is not applied during insertion.* The catheter is pulled back 0.5 to 1.5 cm and intermittent suction is applied while the catheter is withdrawn with a rotating motion. The suction procedure is limited (from insertion of the catheter to complete withdrawal) to less than 10 seconds, and application of the vacuum is limited to less than 5 seconds.
6. The patient's heart rate, respiratory rate, pulse oximetry readings, color, and ECG tracing are monitored during and after the procedure. Suctioning is discontinued

immediately if bradycardia, cyanosis, marked desaturation, or cardiac dysrhythmias occur.

7. The catheter is removed and the patient is immediately reoxygenated and ventilated (as in Step 3) before the catheter is flushed and the procedure is repeated. The patient is allowed adequate time to "recover" from each suctioning attempt (at least 1 minute). The need for further suctioning depends on the patient's clinical status. Most patients can tolerate the catheter being passed three times; however, some patients become stressed after only one suction attempt.
8. The same catheter is used to suction the nares and mouth. *This catheter is not reintroduced into the trachea.*
9. The amount, color, and consistency of the secretions removed, as well as any changes in breath sounds, are noted.
10. Ten to 15 minutes are allowed after suctioning before an arterial or capillary blood gas sample is obtained.

Nasotracheal Suctioning

1. Equipment is assembled and vacuum pressure is set as previously described in the section on endotracheal suctioning.
2. The patient is preoxygenated for 2 minutes prior to suctioning. An oxygen mask may be held to the patient's mouth during the procedure. During suctioning of a patient receiving oxygen via nasal cannula, a prong may be kept in the nostril not being suctioned.
3. The catheter is lubricated with sterile water or a small amount of a water-soluble substance. Under sterile technique (as described previously with endotracheal suctioning) and with the catheter held 2 to 3 inches from the tip of the nose, the catheter is inserted in a patent nostril and advanced in a downward, arcing motion until resistance is met. *Vacuum is not applied during insertion.* The catheter is pulled back 0.5 to 1.5 cm, and intermittent suction is applied while the catheter is withdrawn. The suction procedure (from insertion of the catheter to complete withdrawal) is limited to less than 10 seconds, and application of the vacuum is limited to less than 5 seconds.
4. The remainder of the procedure for nasotracheal suctioning is the same as that for endotracheal suctioning.

Closed Suction Systems

A closed tracheal suctioning device is placed between the ETT and ventilator circuit. These systems are designed to allow minimal disruption during mechanical ventilation and to prevent hypoxia and the loss of PEEP. A closed suction system consists of a closed lock and suction control valve,

TABLE 11–10 Complications Associated With Suctioning

Hypoxemia
Bleeding
Mucosal trauma
Trauma to the nose
Coughing
Gagging
Vomiting
Laryngospasm
Bronchospasm
Vagal stimulation—bradycardia, hypotension
Cyanosis
Infections
Cardiac dysrhythmias
Exacerbation of increased ICP
Atelectasis
Pneumothorax (risk highest in neonates)
Occlusion of ETT or tracheostomy with catheter

ICP, intracranial pressure; ETT, endotracheal tube.

an irrigation port, and a catheter within a protective sleeve. Sterile saline is instilled into the irrigation port to rinse the catheter and connecting tube. The sheathed suction catheter is then passed through a seal (which prevents the fluid from entering the ETT) into the ETT. Markings on the suction catheter aid in determining the approximate depth of suctioning. Suctioning technique follows that of traditional endotracheal suctioning. The system should be changed every 24 hours. The airway may be damaged or occluded if the catheter is not pulled back fully into the correct position.

Complications

Complications associated with nasotracheal and endotracheal suctioning are listed in Table 11–10.

Bibliography

Albarran-Sotelo R, Flint LS, Kelly KJ (eds): Instructors' Manual for Basic Life Support. Dallas, American Heart Association, 1990.

American Association for Respiratory Care: Clinical practice guideline: Endotracheal suctioning of mechanically ventilated adults and children with artificial airways. Respir Care 1993; 38:501.

Berry FA, Yemen TA: Pediatric airway in health and disease. Pediatr Clin North Am 1994; 41:153.

Chameides L (ed): American Heart Association and American Academy of Pediatrics: Textbook of Neonatal Resuscitation. Dallas, American Heart Association, 1990.

Chameides L (ed): American Heart Association and American Academy of Pediatrics: Textbook of Pediatric Advanced Life Support. Dallas, American Heart Association, 1988.

Centers for Disease Control, Division of Injury Control, Center for Environmental Health and Injury Control: Childhood injuries in the United States. Am J Dis Child 1990; 144:627.

Eisenberg M, Bergner L, Hallstrom A: Epidemiology of cardiac arrest and resuscitation in children. Ann Emerg Med 1983; 12:672.

American Heart Association, Emergency Cardiac Care Committee and Subcommittees: Guidelines for cardiopulmonary resuscitation and emergency cardiac care. JAMA 1992; 268:2251.

Fisher DE, Paton JB: Resuscitation of the newborn infant. *In* Klaus MH, Fanaroff AA (eds): Care of the High-Risk Neonate, 4th ed. Philadelphia, WB Saunders, 1993, pp 38–61.

Keep PJ, Manford ML: Endotracheal tube sizes for children. Anaesthesia 1974; 29:181.

Melker RJ, Banner MJ: Ventilation during CPR: Two-rescuer standards reappraised. Ann Emerg Med 1985; 14:397.

Proehl JA: Adult Emergency Nursing Procedures. Boston, Jones and Bartlett, 1993.

Skale N: Manual of Pediatric Nursing Procedures. Philadelphia, JB Lippincott, 1992.

Torphy DE, Minter MG, Thompson BM: Cardiorespiratory arrest and resuscitation of children. Am J Dis Child 1984; 138:1099.

APPENDIX

Laboratory Values

Abbreviations

CBC–Complete blood count
WBC–White blood cell count
RBC–Red blood cell count
PT–Prothrombin time
PTT–Partial thromboplastin time
BUN–Blood urea nitrogen

TABLE 1 Values for Common Blood Chemistry Components

TEST	NORMAL RANGE		PANIC VALUE*
Ammonia (μmol/L)	Premature:	100–130	>130
	Jaundice:	100–150	>150
	Newborn:	65–105	>107
	Infant:	55–90	>90
	Child:	20–55	>57
	Adult:	13–30	>35
BUN (mEq/L)	Newborn:	8–30	
	Infant:	5–15	>35
	Child:	15–35	
	Adult:	10–20	
Calcium (total) (mEq/L) (albumin corrected)	Newborn:	6–10	
	Infant:	7–12	<6 >13
	Child:	8–11	
	Adult:	8–11	
Calcium (ionized) (mEq/L)		2.1–2.6	
Chloride (mEq/L)	Newborn:	95–110	
	Infant:	96–106	<75 >120
	Child:	98–108	
	Adult:	98–108	
Glucose (mg/dl)	Newborn:	20–110	<20 >400
	Infant:	20–110	<20 >400
	Child:	60–105	<60 >400
	Adult:	70–110	<70 >400
Lactic acid (mEq/L)		0.5–2	>2.5
Magnesium (mEq/L)	Newborn:	1.7–2.6	
	Infant:	1.2–2.7	<1.2 >3.7
	Child:	1.4–1.8	
	Adult:	1.2–1.9	

TABLE 1 Values for Common Blood Chemistry Components *Continued*

TEST	NORMAL RANGE		PANIC VALUE*	
Potassium (mEq/L)	Newborn:	4.5–7.5		
	Infant:	4–6.2	<3	>7.5
	Child:	3.7–5.6		
	Adult:	3.5–5.2		
Sodium (mEq/L)	Premature:	128–140		
	Newborn:	132–160	<120	>155
	Infant:	133–145		
	Child:	138–145		
	Adult:	135–150		
Serum osmolality (mOsmol/L)		270–285		
Sweat chloride (mEq/L)†	Negative:	0–40		
	Suspect:	41–60		
	Positive:	>60		

* Unless specified, panic values are listed as values outside the normal range for all ages listed.
† Sweat chloride test indicated for diagnosis of cystic fibrosis and attained by cutaneous electrophoresis.
BUN, blood urea nitrogen.

TABLE 2 Blood Products, Proteins, and Coagulation Times

TEST	NORMAL RANGE	
Blood Products		
Alpha1-antitrypsin (mg/dl) (inhibition potential)	All ages:	0.8–1.6
Bilirubin (mg/dl) (direct)	Newborn:	0–2
	Child-adult:	0–0.4
Bilirubin (mg/dl) (total)	Cord:	<4
	Premature	
	<1 day:	<2
	1–2 days:	<8
	2–4 days:	<12
	<5 days:	<16
	>5 days:	<1
	Full-term	
	<1 day:	<2

Table continued on following page

TABLE 2 Blood Products, Proteins, and Coagulation Times *Continued*

TEST	NORMAL RANGE	
Blood Products		
Bilirubin (mg/dl) (total)	1–2 days:	<6
	2–4 days:	<8
	<5 days:	<12
	>5 days:	<1
Erythrocyte sedimentation rate (ml/hour)	Newborn:	0–2
	Infant-child:	3–13
	Adult female:	15–25
	Adult male:	10–15
Hematocrit (%)	Newborn:	48–72
	Infant:	28–42
	Child:	38–49
	Adult female:	36–46
	Adult male:	37–49
Hemoglobin (g/dl)	Newborn:	14–23
	Infant:	9–14
	Child:	12–15
	Adult female:	15–16
	Adult male:	12–16
Platelets (per mm^3)	Newborn:	90,000–475,000
	Infant-adult:	150,000–450,000
RBC (ml/mm^3)	Premature:	5.1–6.4
	Newborn:	4.3–7.1
	Child:	3.9–5.5
	Adult female:	4.2–5.4
	Adult male:	4.6–6.2
WBC (per mm^3)	Newborn:	9000–30,000
Neutrophils (%)		~61
Lymphocytes (%)		~31
	Infant:	5000–19,000
Neutrophils (%)		~40
Lymphocytes (%)		~60
	Child:	3600–13,000
Neutrophils (%)		~35
Lymphocytes (%)		~60
	Adult:	5000–10,000
Neutrophils (%)		~60
Lymphocytes (%)		~30
Coagulation Times		
PT (seconds) (one-stage)	Newborn:	<17
	Child-adult:	<11–14

TABLE 2 Blood Products, Proteins, and Coagulation Times *Continued*

TEST	NORMAL RANGE	
Coagulation Times		
PTT (seconds)	Premature:	<120
	Newborn:	<90
	Child-adult:	<24–40
Thrombin time (seconds)	All ages:	Control time ± 2

RBC, red blood cell count; WBC, white blood cell count; PT, prothrombin time; PTT, partial thromboplastin time.

TABLE 3 Common Cardiopulmonary-Related Drug Levels

DRUG	RANGE
Digoxin (ng/ml)	0.8–2.2
Dilantin (μg/ml)	10–20
Ethanol (mg/dl)	<50 >300 coma
Phenobarbitol (μg/ml)	15–40 >60 coma
Salicylate (mg/dl)	2–30 >70 lethal
Theophylline (bronchodilator) (μg/ml)	10–20
Theophylline (respiratory stimulant) (μg/ml)	8–15

TABLE 4 Urinalysis Observations and Values

TEST	NORMAL RANGE	
pH	Newborn:	5–7
	Other ages:	5–9
Color	Pale yellow to yellow	
Clarity	Clear	
Specific gravity	Newborn:	1.002–1.02
	Other ages:	1.012–1.022
Volume (ml/day)	1–2 days:	15–60
	Neonatal:	100–400
	Infant:	250–500
	Child:	500–1000
	Other ages:	500–1800

Bibliography

Brown RE (ed): Laboratory Values: The Pediatric Range. Little Rock, Arkansas Children's Hospital, 1980.

Mabry CC: Reference ranges for laboratory tests. *In* Behrman RE, Vaughn VC, Nelson WE (eds): Textbook of Pediatrics, 13th ed. Philadelphia, WB Saunders, 1987, pp 1535 1558.

Rowe PC: Laboratory values. *In* Oski FA, DeAngelis CD, Feigin RD, Warshaw JB (eds): Principles and Practice of Pediatrics. Philadelphia, JB Lippincott, 1990, pp, 1973 1980.

Tietz NB (ed): Clinical Guide to Laboratory Tests. Philadelphia, WB Saunders, 1993.

Tunik MG, Young GM: Status epilepticus in children, the acute management. Pediatr Clin North Am 1992; 39:1007 1030.

Index

Note: Page numbers in *italics* indicate illustrations; those followed by t indicate tables.

ISBN 0-7216-6740-6